The History of

Wills Eye

1832-2007

The History of

Wills Eye 1832-2007

William Tasman, M.D.

Ophthalmologist-in-Chief, Wills Eye; Professor and Chairman,
Department of Ophthalmology, Jefferson Medical College of Thomas Jefferson University;
Consultant, Pennsylvania Hospital, Philadelphia, Pennsylvania.

To Joan and Ed Driscoll
Two wonderful friends!
Sincerely,
Alice Lea & Bill Tasman
July 26, 2007

Valley Press Inc., Bala Cynwyd, Pennsylvania

Library of Congress Cataloging-in-Publication Data

Tasman, William.
The History of Wills Eye
1. Wills Eye Hospital (Philadelphia, Pa.)
2. Hospitals, Ophthalmic — Pennsylvania—Philadelphia — History. I. Title.
DNLM: 1. Wills Eye Hospital (Philadelphia, Pa.).
2. Hospitals, Special — history —Pennsylvania.
3. Ophthalmology — history — Pennsylvania.
WW 28 AP4 P5W7T RE30.P4T37 1987
362.1'977'0974811 87-17050

ISBN 978-0-9725812-2-6 (previously ISBN 0-9725812-0-0 and ISBN 0-397-50918-9)

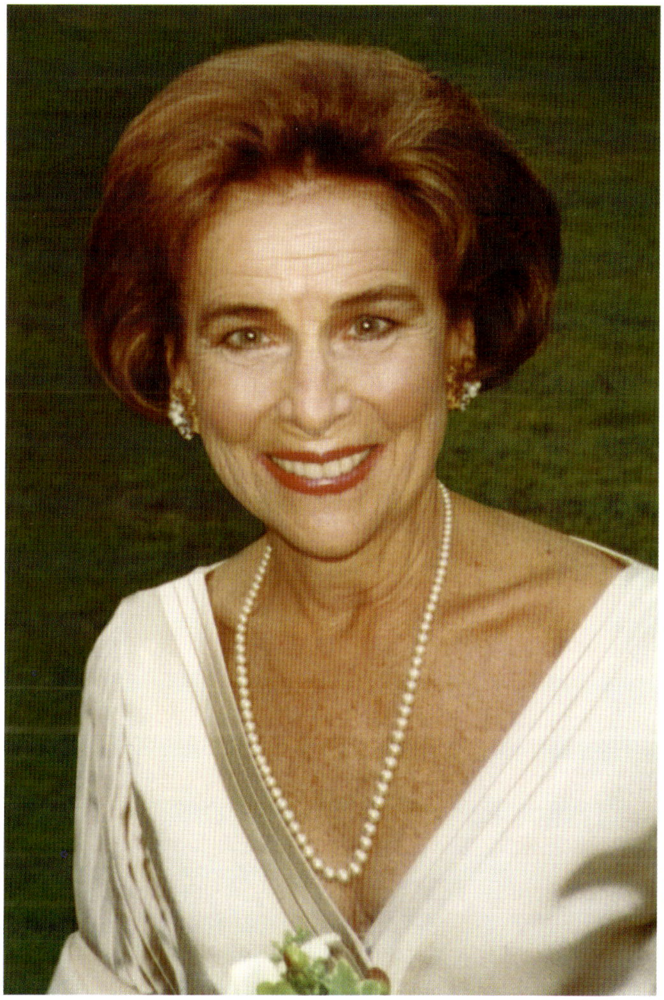

To my loving wife,
Alice Lea
In grateful appreciation of her tireless efforts
on behalf of Wills Eye

and to all of the Wills spouses who continue
to support us year after year.

Contents

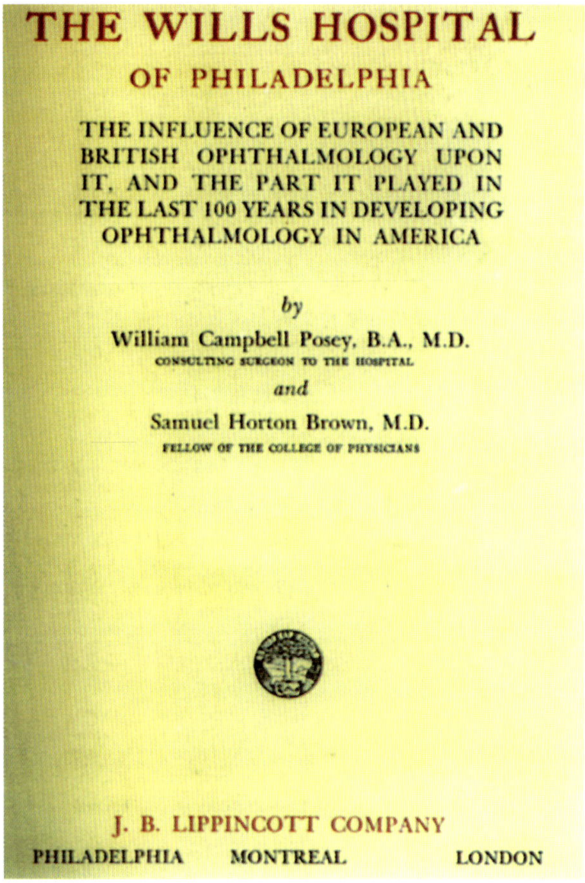
THE WILLS HOSPITAL
OF PHILADELPHIA

THE INFLUENCE OF EUROPEAN AND BRITISH OPHTHALMOLOGY UPON IT, AND THE PART IT PLAYED IN THE LAST 100 YEARS IN DEVELOPING OPHTHALMOLOGY IN AMERICA

by

William Campbell Posey, B.A., M.D.
CONSULTING SURGEON TO THE HOSPITAL

and

Samuel Horton Brown, M.D.
FELLOW OF THE COLLEGE OF PHYSICIANS

J. B. LIPPINCOTT COMPANY
PHILADELPHIA MONTREAL LONDON

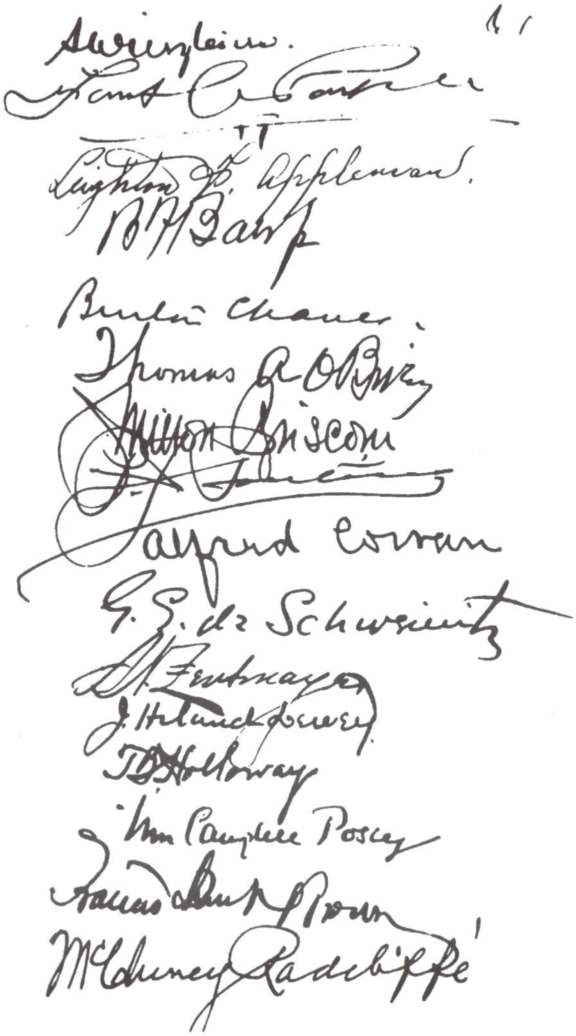

The top photograph at left shows the title page from the 1931 History of Wills Hospital. *Below are signatures from my father's copy of that book. Among them are those of Doctors deSchweinitz, Holloway, Zentmayer, and Posey.*

In their preface Posey and Brown comment on how the Wills "witnessed the birth of ophthalmology — its emergence as a branch of general surgery into the highly developed and specialized science of today." Seventy-one years later, and 168 years since Wills opened its doors in 1834, those words are as true today as they were in 1931.

Posey and Brown further point out that "no other institution in America, perhaps, has been of so great influence in the education of physicians in that branch of medicine, and through its students its influence has spread far and wide." Again, true in 1931, and truer even today. At the beginning of the twenty-first century, Wills remains committed to remaining a preeminent leader in quality patient care, research, and education.

William Tasman, M.D.

Wills Eye Hospital
Honoring
Dr. William Tasman

The Union League of Philadelphia
The Thirtieth Day of October
Two Thousand and Seven

MENU

Salad

Baby Arugula and Spinach
With Crumbled Stilton Cheese and Toasted Walnuts
Drizzled with Maple Vinaigrette

Entree

Filet Mignon in Cabernet Demi Glace
And
Salmon in Tarragon

Oven Roasted Potatoes
Grilled Baby Vegetables

Dessert

Chocolate Cake with Chocolate Mousse Filling
And Fresh Berries

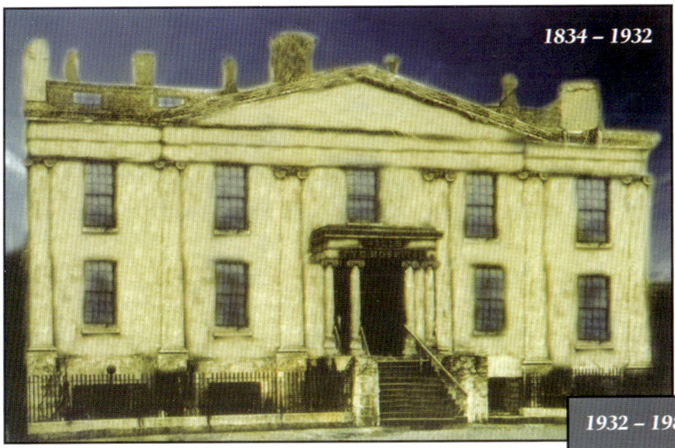
1834 – 1932

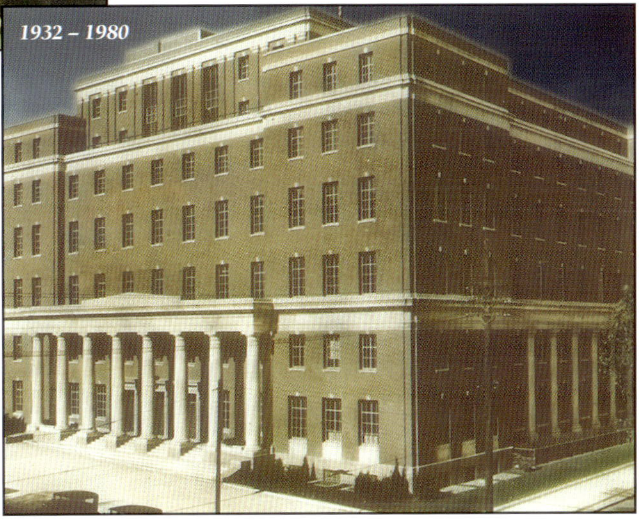
1932 – 1980

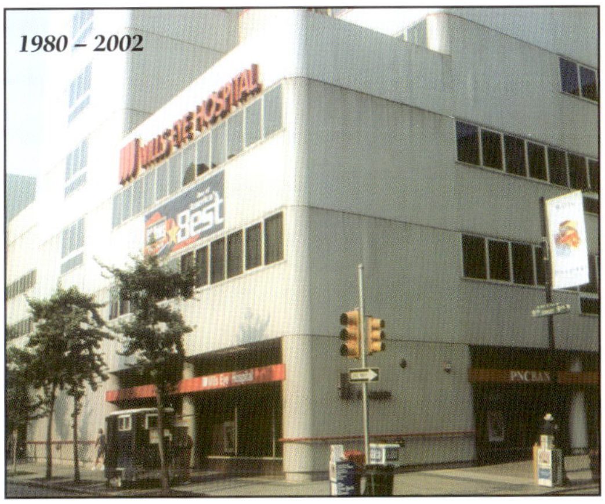
1980 – 2002

The Homes of Wills Eye

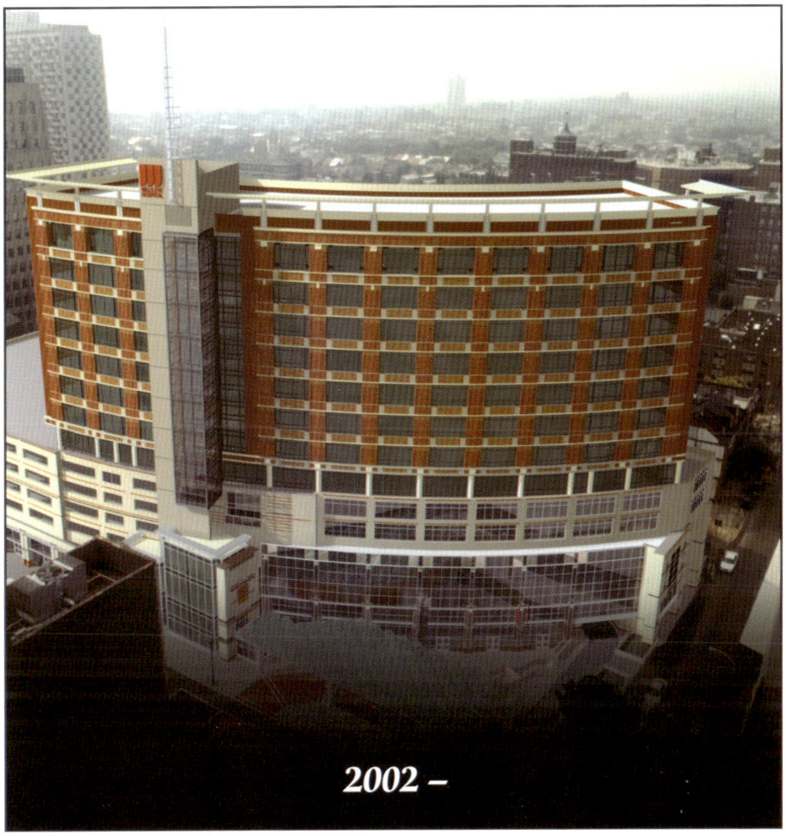
2002 –

Preface

It has been five years since the fourth edition of *The History of Wills Eye Hospital* was published. A lot has happened over those intervening years, and in this updated version of the fourth edition the goal is to review some of those changes, and, since history is ongoing, to update the appendices. As I stated in the preface for the fourth edition in 2002, Wills remains strong and committed to its quality patient care, unparalleled residency and fellowship training. This is due to a huge collaborative effort of our doctors under the leadership of the contemporary service chiefs listed below.

William Tasman, M.D.
Ophthalmologist-In-Chief and Professor
and Chairman Department of Ophthalmology
Jefferson Medical College 1985 – 2007

Cataract and Primary Eye Care Service
Raymond E. Adams, M.D., 1987 – 2001
Robert S. Bailey, M.D., 2001 – Present

Cornea Service
Peter R. Laibson, M.D., 1970 – 2002
Elisabeth J. Cohen, M.D., 1999 – Present

Glaucoma Service
George L. Spaeth, M.D., 1968 – 2007
L. Jay Katz, M.D., 2007

Neuro-Ophthalmology Service
Peter J. Savino, M.D., 1983 – Present

Oculoplastic Service
Joseph C. Flanagan, M.D., 1981 – 2007
Robert B. Penne, M.D., 2007

Oncology Service
Jerry A. Shields, M.D., 1978 – Present
Carol L. Shields, M.D., 1988 – Present

Pediatric Ophthalmology Service
Joseph H. Calhoun, M.D., 1980 – 2007

Retina Service
William Benson, M.D., 1992 – 2003
Gary C. Brown, M.D., 2003 – Present

The History of Wills Eye 1832 – 2007

Introduction

Wills Eye has been an international leader in the field of ophthalmology since 1834. The nation's oldest and largest eye care facility, Wills is a non-profit institution administered by the Philadelphia Board of Directors of City Trusts.

Before Wills was founded in 1832, the care of eye diseases was regarded as but one of the many general surgical responsibilities. Ophthalmology was not yet established as a separate branch of medicine and little specialized training in the field existed. The $116,000 bequest by Philadelphia Quaker merchant James Wills, Jr., which led to the founding of Wills Eye Hospital, would have unforeseen consequences for medical science. As a specialty institution from its inception and a rarity for its time, Wills developed momentum early on as a pioneer in the prevention and treatment of eye diseases.

The first Wills Eye Hospital, a 70-bed institution, was located on Logan Square in Philadelphia. It was here that the nation's first program to train ophthalmologists was developed in 1839. Wills physicians played prominent roles in disseminating the knowledge of the great European eye surgeons, founding leading ophthalmology journals and lecturing to the medical community. The number of patients treated increased dramatically over the years and in 1932 the Hospital relocated to large quarters at 16th and Spring Garden Streets where it remained for nearly 50 years.

This second facility was designed with private and semi-private rooms so that doctors could admit their private patients in addition to clinic patients. Over the years the ward system was phased out, and as the trend toward outpatient care increased Wills decreased its inpatient beds and enlarged its outpatient treatment areas.

Subspecialty services dealing with specific eye diseases or parts of the eye such as the retina and cornea evolved in the 1960s. Wills' commitment to research, present from the Hospital's inception, was formalized in 1952 when the Department of Research was established. In 1972 Wills became formally affiliated with Jefferson Medical College of Thomas Jefferson University and twenty-eight years later Wills still serves as Jefferson Medical College's Department of Ophthalmology.

Wills once again relocated in 1980 to a modern eight-story facility at Ninth and Walnut Streets in Center City. The architecturally award-winning 120-bed facility nearly doubled the size of the Hospital's previous building, provided increased room for outpatient services, and was equipped with state-of-the-art ophthalmic technology.

Over the years Wills physicians have been pioneers in many areas of eye care. Among their achievements have been the first intraocular lens implant in the United States, the development of widely used cataract surgery techniques, and the authorship of texts now considered classics in the field of ophthalmology.

In keeping with changes in the delivery of health care Wills diversified to include geropsychiatry and neurosurgery while developing a widespread network of surgicenters throughout the Delaware Valley, the crowning glory of which is the newest Wills Hospital between 8th and 9th Streets on Walnut Street.

Chapter 1

The Founding of Wills Eye Hospital

Many individuals have contributed to Wills Eye Hospital's reputation as one of the outstanding centers for eye care in the world. The funds necessary for growth and development were contributed by Philadelphia's leading philanthropists. Our staff not only has made countless advances in ophthalmology but also has been active in civic and cultural affairs. Indeed, many aspects of American history are reflected in the history of the Wills Eye Hospital.

Wills Eye Hospital owes its beginning to the Quaker tradition of charity. James Wills, Jr., founder of the hospital, was born in Philadelphia in 1777, just one year after the signing of the Declaration of Independence (Fig. 1-1). His father, James Wills, Sr., was born in 1748 and had come to this country from England, probably to escape religious persecution. Details about the senior Wills' background are sketchy, but we do know that he was a member of the Philadelphia Monthly Meeting and for a time worked for Anthony Benezet. Benezet's family, French Huguenots, had been subjected to religious persecution in France and had fled to England, where they had joined the Society of Friends. Later, the family came to the United States, where Benezet immediately became active in programs to overcome racial prejudice. He established a school for blacks while teaching at the William Penn Charter School. Testimony to the love Benezet had for his fellow man was never more evident than at his

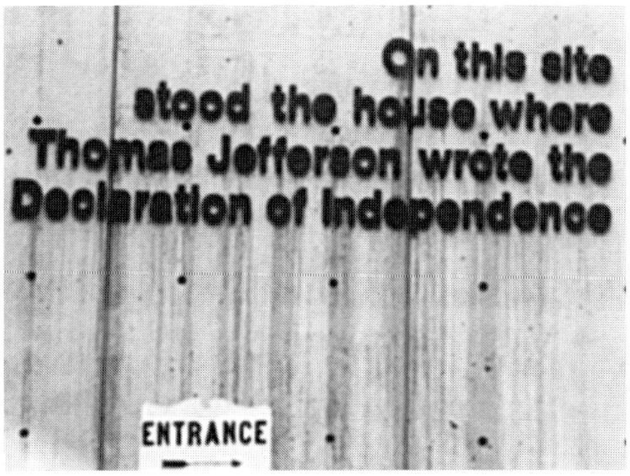

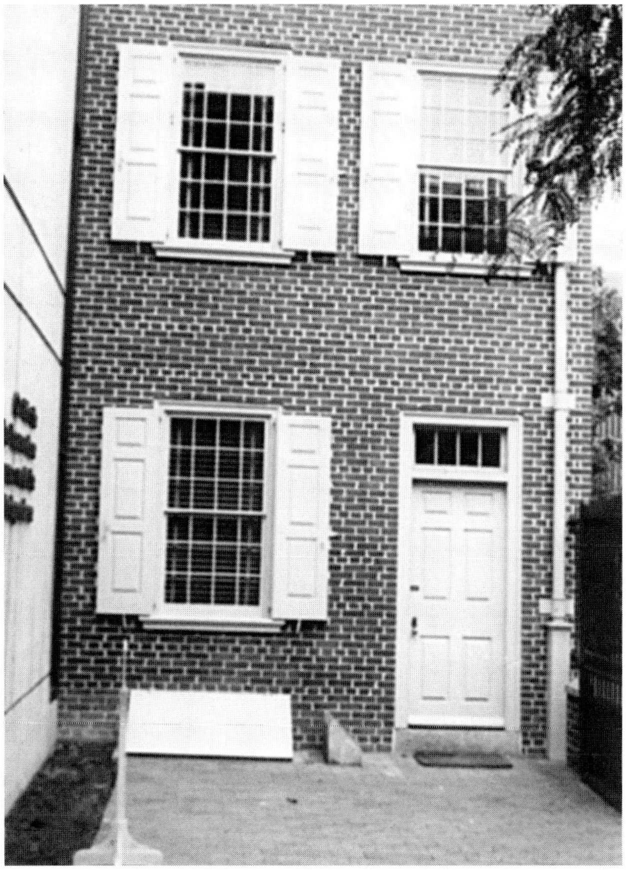

FIGURE 1-1
Site of the Graff House at 7th and Market Streets (four blocks from the present Wills) where Jefferson wrote the Declaration of Independence.

funeral, when rich and poor alike gathered to honor this charitable man in one of the largest funerals ever to take place in the City of Brotherly Love.

Previous reports suggest that James Wills, Sr. probably worked for Benezet as his coachman. However, it was unlikely that Benezet ever had a coach, so this is doubtless erroneous (Fig. 1-2). Nonetheless, Wills' friendship with Benezet probably had a great influence on Wills' later philanthropies, for which the money was earned in business. In 1791, with a stake of only $10, he opened his first store on Chestnut Street near Front Street.

Wills senior married Hannah Roberts. The Roberts family was apparently quite well-to-do, and the newlyweds were socially ostracized by the bride's friends because they suspected that she had married beneath her station. However, as it became obvious that Wills was a born businessman, he became accepted in the "proper" social circles.

Business prospered, and in 1800 Wills and his son, James, moved their store to 84 Chestnut Street (just above Third Street), which was, at the time, considered "West Philadelphia" (Fig. 1-3). Shortly thereafter they purchased buildings on either side of No. 84 (82 and 86 Chestnut Street) (Fig. 1-4, 1-5 and 1-5A).

Hannah Wills, James's mother, died between 1802 and 1809, and Wills Sr. died on April 23, 1823, at the age of 75. His obituary appeared in the paper on April 25.

Little is known about James Wills, Jr. He never married, and he continued his father's business until his premature death in 1825 at the young age of 48. His death was sudden, and his obituary appeared in *Poulson's American Daily Advertiser* on January 25, 1825 (Fig. 1-6). James had added to his father's estate while spending little money on himself. His yearly expenses were estimated at $400, while his benefactions amounted to $1,500.

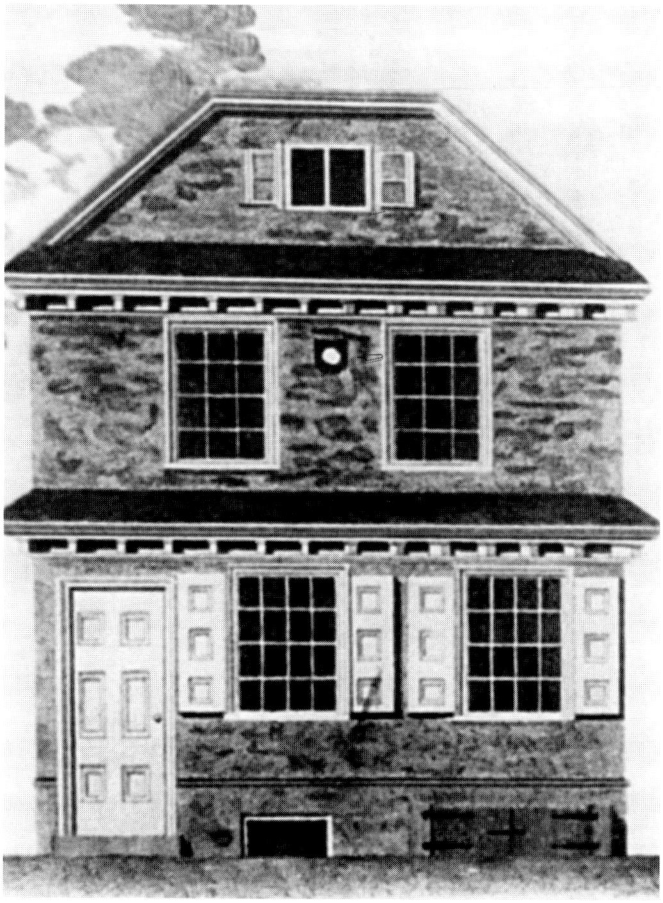

FIGURE 1-2
Home of Anthony Benezet. (Courtesy of Pennsylvania Historical Society)

According to his will, which was dated May 5, 1823 and came to probate January 26, 1825, his estate at the time of his death was approximately $116,000 (Fig. 1-7). With the exception of a few minor grants to places such as the Friends asylum for the insane and other worthwhile charities, the bulk of his wealth went to "the Mayor and Corporation of the City of Philadelphia for the time being and their successors in office forever in trust for the purchase of sufficient plot of ground in the City of Philadelphia, or in the neighborhood thereof, and thereon to erect or cause to be erected suitable building and accommodations for a[n] hospital or asylum to be denominated—The Wills Hospital for the relief of the indigent blind and lame."

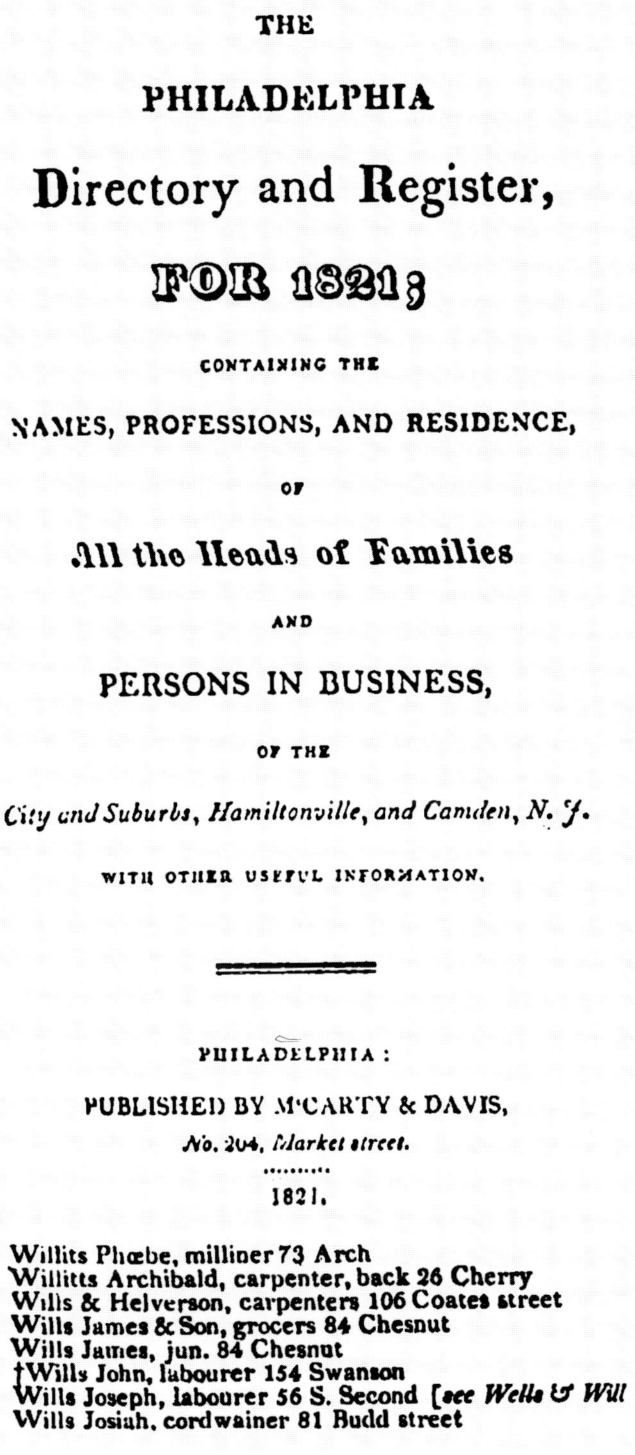

THE

PHILADELPHIA

Directory and Register,

FOR 1821;

CONTAINING THE

NAMES, PROFESSIONS, AND RESIDENCE,

OF

All the Heads of Families

AND

PERSONS IN BUSINESS,

OF THE

City and Suburbs, Hamiltonville, and Camden, N. J.

WITH OTHER USEFUL INFORMATION.

PHILADELPHIA:

PUBLISHED BY M'CARTY & DAVIS,

No. 204, Market street.

1821.

Willits Phœbe, milliner 73 Arch
Willitts Archibald, carpenter, back 26 Cherry
Wills & Helverson, carpenters 106 Coates street
Wills James & Son, grocers 84 Chesnut
Wills James, jun. 84 Chesnut
†Wills John, labourer 154 Swanson
Wills Joseph, labourer 56 S. Second [*see Wells & Will*
Wills Josiah, cordwainer 81 Budd street

FIGURE 1-3
The grocers of Chestnut Street were included in the Philadelphia Directory and Register.

As so frequently happens, however, previously-unheard-of heirs came forward to contest the will. Even in the 1800s, cases tended to drag on in the courts. It was not until March 21, 1831, that the Supreme Court of Pennsylvania finally decided in favor of the corporation of the City of Philadelphia, and the existence of the Wills Hospital became assured.

As it turns out, the delay was serendipitous: at the time of the bequest the sum available to establish a hospital was $108,395.35; however, in the interim, interest accrued, so that by the time work was ready to proceed on the hospital, funds available had risen to $122,548.57.

There has been much speculation about why James left his fortune as he did. One theory is that Wills became acquainted with Joseph Parrish, also a Quaker and one of the leading physicians and most prominent citizens in Philadelphia. Parrish would have known about the importance of establishing such an institution and no doubt would have transmitted his feelings to James. Further evidence of Parrish's influence over James is that all the other legacies left by Wills Jr. were to charities of particular interest to Parrish. A sum of $5,000, for example, went to the Friends asylum in Frankford, where Parrish served as one of the first attending physicians.

The City Council selected a plot between Eighteenth and Nineteenth Streets and between Race (then known as Sassafras) and Vine Streets, facing Logan Square, for the new hospital. The cost of the ground was $20,000, not quite as good a deal as Peter Minuit's $24 buy of Manhattan Island, but considerably less than the more than $1 million the ground was worth in 1930 and a mere fraction of what that block commands today. Cost of the building was estimated at $57,203.69, which left a balance of $45,344.88. All in all, even taking into account inflation over the years, the cost was

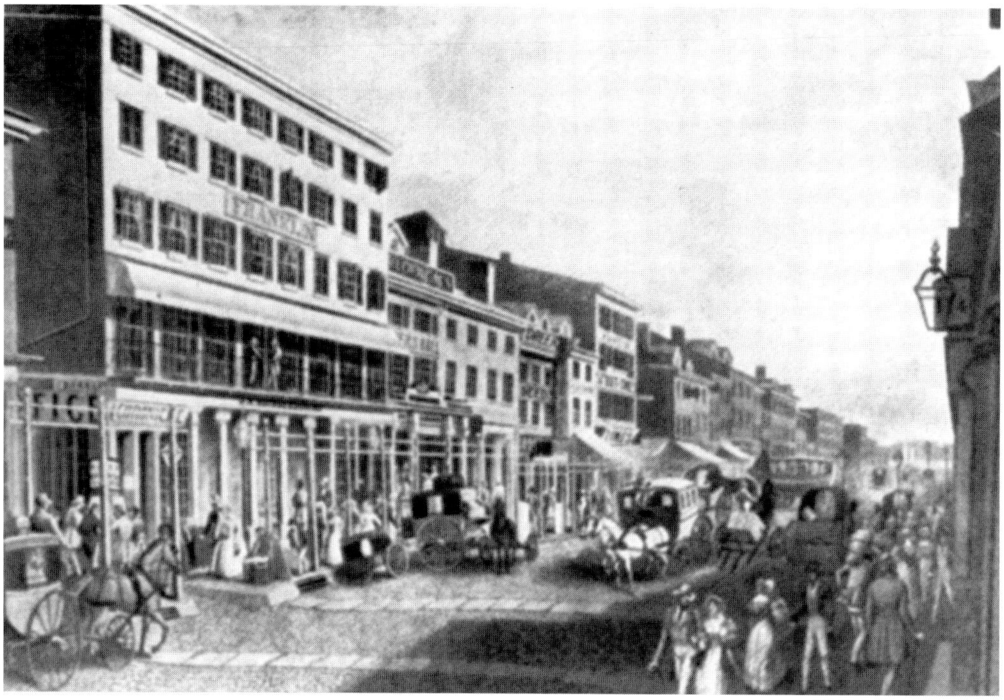

FIGURE 1-4
Chestnut Street in the 1820s between Third and Fourth near Wills Grocery. (Courtesy of Pennsylvania Historical Society)

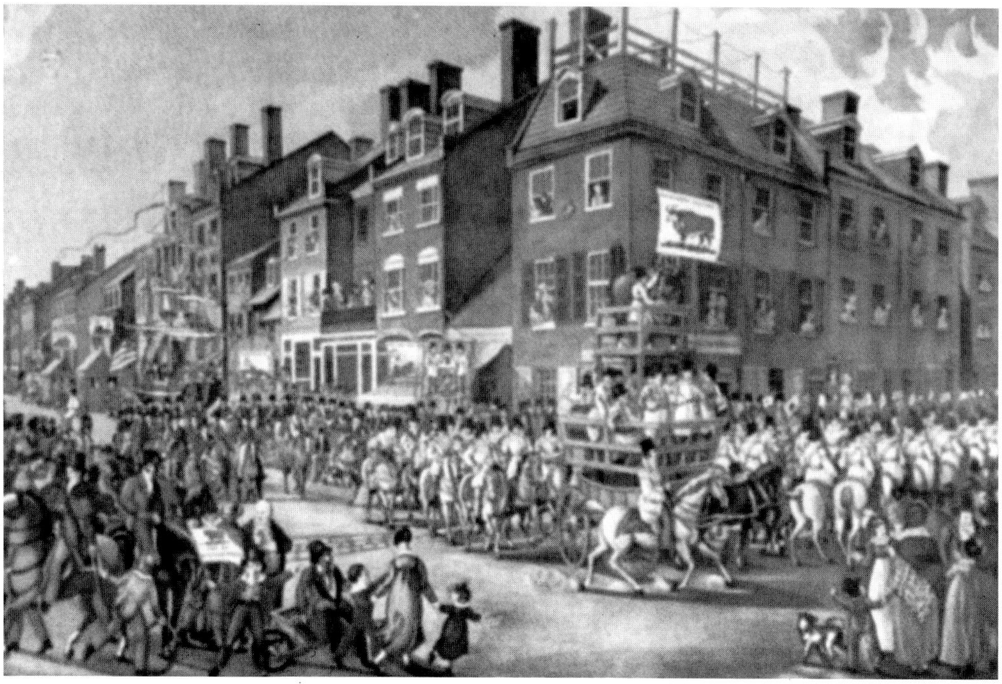

FIGURE 1-5
Parade at the southeast corner of Fourth and Chestnut Streets in the 1820s. (Courtesy of Pennsylvania Historical Society)

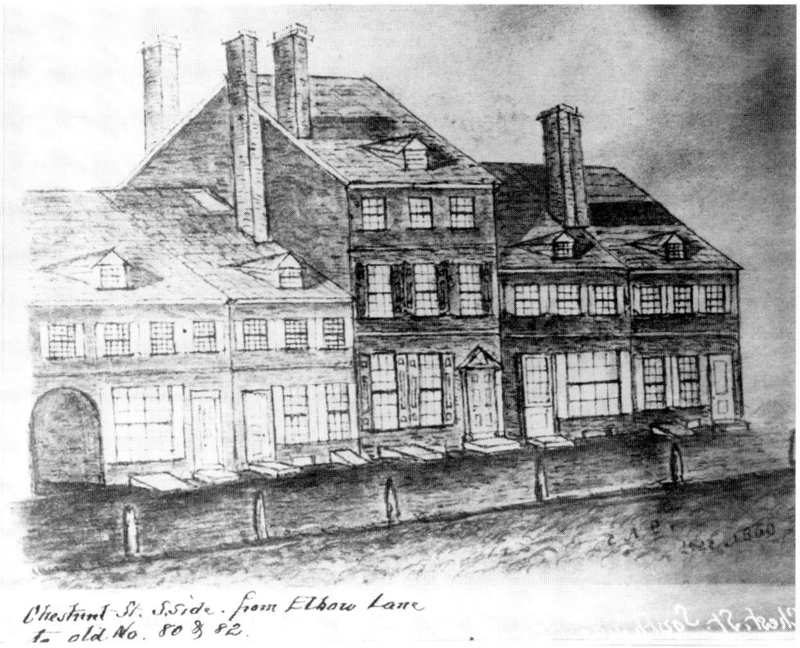

FIGURE 1-5A
Two homes, 80 and 82 Chestnut St., owned by James Wills, presumably adjacent to the grocery.
(Courtesy of the Free Library of Philadelphia)

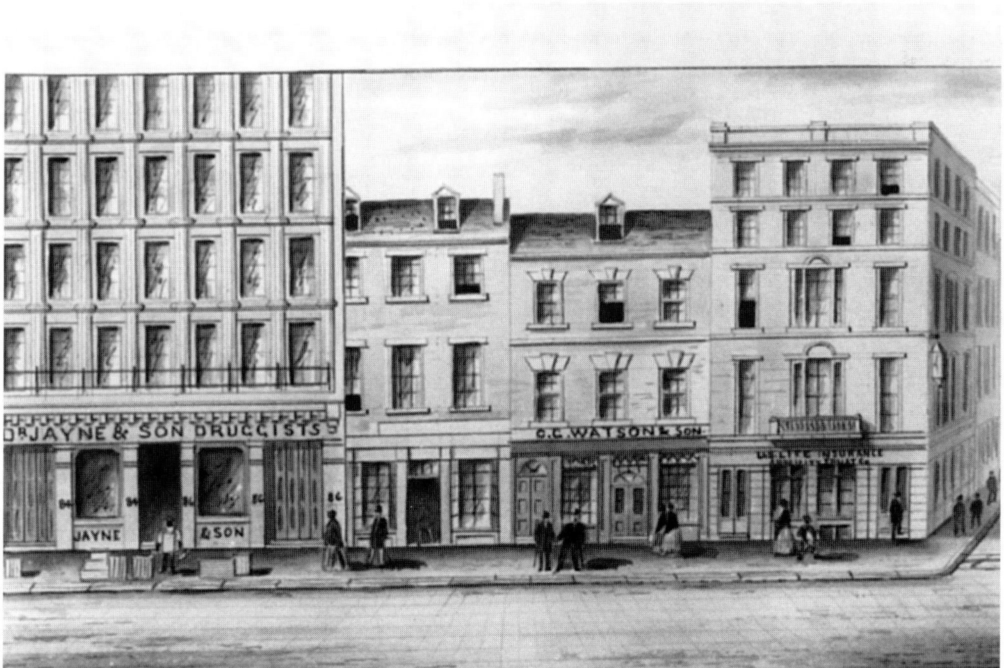

FIGURE 1-5B
By 1851, Wills Grocery at 84-86 Chestnut had been replaced by Jayne & Son Druggists.
(Courtesy of Pennsylvania Historical Society.)

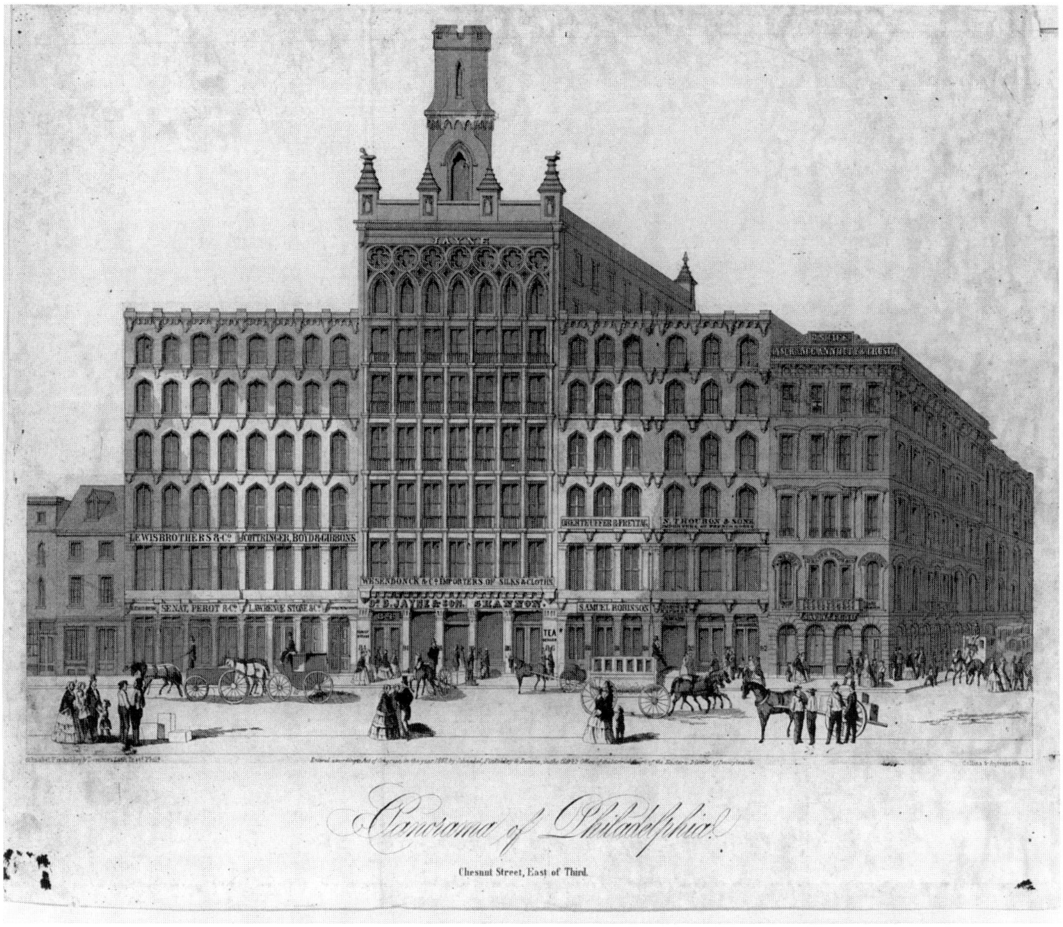

FIGURE 1-5C
Jayne Building years later (Courtesy of the Free Library of Philadelphia)

significantly lower than that of the 1980 Wills Eye Hospital—over $26 million—and the present Wills—$50 million.

Logan Square, one of the four original squares laid out by William Penn and the site of the first Wills Hospital, was named in honor of James Logan, William Penn's secretary, by an act of City Council in 1825. All of these four squares were originally set aside as open spaces for air, a designation similar to that made for the land upon which Moorfields Eye Hospital in London is built.

At that time, streets west of Broad Street were not paved and it was common to see cattle pasturing on nearby lands. Logan Square was also the site of a public hanging in 1823. A map of Philadelphia from 1840 shows that the Wills Hospital was the only building built upon the ground bounding that square. The Cathedral of Saints Peter and Paul at the corner of Eighteenth and Race Streets was not started until 1846 and took several years to complete. Today the Four Seasons Hotel is located on the site of the original Wills Hospital.

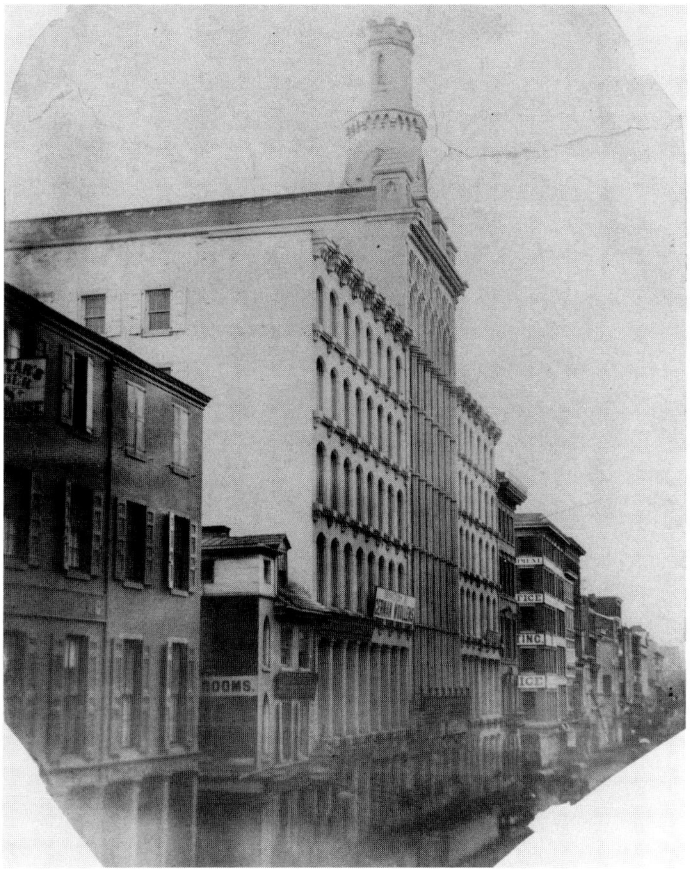

FIGURE 1-5D

The Jayne Building as it appeared in 1929 (Courtesy of the Free Library of Philadelphia)

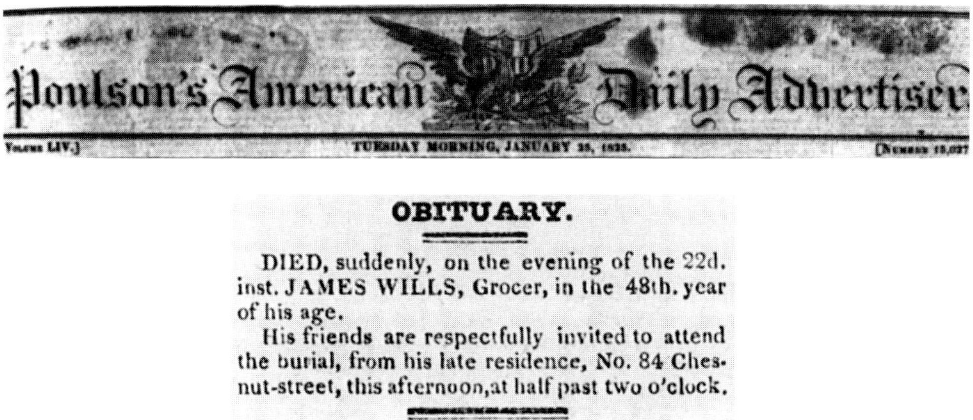

Poulson's American Daily Advertiser

VOLUME LIV.] TUESDAY MORNING, JANUARY 25, 1825.

OBITUARY.

DIED, suddenly, on the evening of the 22d. inst. JAMES WILLS, Grocer, in the 48th. year of his age.

His friends are respectfully invited to attend the burial, from his late residence, No. 84 Ches-nut-street, this afternoon, at half past two o'clock.

FIGURE 1-6

Obituary of James Wills, Jr., as it appeared in Poulson's American Daily Advertiser *on January 25, 1825. This is all we know about the sudden death of James Wills, Jr. Cause of death and, indeed, his style of living and even his appearance remain mysteries forever.*

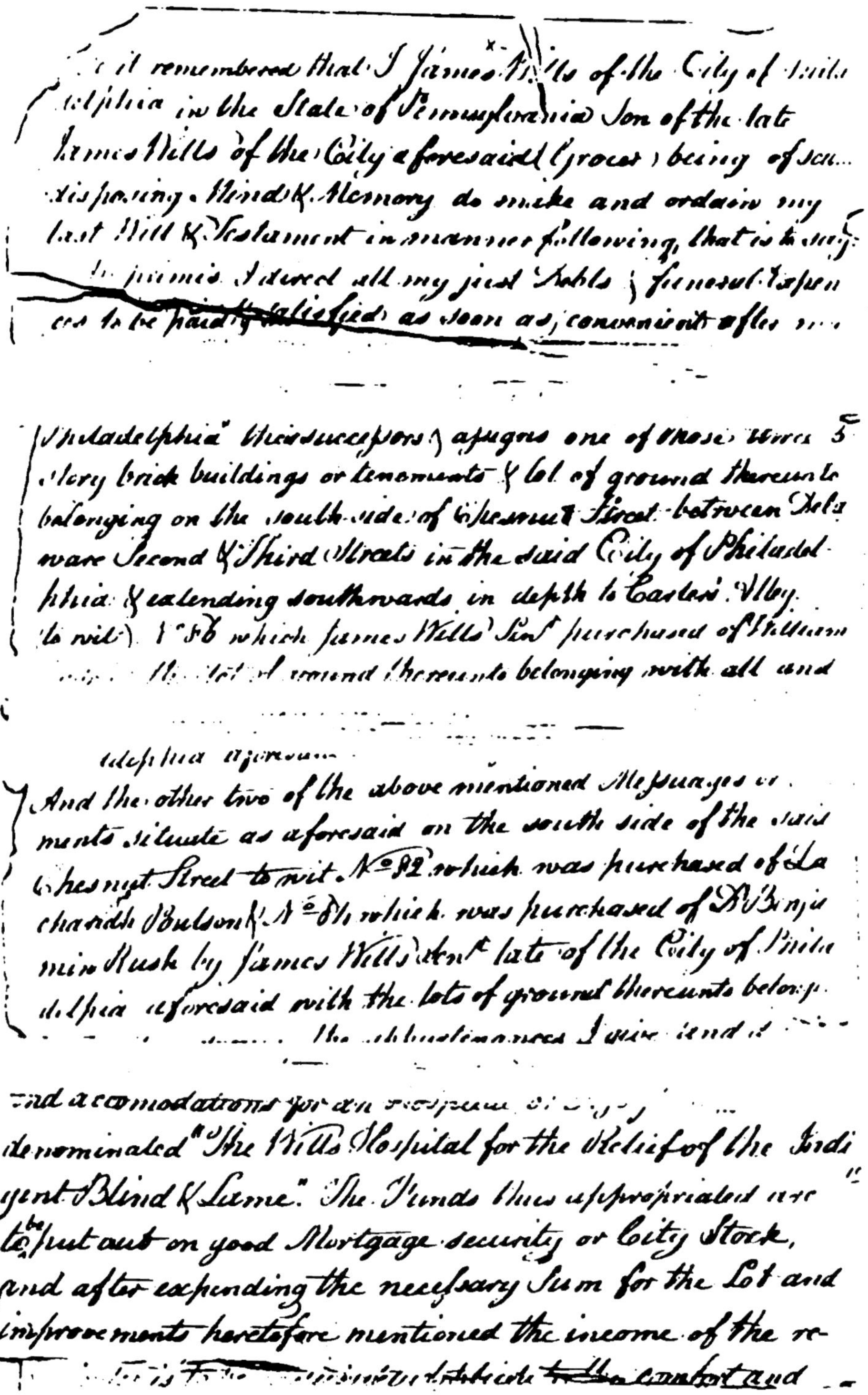
[illegible] it remembered that I James Wills of the City of Phila-
delphia in the State of Pennsylvania Son of the late
James Wills of the City aforesaid Grocer, being of sou[nd]
disposing Mind & Memory do make and ordain my
last Will & Testament in manner following, that is to say:
Imprimis I direct all my just Debts & funeral Expen
ces to be paid & satisfied as soon as convenient after m[y]

Philadelphia their successors & assigns one of those three 5
story brick buildings or tenements & lot of ground thereunto
belonging on the south side of Chesnut Street between Dela
ware Second & Third Streets in the said City of Philadel-
phia & extending southwards in depth to Carter's Alley
to wit No 86 which James Wills Senr purchased of William
[illegible] the lot of ground thereunto belonging with all and

[illegible]delphia aforesaid [illegible]
And the other two of the above mentioned Messuages or [illegible]
ments situate as aforesaid on the south side of the said
Chesnut Street to wit No 82 which was purchased of La
chariah Paulson & No 84 which was purchased of Dr Benja
min Rush by James Wills Senr late of the City of Phila
delphia aforesaid with the lots of ground thereunto belong[ing]
[illegible] the appurtenances I give and [illegible]

and accomodations for an Hospital [illegible]
denominated "The Wills Hospital for the Relief of the Indi
gent Blind & Lame." The Funds thus appropriated are
to be put out on good Mortgage security or City Stock,
and after expending the necessary Sum for the Lot and
improvements heretofore mentioned the income of the re-
[illegible] the comfort and

FIGURE 1-7
The last will and testament of James Wills, Jr.

Chapter 2

The First Hospital Building

The next question was to determine the builder and the design of the hospital. This decision was placed in the hands of a committee composed of men from City Council all of whom were eminent Philadelphians: Messrs. Daniel Groves, Joshua Lippincott, and John Moss. Their first meeting was on April 20, 1832. Incidentally, the minutes shown in Fig. 2-1 point out that a James Walker offered to serve as superintendent of the new hospital for the sum of $30 a month, considerably less than the current rate. Another candidate, Samuel Steal, also volunteered to serve at this low rate. It must have been considered quite an honor to work for this newly founded institution.

To select a design for the new hospital, the committee sponsored a competition, to be judged by William J. Duane, Joshua Lippincott, John R. Neff, and the president of the Bricklayers Company, Daniel Groves, who had recently been elected to the council on October 11th. Risley, a famous Will surgeon, named others appointed to the committee (probably from Common Council): Joseph Worrell, R. McMullin, R.M. Huston, B.H. Yarnall, and Enoch Robbins, another member of the Bricklayers Company.

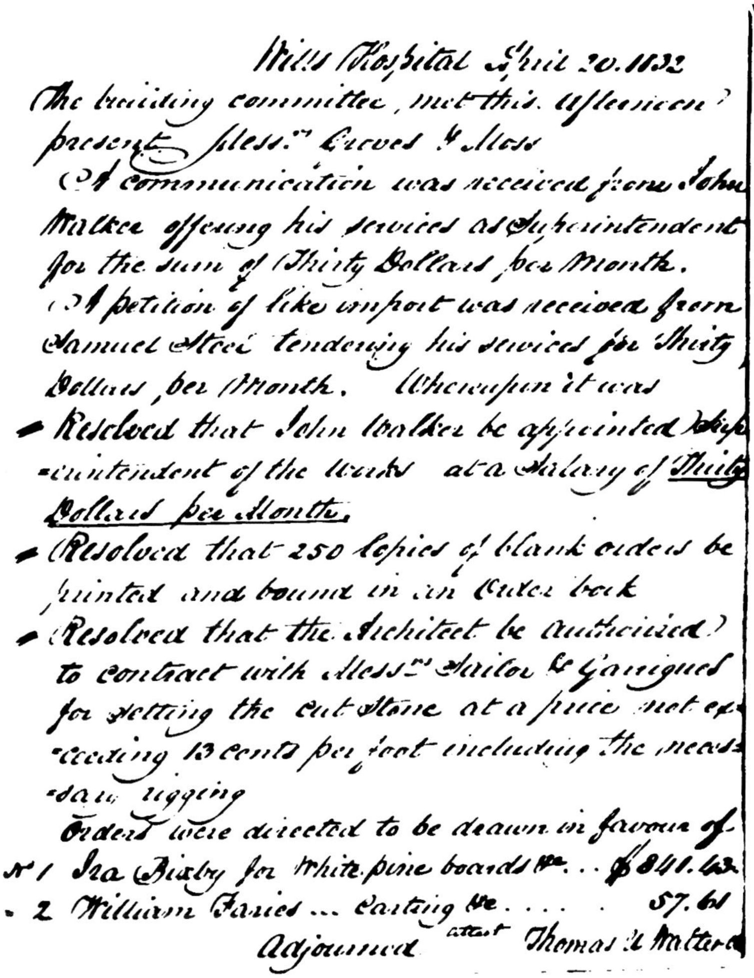
Wills Hospital April 20. 1832
The building committee, met this afternoon
present Messrs. Groves & Moss
A communication was received from John
Walker offering his services as Superintendent
for the sum of Thirty Dollars per Month.
A petition of like import was received from
Samuel Steel tendering his services for Thirty
Dollars per Month. Whereupon it was
Resolved that John Walker be appointed Super-
intendent of the works at a Salary of Thirty
Dollars per Month.
Resolved that 250 copies of blank orders be
printed and bound in an Order book
Resolved that the Architect be authorised
to contract with Messrs. [illegible]
for setting the cut stone at a price not ex-
ceeding 13 cents per foot including the neces-
sary rigging
Orders were directed to be drawn in favour of
No 1 Ira Bixby for White pine boards &c. . . $841.43
" 2 William Davies ... Casting &c. 57.61
Adjourned attest Thomas U. Walter

FIGURE 2-1
The first committee meeting minutes of the Wills Hospital, April 20, 1832, written in longhand and signed by Thomas U. Walter.

Several rising young architects competed in the contest: John Haviland, John C. Trautwine, William Rodrigue, George Seneff, and Thomas Ustick Walter all submitted designs for the hospital. The committee met on December 29 to reach a decision. After careful review, to Walter went the first prize of $100; to Trautwine, second prize of $50; and to Rodrigue, Seneff, and Haviland, $25 each (although, as Baigell points out, Haviland recorded receiving no less than $100, which may have been payment for his first, presumably solicited design presented in June). The results were published in the *Philadelphia Gazette and Daily Advertiser* on January 6 and were reprinted in *Poulson's American Daily Advertiser* the next day.

The original drawings Walter submitted have been lost. However, among his papers are fragments of a letter accompanying the design which, when pieced together, reads as follows:

Gentlemen:

I herewith submit for your consideration a design for an "Asylum for the Lame and Blind," see [drawing] no. 1. By reference to the plan of Principal story you will observe that I have placed all the living rooms or dormitories in wings contiguous to the Centre building, in which I have made arrangement for the Dining Room, Meeting Room etc. My object in making this disposition is, in the first place, to obtain the greatest accommodation at the least expenditure, [and] secondly, to have a dining room on the principal floor which in my opinion is a desideratum of considerable importance. The dining room in the Widows Asylum [by Strickland, 1819-1820] is in the Basement Story and from information received from the matron this arrangement completely destroys the comfort of the house.

Another object of importance gained by the disposition I have made, is the approach to all the dormitories, stairways, dining rooms, etc. from a straight passage or Corridor, which makes the establishment peculiarly adapted to the accommodation of the Blind. You will observe also that this manner of building ensures a free circulation of Air thro' all the rooms (see no. 2). I have made the dormitories 10 x 15 ft., supposing this to be sufficiently large for 2 persons. There are 40 dormitories. Consequently the building will contain 80 persons with the necessary accommodations for Steward, Matron, Physicians, Attendants, Kitchen, Washing Room, Ironing Room, Bath room, a room for Religious meeting, etc. In designing an edifice of this kind, it is necessary to have reference to a future enlargement of the establishment. With the design I offer for your consideration this may be advantageously effected. The Wings may be extended to any required distance and flanked by two end buildings symmetrical with the center, and, should the accommodations thus obtained prove insufficient at any future period, other ranges of dormitories may be constructed extending from each corner building at right angles with the front.

Walter's career had started out rather inauspiciously. Initially he was a bricklayer. However, taking advantage of architecture courses offered at the Franklin Institute, he ultimately became one of Philadelphia's leading architects. The high point in his professional life came in 1842, when he was appointed to the faculty of the Franklin Institute as professor of architecture. He also laid out the plans for Girard College and assisted Charles Pierre L'Enfant in designing the wings of the Senate and House of the United States Capitol in Washington, D.C.

Walter's design of Wills Hospital was one of his first efforts. The committee considered him a novice, a fact that became evident in its report giving the reasons for its choice. They stated that judgment had been made from "consideration of all circumstances connected with the legacy and the object, and not strictly from a regard of mere architectural merit. The fund is too limited to warrant such structures as some of the plans represent, so that economy as well as adequacy have been regarded in preference to display or beauty."

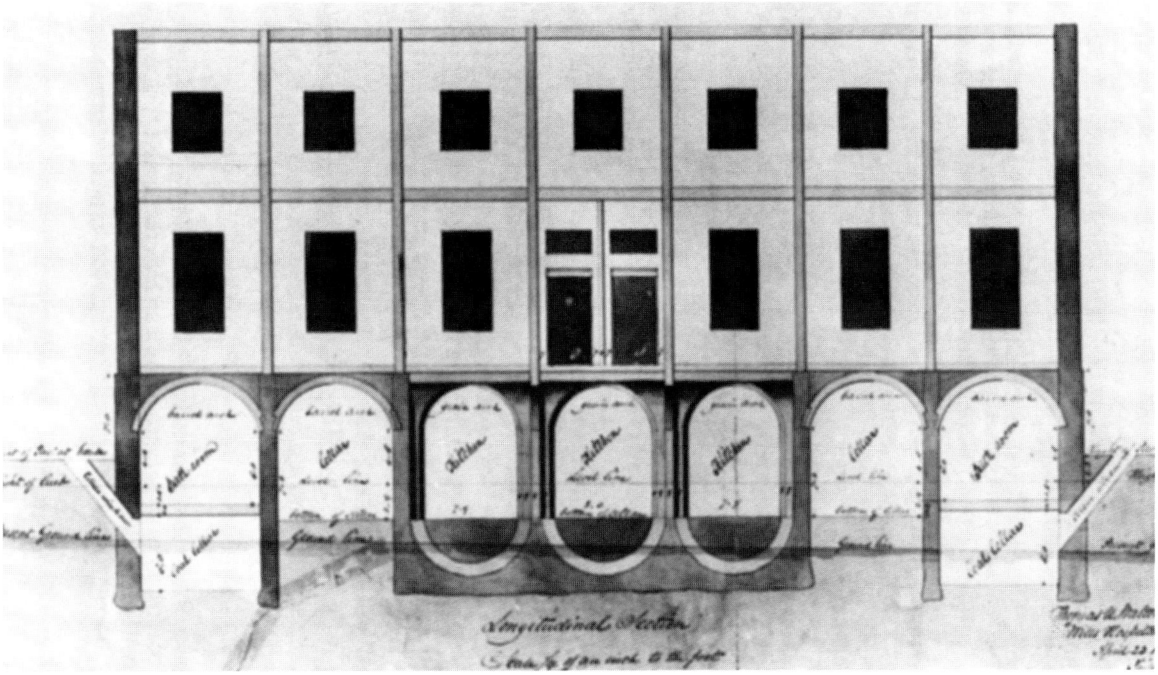

FIGURE 2-2
Plans for the original Wills Eye Hospital on Logan Square. (Courtesy of the Athenaeum of Philadelphia, private collection.)

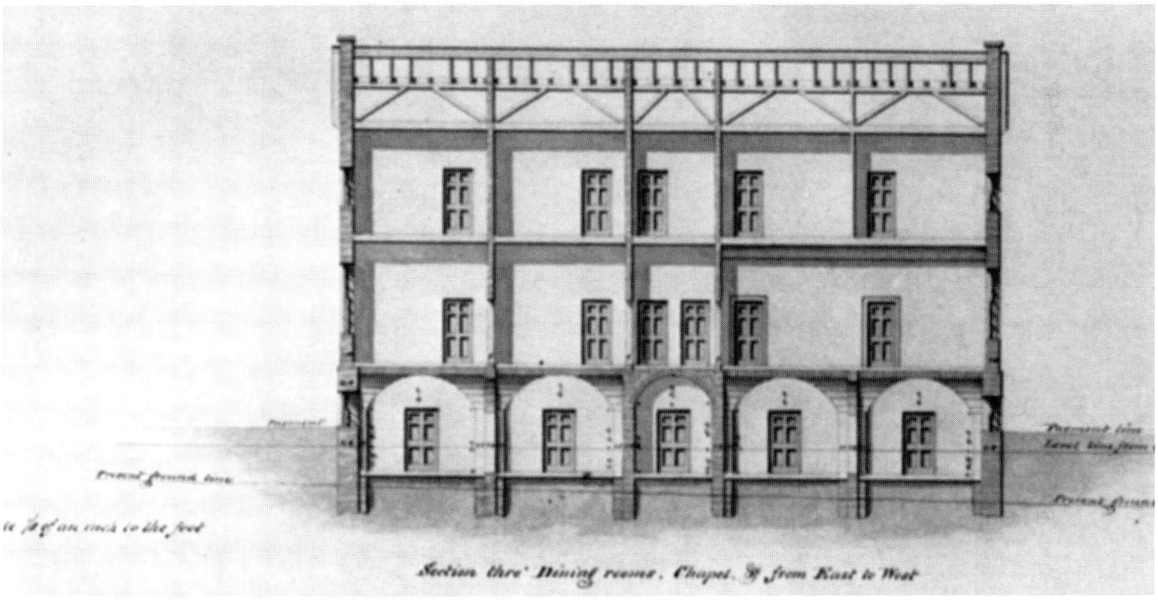

FIGURE 2-2A

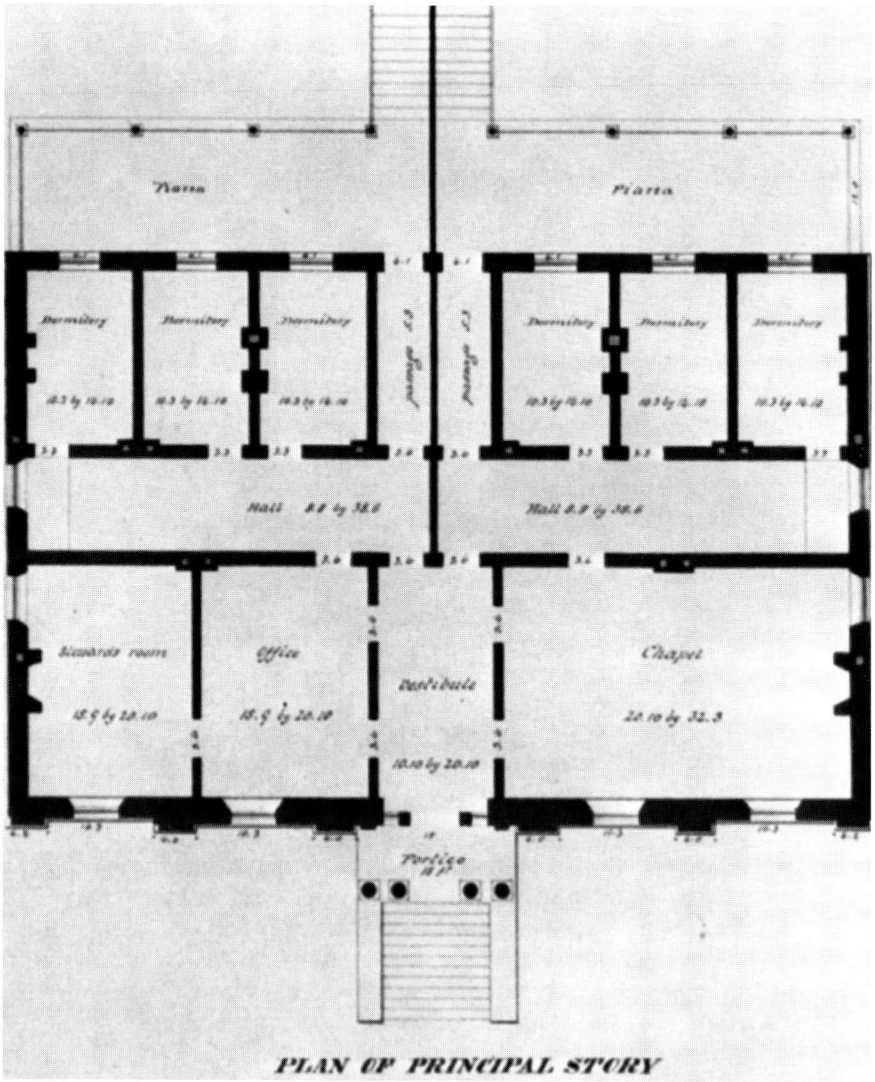

FIGURE 2-2B

Final plans for the hospital were submitted to the city council and were approved by them on January 13, 1833 (Figs. 2-2, 2-2A and 2-2B). The minutes of the Select Committee of Philadelphia state that plans and estimates for the new hospital were received on June 6, 1831. According to Hazard's Register (IX, 1), they were submitted by Haviland and Strickland. The committee, however, did not find them satisfactory, and they had to be redone.

There is some question as to when the cornerstone of the hospital was actually laid. The earlier *History of Wills Eye Hospital* states that it was April 2, 1832, but there is some doubt about whether this date is accurate, since the hospital building committee appointed by Philadelphia City Council did not meet until April 20, 1832 (Fig. 2-1). We are sure, however, that the hospital was completed by 1834.

The completed building was 80 feet long and 50 feet deep. On the south side there was a piazza approximately12 feet wide. The hospital was built to accommodate approximately 70 patients and consisted of three stories: basement, first floor, and second floor, with an attic 24 feet wide and 80 feet long. The roof was made of copper, and the lot was surrounded by a cut stone fence 2 feet high, upon which was placed an iron railing. The front of the building on Race Street was made of sandstone and featured six ionic pilasters (Fig. 2-3). Surrounding the front door was a Grecian ionic portico consisting of four columns (Figs. 2-4 and 2-4A).

The hospital opened on March 3, 1834, and Joseph R. Ingersoll gave the dedication address. In the midst of all the preparations, however, the hospital founders began to question the intentions of James Wills. Was the institution to be a hospital for the treatment of the blind or lame or should it become an asylum for the incapacitated? Fortunately, the committee voted in favor of continuing as a hospital, because it was their feeling that an asylum could care for only 12 to 15 people, while a hospital could treat thousands.

On April 1, 1834, the hospital committee reported that the Wills Hospital had opened in March 1834 (Fig. 2-5). The report shows that ten patients were admitted for medical or surgical care, while ten others were apparently turned away because it was felt that they could not be helped.

Isaac Parrish (Joseph's son) performed the first cataract operation at Wills Hospital, a fact recorded in the report of April 1, 1834 (Fig. 2-5). At the time of the report, the outcome of the surgery was not known, but Rodman Paul and Charles Stout were optimistic that the operation would be successful.

As expected, the expenditures of the day were somewhat less than we encounter today. Only $247.36 was spent in the month covered by the report: this included bread and milk, as well as medicines, which were felt would last "several months." The committee then recommended that $20, in addition to the $5.37 already in the hands of the steward, be appropriated for current expenses during the month of April. Of interest, too, is a notation in the final paragraph that alterations be made to the south portico of the building to prevent deterioration of the plaster from rain. As with all new buildings, past and present, defects creep up even shortly after completion.

The City Council of Philadelphia managed the hospital until 1869, when the Board of Directors of City Trusts took over. While still under the aegis of City Council, a board of managers composed of 18 members, none of whom were members of the council, were charged with the responsibility of managing Wills Hospital. In addition, there were five presidents of the board of managers during the period before 1869; three of them were physicians. The first, of course, was Dr. Joseph Parrish, who served from December 2, 1833, to March 2, 1840. He was succeeded by Dr. Frederick Eringer, who resigned in 1843, to be followed by Dr. J. Rodman Paul, who served from 1843 to 1864, when he resigned. Next in line was Dr. Andrew Nevinger, who served for only a little over a year and was not reappointed. The final president during this period was Charles Ellis (not a physician), who assumed that position in December 1865 and then went on to become a member of the Board of Directors of City Trusts.

The name Wills Hospital, by the way, was never officially changed to Wills Eye Hospital. Despite this the sign over the original Logan Square building clearly reads Wills Eye Hospital. When a third story was added, the name on the building reverted to Wills Hospital, and this same designation was continued at 16th and Spring Garden where the name Wills Hospital is carved in stone above the pillars and can still be seen today.

However, Wills Hospital's reputation for quality eye care has led to it commonly being called Wills Eye Hospital. This is confirmed by maps of the city from 1875 showing the building on Logan Square as Wills Eye Hospital. Advertisements for a course of lectures on ophthalmic surgery in 1869 referred to Wills

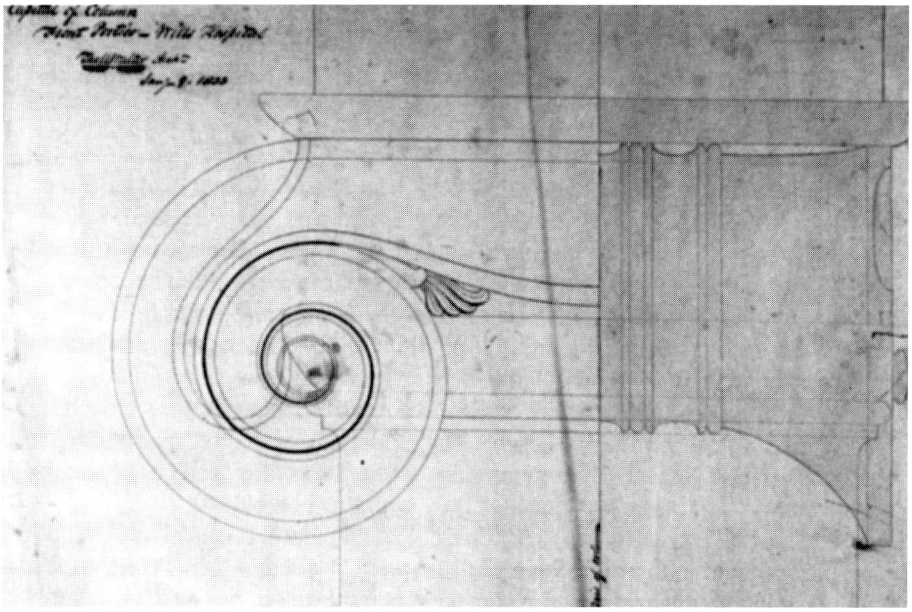

FIGURE 2-3
Drawing of column, front portico, Wills Hospital. (Drawing in possession of Girard College).

Ophthalmic Hospital, while notice for another course on practical ophthalmoscopy conducted in 1873 reverted back to Wills Hospital.

Since 1932, however, the name Wills Eye Hospital seems to have taken hold as evidenced by the many newspaper clippings reporting on the hospital and the large red letters on the Ninth Street side of the present building.

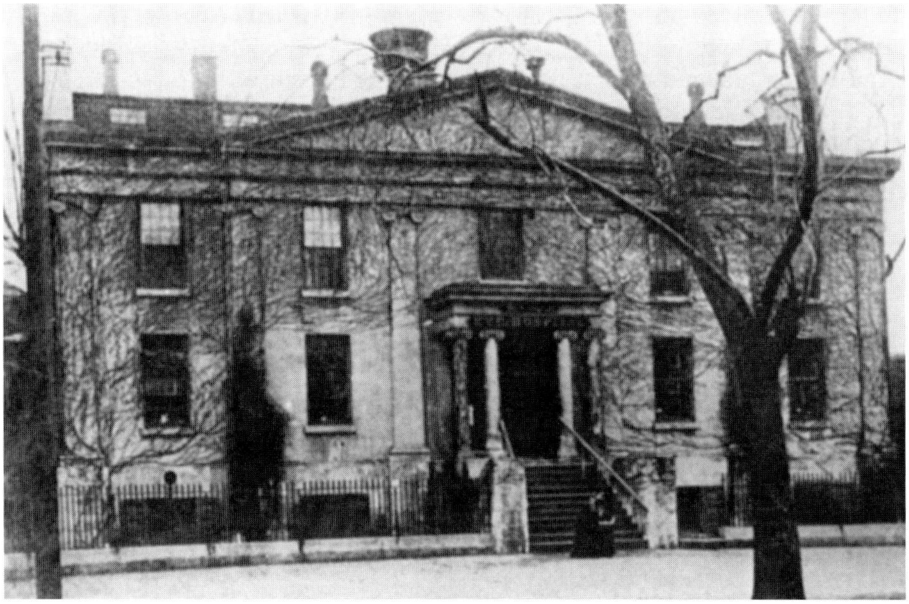

FIGURE 2-4
Wills Hospital, created as an asylum for the indigent blind and lame. Located on Logan Square, it reflected the architectural style of the 19th century.

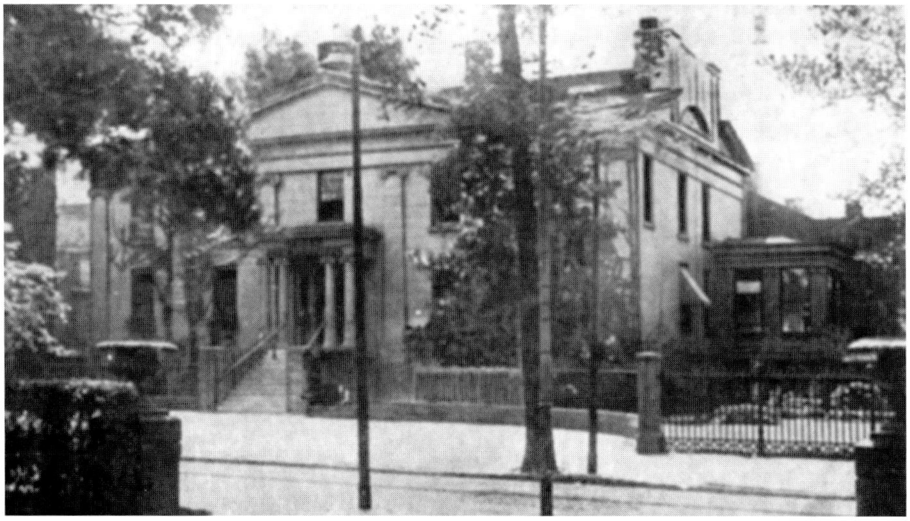

FIGURE 2-4A
Wills Eye Hospital, Race Street between 18th and 19th (Logan Square), Philadelphia, PA.

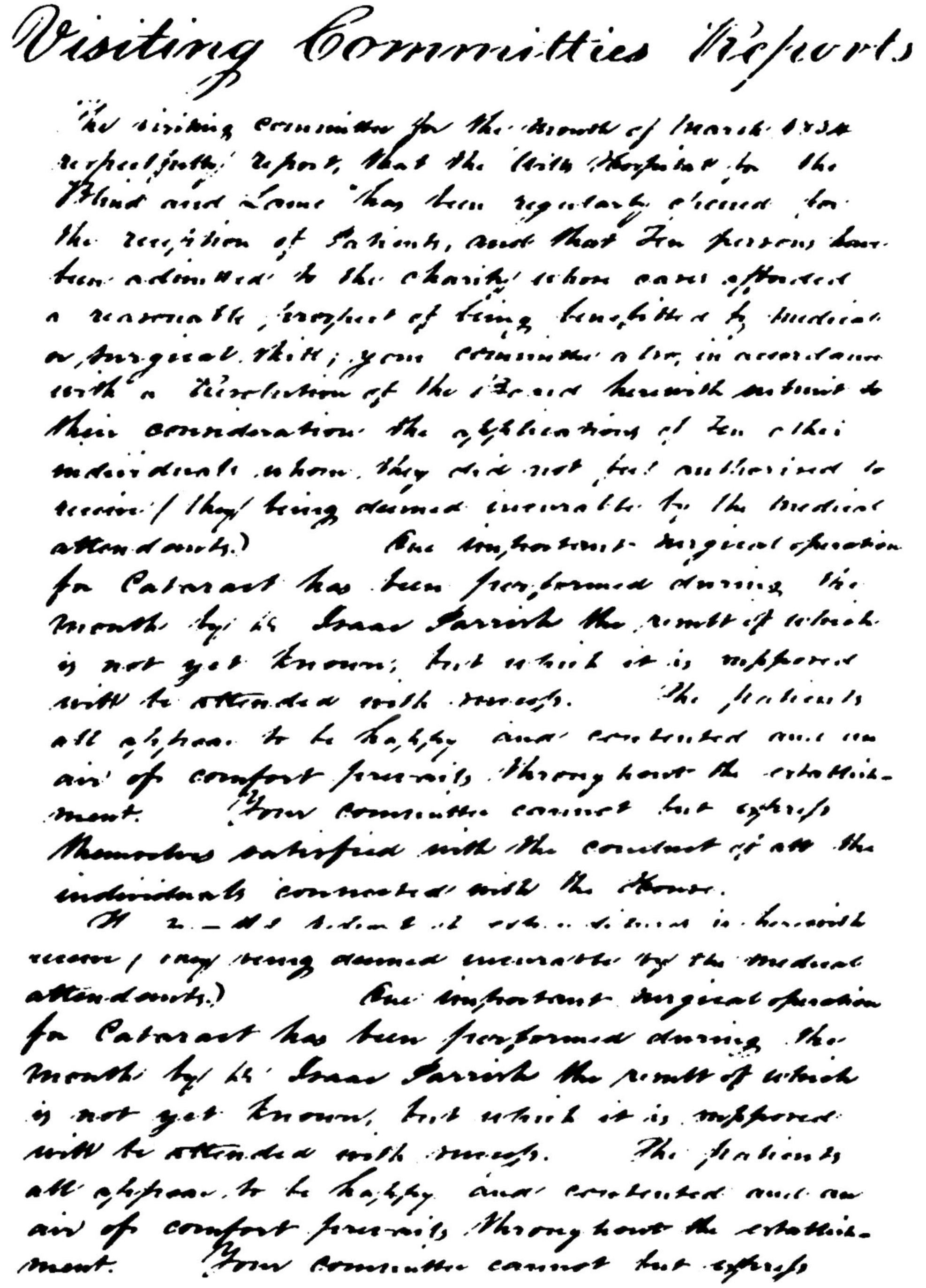

Visiting Committees Reports

The visiting committee for the month of March 1834 respectfully report, that the Wills Hospital for the Blind and Lame has been regularly opened for the reception of Patients, and that ten persons have been admitted to the charity whose cases afforded a reasonable prospect of being benefitted by medical or surgical skill; your committee also, in accordance with a Resolution of the Board herewith submit to their consideration the applications of ten other individuals whom they did not feel authorized to receive (they being deemed incurable by the medical attendants.) One important surgical operation for Cataract has been performed during the month by Dr Isaac Parrish the result of which is not yet known, but which it is supposed will be attended with success. The patients all appear to be happy and contented and an air of comfort prevails throughout the establishment. Your committee cannot but express themselves satisfied with the conduct of all the individuals connected with the House.

receive (they being deemed incurable by the medical attendants.) One important surgical operation for Cataract has been performed during the month by Dr Isaac Parrish the result of which is not yet known, but which it is supposed will be attended with success. The patients all appear to be happy and contented and an air of comfort prevails throughout the establishment. Your committee cannot but express

FIGURE 2-5

Excerpts from the minutes of the visiting committee report, March 1834. The minutes refer to the first cataract operation at the Wills.

Chapter 3
The Early Surgeons

Isaac Parrish was born in Philadelphia in 1811. Son of the first president of the board of managers of Wills Eye Hospital, Joseph Parrish, he was one of 11 children and was educated in a Friends school. He later matriculated at the University of Pennsylvania and was graduated with a medical degree in 1832. After further training at the Philadelphia Hospital, he became one of the first surgeons at the Wills Eye Hospital at the young age of 23. He is credited with performing its first cataract operation. He also lectured extensively on ophthalmology and was generally well liked by his colleagues.

Parrish was very active in the Society for the Abolition of Slavery and was also interested in improving the plight of prisoners. He was still a young man when he died in 1852 of dysentery, which he contracted from his eldest son, who had been ill for several weeks. Both father and son died in the same hour. This tragedy deprived society of a dedicated individual who undoubtedly would have made even greater contributions to mankind had he lived longer.

As an aside, the Parrish family includes a well-known artist of the day. Maxfield Parrish was Isaac Parrish's great-nephew, son of Stephen Parrish, who was the son of Dillwyn Parrish, Isaac Parrish's brother. Maxfield Parrish's chemistry notebook from Haverford College testifies to his playfulness and good spirit (Fig.3-1). The same spirit is evident in his mural of "Old King Cole," originally the bar mural of John Astor's Knickerbocker Hotel in New York City and now displayed in the St. Regis barroom (Fig. 3-2).

Squier Littel

Squier Littel was another of the four surgeons appointed to Wills Eye Hospital. Squier Littel was born in Burlington, New Jersey, in 1803. His ancestors had come from London, England, and had settled initially in Newberry, Massachusetts, in 1630. From that point, the family scattered throughout the East and Midwest.

Both of Littel's parents died while he was a young child, so he was adopted by an uncle, Dr. Squier Littel, of Butler, Ohio. Inspired by his uncle to enter medicine, he came to Philadelphia in 1821, where he studied under the guidance of Dr. Joseph Parrish. He entered medical school at the University of Pennsylvania and was graduated in 1824. His graduation thesis was entitled "Inflammation."

Squier Littel was an adventurous soul and was soon lured to Buenos Aires by the prospect of a South American adventure. Disillusioned and homesick, he stayed for only about four months before returning to Philadelphia by way of Chile, Peru, and Ecuador. On his return to Philadelphia, Littel became an active member of a committee to revise and correct an edition of the *Book of Common Prayer*. He also was editor of "The Banner of the Cross," one of the most influential church papers of the times, and wrote poetry and metrical translations of medieval hymns.

Littel's contributions to medicine were many and varied. They included editorship of three volumes of the *Journal of Foreign Medicine* as well as contributions to the American *Journal of*

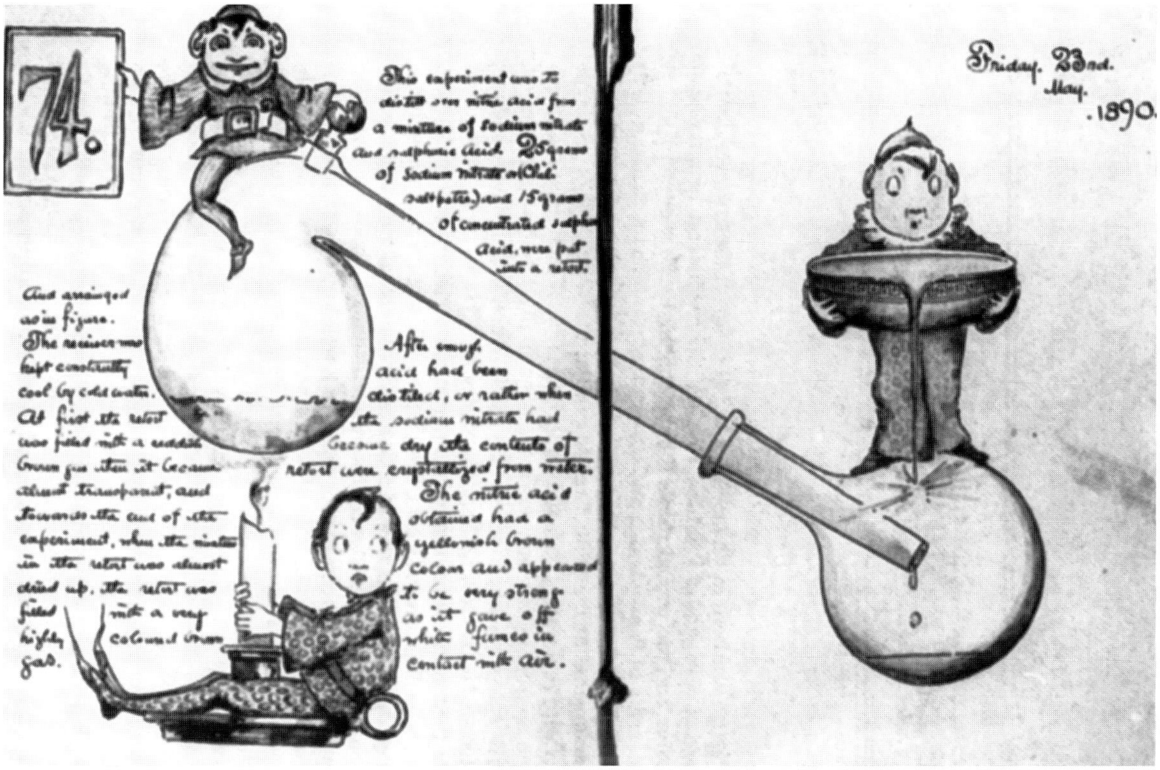

FIGURE 3-1
There are different ways to approach chemistry, as Maxfield Parrish, great-nephew of Isaac Parrish, shows. Elves clutch the Bunsen burners and slide down the beakers he used in his chemistry experiments. Unfortunately, his artwork did not earn him any points in chemistry. His grade for the course was only 68!

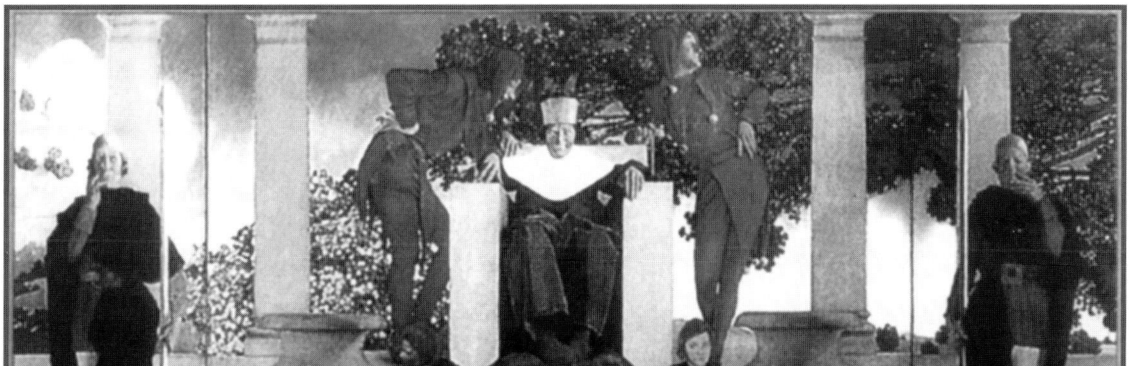

FIGURE 3-2
Maxfield Parrish painting over the bar in the St. Regis Hotel, NYC.

Medical Sciences. He also wrote a textbook entitled *A Manual of Diseases of the Eye*, which was published in 1837. This was a clearly written, concise work that was later revised in 1838 by Hugh Houston, a member of the Royal College of Surgeons in London.

In 1854, he edited an American edition of H. Hayes Waldman's *Operative Ophthalmic Surgery*. This innovative text recommended chloroform over ether and suggested its use for patients of all ages as an agent that would "tranquilize the mind, deaden the sensibility . . . , while to the operator it assured complete command of the patient." As it turned out, however, general anesthesia was not the great boon to the ophthalmic surgeon that it was to the general surgeon. Too often, vomiting and retching impeded or complicated the recovery following ocular surgery. There was no way, certainly, for Littel to have known this, and there is no doubt that he was very concerned about making advancements in the field of ophthalmology.

It is reported that late in life he developed choroiditis and failing sight before he died of cardiorenal problems at the age of 83. His contributions to the Wills Eye Hospital also included his son-in-law and assistant, Dr. A.D. Hall, who served as an active member on the Wills Eye Hospital staff.

Isaac Hays

The third representative to the staff of the Wills Eye Hospital was Isaac Hays. Hays was the only Jewish physician on the staff. He was born in 1796 and on his mother's side was a descendant of the well-known Gratz family. His aunt, Rebecca Gratz, was the model for Rebecca in *Ivanhoe*.

How Rebecca Gratz of Philadelphia became the model for Scott's Rebecca is a story worth telling. Rebecca Gratz had become a good friend of Tilly Hoffman, a daughter of a New York judge, and had visited her numerous times in New York City. Unfortunately, Tilly developed tuberculosis, from which she died at the age of 18. During her illness, she was visited many times by Rebecca, who thereby made the acquaintance of another visitor, Washington Irving. Irving was in love with Tilly and spent many hours at her bedside. He was charmed by Rebecca's beauty and grace. After Tilly's death, Irving met Walter Scott during a trip to Europe. Coincidentally, Scott told Irving that he was planning a book that included some Jewish characters. Irving, remembering the beauty and character of Rebecca Gratz, described her to Scott, who subsequently created the famous heroine of *Ivanhoe*. Had this book been written today rather than in the 19th century, it is very possible that Wilfred of Ivanhoe might have chosen to marry Rebecca rather than Rowena. The prospect of interfaith marriage at that time, of course, was extremely unlikely.

Upon completion of his novel, Scott wrote to Irving and asked "What do you think of your Rebecca—did I follow the pattern?" The answer was yes.

Isaac Hays' father had been a successful merchant who had hoped that his son would follow in his footsteps. However, Isaac was more interested in medicine, and he graduated from the University of Pennsylvania Medical School in 1820. Initially engaged in general practice, he began more and more to devote himself to the study and treatment of diseases of the eye. With Squier Littel, he became one of the pioneers in American ophthalmology. Like Littel, he was a good writer and ultimately became editor of the *American Journal of Medical Sciences*.

Isaac Hays married Sarah Minus, and their son, Isaac Minus Hays, also became a physician and later joined his father in practice; father and son were coeditors of the *American Journal of Medical Sciences* for 75 years. As editor, Hays had the right to refuse any manuscript. However, he was a courteous gentleman, and it became well known that a casual greeting to someone who had submitted a manuscript usually meant that the paper had been accepted, while obsequious behavior meant that the paper had been turned down. By such contact Hays hoped to lighten the blow of rejection.

Some landmark papers that appeared in the *Journal* included Horner's original description in 1824 of the small muscles at the internal commissure of the eyelids, as well as an ingenious operation described by Horner for correction of ectropion of the lower lid.

Hays became a close friend of Joseph Parrish and continued as a surgeon at the Wills Eye Hospital until 1854, when pressures of his editorship forced him to resign. However, he continued to contribute quarterly reports of the work done on his service at the Wills Eye Hospital; these were published in the *American Journal of Medical Sciences.*

Isaac Hayes was also very interested in natural history and contributed many articles in this field. One of them was a masterful work on the mastodon. As a result of this interest, he was made president of the Academy of Natural Sciences in Philadelphia in 1865. He also became an honorary member of the American Ophthalmological Society at its first meeting in 1864 and received honors from the Medical Society at Hamburg, the Societé Universelle d'Ophthalmologie, and the Congrés Médicale Internationale de Paris. A respected member of the community, he died in 1879 at the age of 83.

George Fox

The final member of the original foursome was George Fox, the youngest son of 13 children born to Samuel Mickel Fox. He was born in 1806 and, like Parrish, was a member of the Society of Friends. He was a graduate of Philadelphia private schools and attended the University of Pennsylvania, receiving his medical degree in 1826. He was another of Dr. Joseph Parrish's distinguished pupils. While a resident physician at the Pennsylvania Hospital, he devised an apparatus for the treatment of fractures of the clavicle. He was not a prolific writer, but he did bring the work of Wills Eye Hospital to the attention of the medical profession by publishing clinical reports in the *American Journal of Medical Sciences* in November 1839.

Though interested in diseases of the eye, he was against sub-specialization and did not wish to be known only as an ophthalmologist. In 1854, he retired and left the city to live in the country. He was a good businessman and had been able to acquire a sizable fortune at a young age, as well as a directorship of the National Bank of Commerce in 1876, a position he held until his death. A philanthropist, he was also active in obtaining a building at Thirteenth and Locust Streets for the College of Physicians. He died in 1882 at the age of 76.

Chapter 4

Wills Eye Hospital in the 19th Century

The 19th century was a good era for Wills Eye Hospital. Physicians famous in their own right and those who fathered famous sons passed through the portals of this growing medical center. Some were known as surgeons, others as pioneers in the technology of ophthalmology; still others had sons who achieved fame in the military or the arts. Their stories are unusual and deserve special attention.

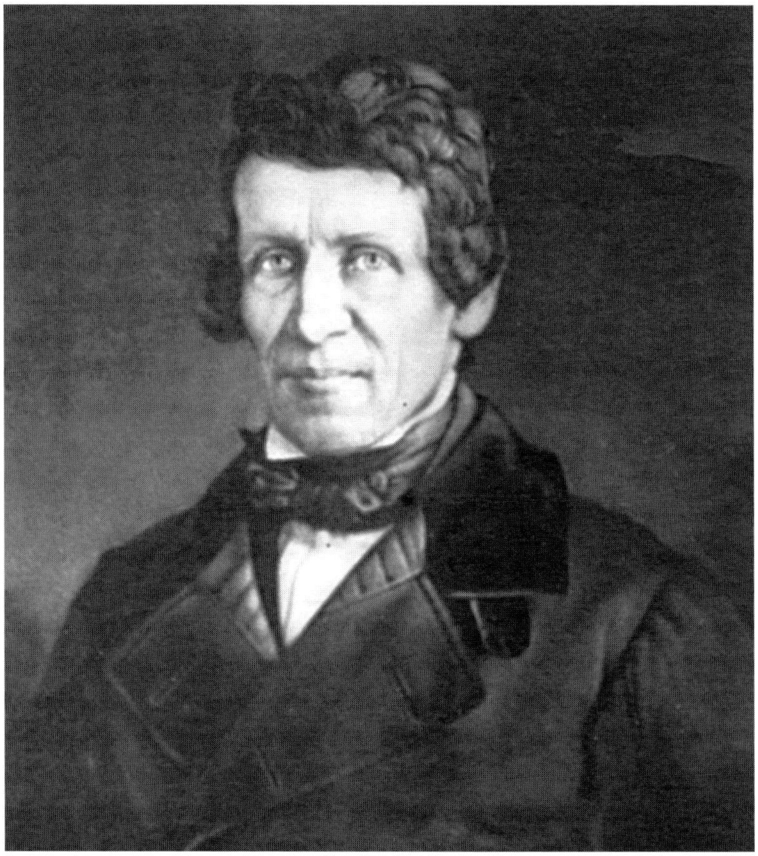

FIGURE 4-1
George B. McClellan.

George B. McClellan

George B. McClellan (Fig. 4-1) was born in Woodstock, Connecticut, on December 23, 1796. McClellan was a famous surgeon as well as the father of General George B. McClellan of Civil War fame. A graduate of Yale University at the age of 15, he later attended the University of Pennsylvania Medical School. He was an enthusiastic student, particularly interested in anatomy. Shortly after graduation from medical school, he and some associates started a private school of anatomy, later known as Jefferson Medical College. One reason that McClellan started a new school was that there were no available positions at the University of Pennsylvania, where he doubtless would have liked to teach. McClellan therefore served as professor of surgery at the new Jefferson Medical College, and his skill as a surgeon and teacher was unsurpassed.

In 1821, McClellan, though a general surgeon, founded still another institution, a hospital for diseases of the eye and ear. Unfortunately, however, this survived for only four years. To add to his bad luck, in 1838 the Jefferson Medical College reorganized and McClellan was not reappointed to the staff.

McClellan was dynamic and active and liked to be in the forefront of his profession. However, he had a bombastic personality and probably talked too much. It is said that at the time of his death he had virtually no friends.

McClellan was interesting indeed since he had some difficulty getting along with people, a trait that eventually led to his being ostracized from the University of Pennsylvania which had been his medical school alma mater. It undoubtedly, as well, probably had a lot to do with his starting Jefferson Medical School. Among other things it has also often been believed that McClellan was involved in one of the first malpractice suits. Actually that is not the case. A suit did occur but it was initiated by George McClellan as plaintiff against Francis S. Beattie, M.D., and the suit was for libel.

Beattie had been in the navy where he served on the U.S.S. Constellation. This ship, now in the inner harbor in Baltimore, served as symbolic flagship for the Atlantic fleet during the Second World War.

Beattie's specialty was obstetrics and when he left the navy he joined Jefferson Medical College where he was on the faculty from 1825 to 1826. Beattie did not get along with some of his peers and was relieved of his teaching duties after 1827. McClellan felt that he had been libeled by Beattie because of several pamphlets Beattie wrote which were critical of McClellan's management of two patients, one a Mr. Kunkle who had been operated for cancer of the jaw and another, Mr. William Davis, who had undergone cataract surgery. In 1827 McClellan countered by suing Beattie for libel (Fig. 4-1A). It is the testimony in this case that has led to the misconception that it was actually a malpractice suit.

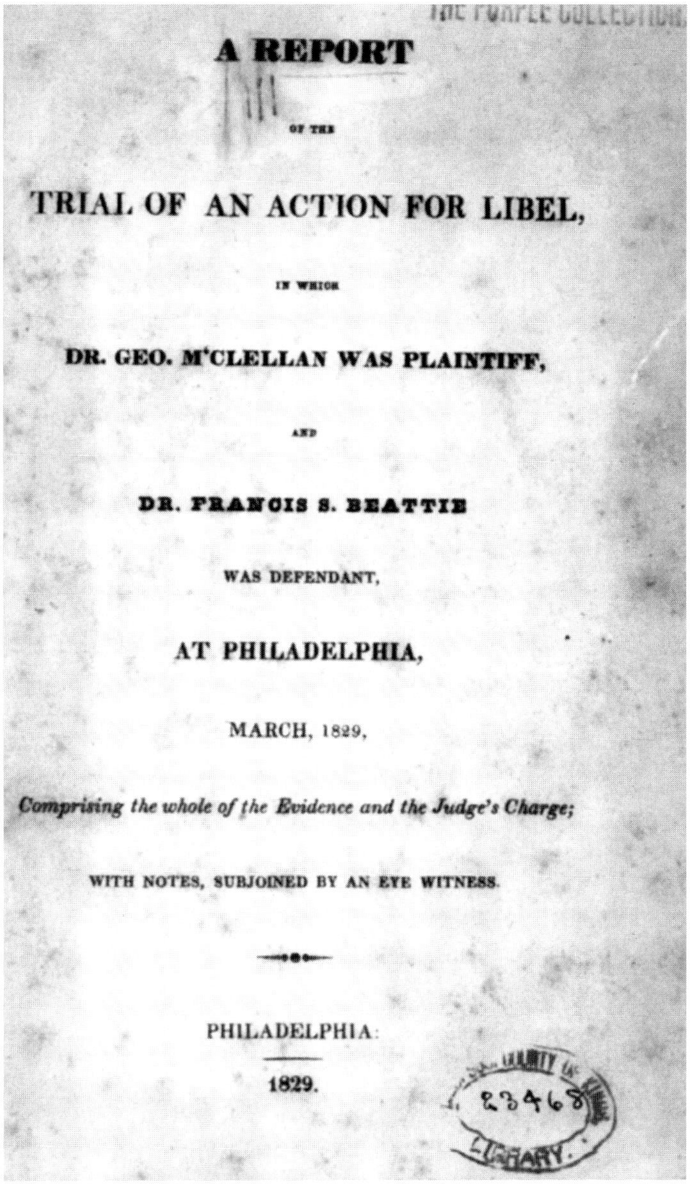
A REPORT

OF THE

TRIAL OF AN ACTION FOR LIBEL,

IN WHICH

DR. GEO. M'CLELLAN WAS PLAINTIFF,

AND

DR. FRANCIS S. BEATTIE

WAS DEFENDANT,

AT PHILADELPHIA,

MARCH, 1829,

Comprising the whole of the Evidence and the Judge's Charge;

WITH NOTES, SUBJOINED BY AN EYE WITNESS.

PHILADELPHIA:

1829.

FIGURE 4-1A
McClellan vs. Beattie (courtesy of the author).

With regard to the cataract surgery Mr. William Davis had had an unsuccessful cataract operation performed by Joseph Parrish on one eye. Parrish later operated on the fellow eye. He incised the anterior lens capsule and divided the nucleus into fragments. The hope in those days was that the lens material would then be absorbed by the aqueous. Indeed, it is fairly well documented that Mr. Davis' lens material did in large part absorb because he began to see. However, he visited Dr. McClellan on one occasion and McClellan advocated removing a nuclear fragment from the anterior chamber. Dr. Parrish had cautioned that this should be left alone, but eventually Davis permitted McClellan to operate. Unfortunately, Mr. Davis lost his remaining sight. Overall, he had spent about seventeen months in Pennsylvania Hospital which is considerably different from the outpatient surgery done today. Although Davis states in the libel suit testimony that the last thing he ever saw was Dr. McClellan, McClellan prevailed in the suit. He had sought ten thousand dollars in damages but was awarded only five hundred. Not unlike today, Beattie appealed and it was not until 1838 that Beattie's appeal was denied and McClellan was awarded the five hundred dollars.

From the standpoint of both Wills and Jefferson it is interesting to point out that McClellan lived at 912 Walnut Street from October 12, 1832, the year it was decided to build Wills Hospital, until May 8, 1847 when he died. Wills, of course, was located at 900 Walnut Street. The numbering of Walnut Street, by the way, changed sometime during the mid 19th century because McClellan's property previously had been numbered 248 Walnut Street. The three story dwelling is pictured (in Fig. 4-1B). In later years its basement housed a barber shop where many Jefferson students got their hair cut.

On May 1, 1974, the Philadelphia Historical Commission granted permission to the redevelopment authority to demolish the structure and that space is now occupied by a corner of the 1980 Wills Eye Hospital. Hutchinson Street runs between Wills and the Bluemle building (Fig. 4-1C), but actually the true Hutchinson Street before the demolition of McClellan's home ran through the current Wawa store on Walnut Street.

McClellan's son, General Brinton McClellan, actually became more famous than his father, although many felt that if the surgeon had been the general, the army would have won more battles and fought more often, thereby shortening the duration of the Civil War. George Brinton McClellan was born in Philadelphia in 1826 and was graduated from the United States Military Academy in 1846, second in his class. He served in the Mexican War and in 1855 went to Europe as a member of the commission to study European military systems. While there, he had the opportunity to

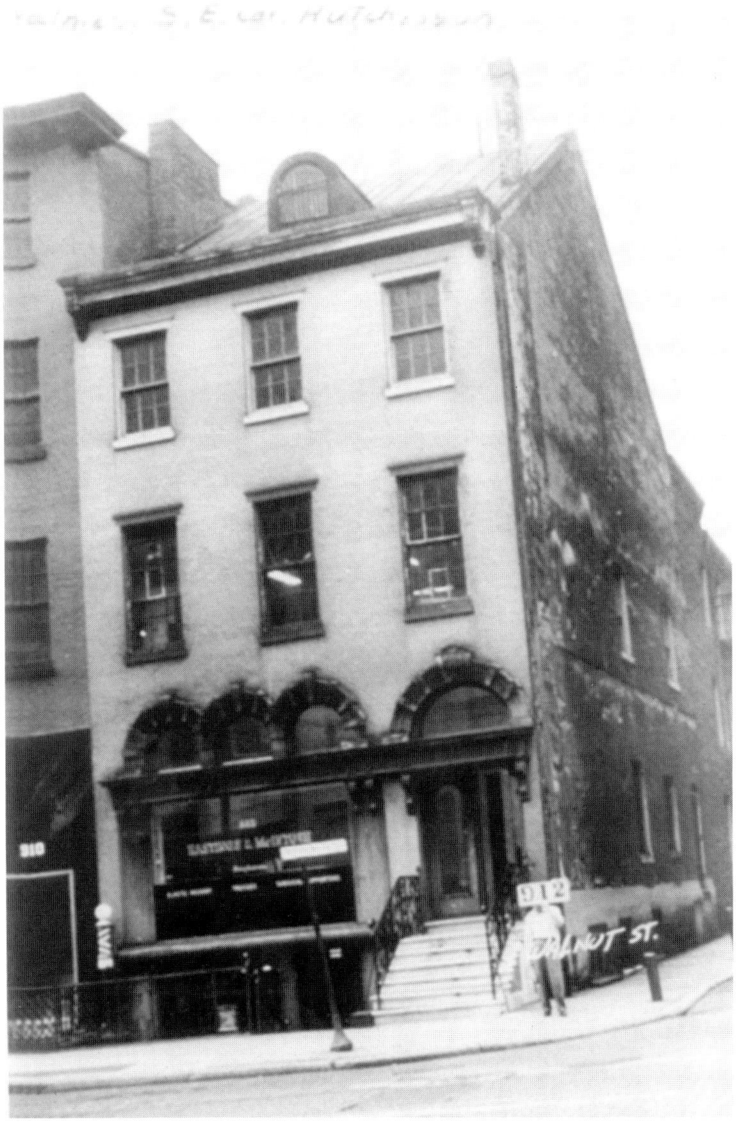

FIGURE 4-1B
McClellan's home. One corner of the 1980 Wills now occupies this space.

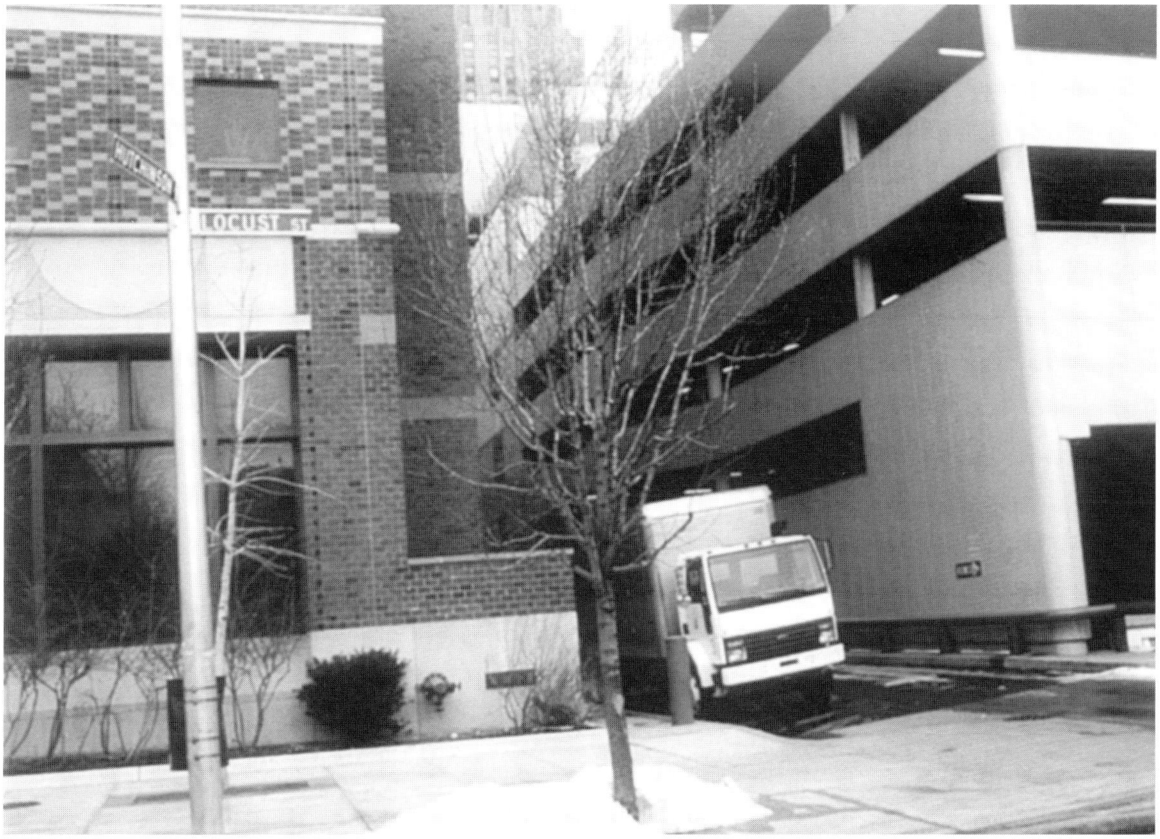

FIGURE 4-1C
Hutchinson Street between the 1980 Wills and the Bluemle Building.

observe part of the Crimean War. In 1857, McClellan resigned from the army and became chief engineer of the Illinois Central Railroad. He was to become its vice president before moving on to become president of the eastern division of the Ohio and Mississippi Railroad.

At the outbreak of the Civil War, McClellan enlisted and became a major general in command of Ohio volunteers. After defeating all the Confederate forces in western Virginia, he was made a major general in the regular United States Army. In the summer of 1861, he took command of the Union Army in the East, which became known as the Army of the Potomac. Under his exemplary leadership, it became one of the best forces in the Union Army. At the height of his career, McClellan was chief of all the armies in the Union. However, despite his proven military skill, President Lincoln thought he was not aggressive enough against the Confederates and relieved him as supreme general in 1862.

McClellan remained in the service as an army commander. In the spring of 1862, he attacked, moving against Richmond from the east in the Peninsular Campaign. Lee retaliated in the Battle of Seven Days and drove him back to Harris' Landing on the James River. Washington authorities transferred McClellan's army to northern Virginia. Most of his troops were placed temporarily under the command of General John Pope, who, in turn, was defeated at the second battle of Bull Run, also called Manassas. McClellan then became commander of all troops in the Washington area. He led his army into Maryland to meet a Confederate invasion and forced the southern army to retreat to Virginia in the Battle of Antietam (September 1862), the bloodiest one-day battle of the Civil War. Lincoln, however, was displeased with

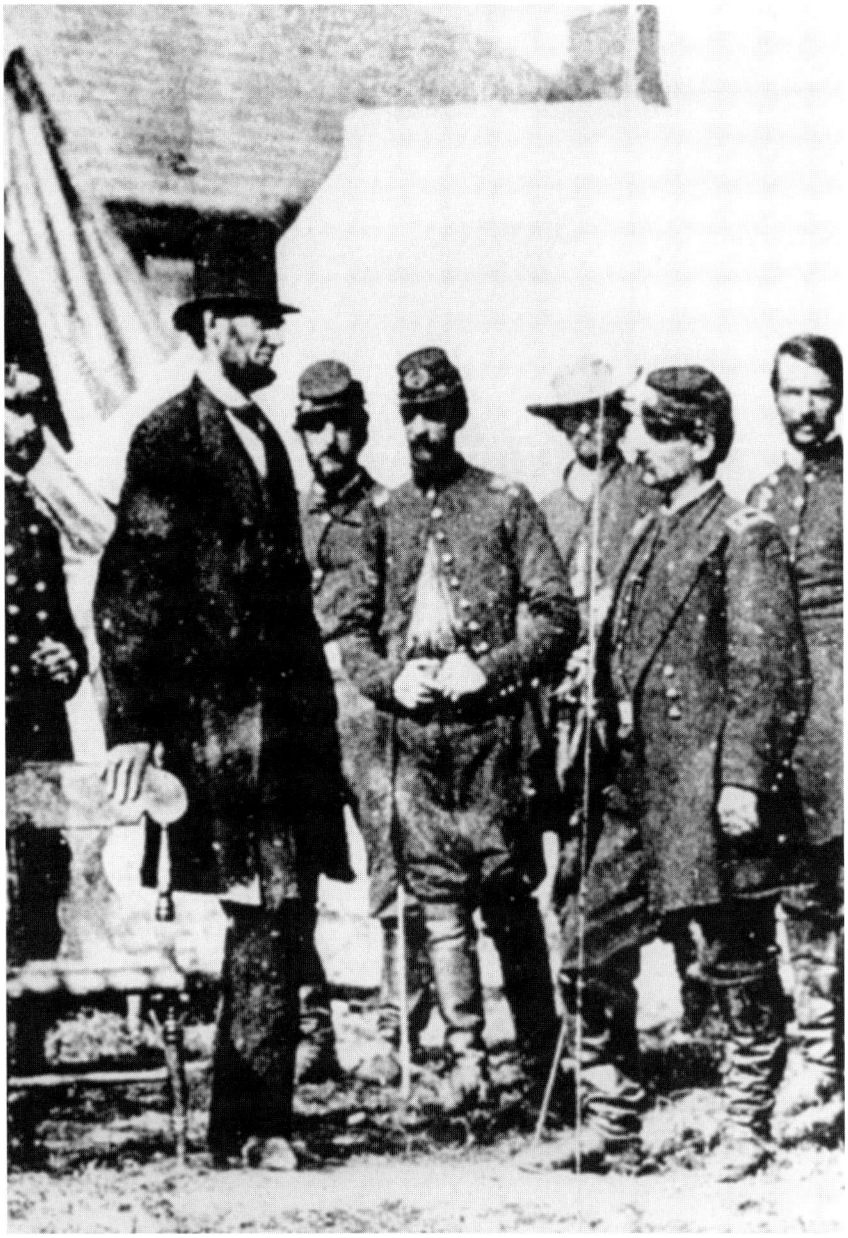

FIGURE 4-2
Abe Lincoln and "Little Mac" George McClellan stand face to face.

McClellan was well liked by his troops, who affectionately called him "Little Mac." A man of short stature, his height of 5'7" or 5'8" contrasted dramatically with President Lincoln, especially when the latter wore his stovepipe hat (Fig. 4-2).

In 1864, McClellan ran unsuccessfully against Lincoln for the presidency. He later became governor of New Jersey serving from 1868 to 1872. His son, also George McClellan, followed in his father's footsteps; associated with Tammany Hall, he also served as a U.S. senator from New York and as mayor of New York.

McClellan's failure to follow up on his victory and to deal Lee and the Confederates a death blow. McClellan was replaced by General Ambrose Burnside, and his military career ended. Nonetheless, Lee respected McClellan as one of the Union's most talented field commanders.

Despite his military career misadventures,

Fitzwilliam Sargent

Fitzwilliam Sargent is better known as the father of a famous artist, John Singer Sargent, than for his accomplishments as an ophthalmologist. Born on May 17, 1829, he was part of an English family of military, political, and artistic accomplishments. Fitzwilliam Sargent, in the tradition of his successful family, graduated from the University of Pennsylvania Medical School by which time he was already on the staff of the Wills Eye Hospital. He is best known for his book entitled *Bandaging and Other Operations of Minor Surgery*, which was published in several editions and was also translated into French and Japanese. He also edited a few books on surgery and, in 1862, while living in France, wrote a pamphlet entitled *England, the United States, and the Southern Confederacy* in defense of the Union cause.

Sargent married Mary Newbold Singer in 1850. She was the talented daughter of a local merchant and had spent much of her early life in Italy. She was artistic and an accomplished musician. At her insistence, Sargent, who had been an attending eye surgeon at Wills Eye Hospital since 1852, resigned in 1854 at the young age of 34, allegedly because of poor health. It is reported that he had earned enough money from his practice to retire at this early age. In any case, his health had to have been better than he supposed because Sargent lived another 35 years. He did not die until he reached the age of 69.

Shortly after his retirement, the family moved to Florence, Italy, where his son, John Singer Sargent, was born in 1856. Fitzwilliam Sargent hoped that his son would enter the U.S. Navy, but Mrs. Sargent and friends persuaded him to nurture the boy's artistic talents. At the age of 13, John went to work in the studio of Carl Welsch in Rome.

His natural gifts were immense. The violinist Joachim observed that "had Sargent taken to music instead of painting he would have been as great a musician as he was a painter." He called him "the van Dyke of our times." His teacher, Carolus-Duran, the foremost portraitist in Paris, offered him the considerable compliment of an invitation to join him in decorating a ceiling in the Louvre. Each incorporated a portrait of the other in the painting. Carolus-Duran lived to regret asking Sargent to participate because he soon found that critical acclaim at the annual Paris Salon (on which depended lucrative portrait commissions for the following year) was lavished more upon the pupil than the teacher.

One of the earliest and most important of Sargent's Salon pieces was exhibited in 1883, under the title "Portrait d'Enfants." This was actually the portrait of the four daughters of the American expatriate artist Edward Boit, painted the year before in the family apartment in Paris. It was the first large painting in which Sargent's personal and peculiar traits manifested themselves.

Basing the composition on "Las Meninas" of Valezquez, which he had copied in Spain (the copy still belongs to his sister's family), it is his first masterwork that shows his passion for objects and materials—the Savonnerie carpet in the foreground and the vast Chinese blue and white vases that add a mysterious timelessness to the work. It was subsequently presented by his sisters to the Boston Museum of Fine Arts.

In 1884, Sargent, continuing in his steady rise to fame, showed a major portrait in the Royal Academy of London summer exhibition. This exhibition brought the same sort of portrait patronage in England as it did in France. Again, his sitter was American, and again the painting had been finished in Paris. But, fortunately for Sargent, his subject, Mrs. Henry White, had moved to London, where her husband was secretary to the U.S. embassy. She had furnished a fashionable mansion in Grosvenor Crescent, where, after the Royal Academy Show, the Sargent portrait was placed in the White Dining Room, a companion to the portrait of Henry White, which had been completed by the more famous and much older Leon Bonnet.

Sargent established a studio in London's Chelsea district in 1885 and was for 40 years the accepted master in Anglo-American portraiture.

In 1888, John Singer Sargent painted Isabella Stewart Gardner, who by her will established the Isabella Stewart Gardner Museum in Boston, Massachusetts. She was extremely friendly with Sargent, as evidenced by a collection of nearly 200 letters from him in her museum. Most are concerned with Mrs. Gardner's various acts of kindness.

Sargent's portrait of Mrs. Gardner shows her in a low-necked black dress against a piece of red and gold brocade (Fig. 4-3). The pattern around her head is fitted with exact symmetry. From each of the two rows of pearls around her waist hangs one of her rubies.

Records indicate that this painting turned out to be something of an ordeal for Sargent. Apparently he completed nine painting before the last was finally acceptable to her. Some sources say that the portrait created considerable scandal in the Boston area and that her husband forbade its showing in his lifetime because of the daringly low-cut neckline.

D. Hayes Agnew

D. Hayes Agnew, the only child of Robert Agnew and Agnes Anderson, was one of the first surgeons to bring fame to Wills Eye Hospital because of his skill as an ophthalmic surgeon. Agnew, like most of Wills' early surgeons, was a graduate of the University of Pennsylvania. He married Margaret Creighton Irwin on November 21, 1841, and in 1843 gave up the practice of medicine to join his brother-in-law in the iron business. The business failed and he returned to medicine, this time in Cochranville.

He was determined to become a surgeon and had cadavers transported from Philadelphia to Cochranville, where, much to the dismay of local villagers, he performed his dissections. One legend about Agnew and his cadavers is that a farmer approached him and asked if he could put the bones from Agnew's cadavers into his fish pond. Subsequently, one of the local fish dealers became well known for the unusually fat eels that he regularly had for sale. The same farmer who had used Agnew's bones in his fish pond asked how the fish dealer had produced so many eels. To his dismay, he learned they came from his very own pond. This and other tales about Agnew ultimately forced him to leave Cochranville.

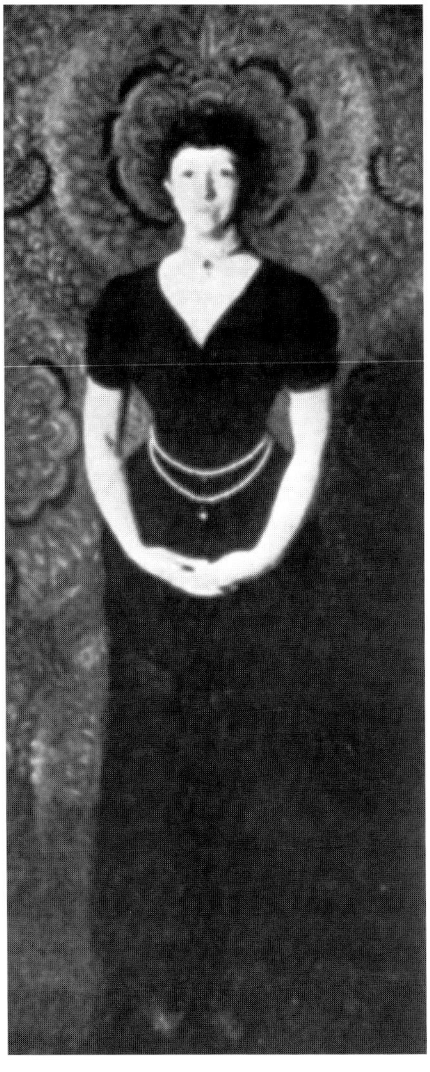

FIGURE 4-3
Sargent's famous portrait of Isabella Stewart Gardner that (in 1888) was considered too "risqué" by her husband.

In 1848, he returned to Philadelphia, where he purchased a school of anatomy for $600. At the time of his purchase there was an enrollment of only nine students, but because of his energies and teaching abilities, students from the University of Pennsylvania and Jefferson Medical School were quick to enroll. When he later sold the school at no profit, the student body had increased to 50 students. In 1862, Agnew became acting surgeon to Satterly Hospital and traveled to Gettysburg, where he treated the wounded after that historic battle.

To increase his skill in eye surgery, Agnew applied for a position at Wills Eye Hospital and was appointed the 13th attending surgeon. He served four years and then was emeritus surgeon until his death. He became a dominant force in medicine in Philadelphia and, indeed, in surgery throughout the United States. He influenced ophthalmology by the Agnew peritomy operation and the Agnew linear cataract extraction. He also developed a flexible canaliculus knife and a double hook for removing the lens nucleus when it could not be expressed spontaneously. Agnew was a severe critic of the couching operation and advised against the linear operation in senile cataracts because of poor early results. His most significant contribution was a three-volume treatise on surgery, including a section on ophthalmology over 140 pages long.

At the height of Agnew's popularity, James Garfield became president of the

United States. Garfield, a Republican, was in many ways a compromise candidate for president. The Republican party at the time was divided into two factions: the "Stalwarts," led by Senator Roscoe Conkling of New York, and the "Half-Breeds," led by Senator James G. Blaine of Maine. These groups quarreled over personal differences and government jobs rather than over political principles. Though Garfield was closer to the Half-Breeds, he tried to walk a fine line between both factions and therefore kept some of the confidence of both sides.

At the Republican National Convention in Chicago, the Half-Breeds tried to nominate Blaine for president, while the Stalwarts backed former President Ulysses S. Grant. Neither Blaine nor Grant could muster enough votes for nomination, so the Half-Breeds turned to Garfield as a dark horse candidate. After 36 ballots, the convention finally chose Garfield. Chester A. Arthur, member of the Stalwart group and Conkling's lieutenant in the Republican regime, was selected as his vice-presidential running mate. In 1880, Garfield defeated his Democratic opponent, Winfield Scott Hancock, by about 40,000 votes (4,453,285 to 4,414,082).

After assuming office, Garfield, who owed his nomination primarily to the Half-Breeds, favored this faction in handing out patronage jobs. He made their leader, Blaine, his secretary of state and appointed several others to important offices. The Stalwarts received only minor positions and their leader, Conkling, tried to stop the Senate from confirming some of the appointments. He failed, however, and was forced to resign from the Senate.

On July 2, 1881, Garfield was about to leave Washington to attend the 25th reunion of his class at Williams College (prior to becoming president, he had been president of his alma mater). As he stood at the railroad station, a stranger stepped out of the crowd and fired two pistol shots at him. Garfield fell, and the assassin cried, "I am a Stalwart and Arthur is president now!"

The assassin, Charles J. Guiteau, was arrested immediately. He held a grudge because Garfield had refused to appoint him as the US consul in Paris. At his trial, Guiteau tried to act like a madman and his attorney argued that he was innocent by reason of insanity. However, a jury found him guilty and he was hanged in 1882.

Garfield lingered for 80 days. While one of the assassin's bullets had merely grazed his arm, the other had lodged in his back. Roentgen had not yet discovered x-rays, and surgeons could not find the bullet. Even Alexander Graham Bell tried, unsuccessfully, to locate it with an electrical device.

Agnew, as one of the outstanding surgeons in the United States, was called into consultation on July 3, two days after Garfield had been shot. He left immediately for Washington in a private train, which made a record run of less than three hours. Agnew was ceaseless in his attention to President Garfield, and it was the opinion of the authorities that Garfield had received the best possible treatment. Undoubtedly, had radiology, antibiotics, and modern surgical techniques existed, Garfield's life might have been saved. Unfortunately, infection set in, and Garfield died at a seaside cottage in Elberon, New Jersey, on September 19, 1881.

Thus, D. Hayes Agnew added to the prestige of Wills Eye Hospital not only through his contributions to ophthalmology but also as a consultant to President James Garfield.

Other Key Surgeons

There were many other respected surgeons who practiced ophthalmology in the 1800s. Richard Levis, a graduate of Jefferson Medical College, was a general surgeon who was known for his personal neatness and habit of entering the operating room without changing clothes. He was probably one of the best-dressed surgeons of the day and took great pride in showing off his cuffs during surgery. He was particularly proud of the fact that even in the bloodiest of operations, he always managed to keep his cuffs spotless. Upon completion of the operation, he would wash his hands, adjust his bow tie, and make rounds on his private patients.

His operative dexterity added to the prestige of the institution. In addition, he is credited with the development of the wire lens loop for delivery of the lens during cataract surgery.

These early surgeons had the difficult task of performing ophthalmic operations with the crudest of techniques and equipment. Wills Eye had, however, always been known for its excellent cataract extractions, as well as for its superb plastic work. Recessions and resections of the rectus muscles for strabismus were unknown. As an alternative, complete tenotomies of the horizontal recti were frequently performed, which, needless to say, frequently made the eyes that turned out turn in, and eyes that turned in turn out. Fortunately, the vertical recti were apparently spared this fate.

The surgical treatment of glaucoma did not begin until 1856, when von Graefe devised the technique of iridectomy. Before this time there were no anesthetics, either local or general. Thus, the surgeon was extremely limited in what he could accomplish.

Two exciting discoveries changed the course of ophthalmic surgery. The first was the development of the ophthalmoscope by Helmholtz in 1851, and the second was the development of the indirect ophthalmoscope by Reute in 1852. Because of these developments, by 1860 ophthalmology had emerged as a recognized subspecialty.

Following the Civil War, it became the fashion for physicians to study in Europe and then return to the United States as ophthalmic specialists. Notable among surgeons who did this were Dyer, Kaiser, Norris, Strawbridge, and Thompson. William Norris and William Thompson, both Wills Eye surgeons, spent five years in Vienna and then came back to teach at the University of Pennsylvania.

Two other surgeons, Hall and Harlan, were elected surgeons at the Wills Eye Hospital, at a time earlier than that of Levis and Agnew. After the Civil War, both confined their work to diseases of the eye. These two, therefore, were probably the first specialists at the Wills Eye who can be considered strictly ophthalmologists. Dyer, Kaiser, McClure, Norris, Thompson, and Strawbridge followed quickly in their stead.

William Fisher Norris and William Thompson

William Fisher Norris lived between 1839 and 1901. His parents came from Quaker stock, and Norristown was named after his family. A member of the Society of Friends, he joined the Union Army, and from July 1 to July 3, 1863, he worked constantly at taking care of the wounded at the Battle of Gettysburg. Later he served at the Douglass Hospital in Washington, and with William Thompson he helped found the Army Medical Museum. He spent five years studying in Vienna under the guidance of Jaeger and later came back to work at Wills Eye Hospital with George Strawbridge. In 1874 he became the first professor of ophthalmology at the University of Pennsylvania, where the present chair of ophthalmology carries both his name and that of Dr. George deSchweinitz. He was president of the American Ophthalmological Society. His comprehensive textbook of ophthalmology was translated into many foreign languages.

Dr. Norris was married to Fräulein Rose Buchmann, a woman he met while a student in Vienna. They had three sons, one of whom died early in life. One of the remaining sons became a teacher and the other a lawyer.

William Thompson, a contemporary of William Fisher Norris, came from Chambersburg, Pennsylvania. A graduate of Jefferson Medical College, he was a lover of music. Like Norris, he served in the Civil War on the staff of General McClellan during the Peninsular campaign and at Antietam. A successful specialist, he was associated with Drs. S. Weir Mitchell and W. W. Keen and participated in many of their projects. One of these was a paper on eyestrain entitled "Eye and its Association with Headache," written with Mitchell and published in 1874. In the preceding year he had written about the diagnosis of brain tumors by use of the ophthalmoscope. An authority on the optics of refraction, he invented several new instruments, including a type of refractor. He was also an authority on color blindness.

Thompson was a contemporary of the famous Philadelphia painter Thomas Eakins. Eakins had always maintained a keen interest in anatomy; in addition to his studies at the Pennsylvania Academy of the Fine Arts, he studied anatomy at the Jefferson Medical College. At one point, he even considered becoming a physician. His famous 1874 painting of the Gross Clinic still hangs at the Jefferson Medical College, although at the time of its unveiling it was severely criticized because of the blood shown on the fingertips of Dr. Gross. Eakins also painted the Agnew Clinic, now at the University of Pennsylvania, and Dr. William Thompson. That painting now hangs in the College of Physicians in Philadelphia. It was painted in 1907, the year Thompson died.

Of interest is the fact that Eakins received only about $15,000 for all of his paintings. Many portraits he simply gave away.

Samuel Doty Risley

Many other Wills surgeons became well known, and certainly one cannot fail to mention Samuel Doty Risley, born in Cincinnati in 1845. Risley grew up in Cincinnati and in Davenport, Iowa. At the age of 17, stirred by the patriotic impulses of the period, he enlisted with the 20th regiment of Iowa volunteers. He enlisted on August 12, 1862, and by January 23, 1863, had been promoted to eighth corporal. He rose to fourth sergeant by May 23, 1865, before being mustered out in Mobile, Alabama, in July of the same year.

His regiment fought at the first big battle at Perrygrove, Arkansas, and later in the siege and capture of Vicksburg and Fort Blakely, Alabama.

After his initial matriculation at Iowa State University in 1865, he entered the medical department at the University of Pennsylvania, from which he graduated in 1870. His interest in the eye led to an appointment at the Wills Eye Hospital in 1871.

Arthur Bedell recalled that Risley was a cordial gentleman who invited Bedell to his country home on the first day they met. Risley is described as a calm, quiet, dignified, and very gracious physician who was wholeheartedly sympathetic to his patients. His office routine was quite formal; when a patient entered, he was expected to place his calling card on a card plate, which was then taken to Dr. Risley's desk and the card placed in the order of receipt. If a patient had no card, his name and address were written on an 8 x 14–inch slate which was placed on the doctor's desk.

Risley worked in an unhurried manner and carried many new ideas to fruition, notably the Risley prism.

George E. deSchweinitz

George deSchweinitz, a consultant to Wills, was one of the truly great American ophthalmologists. Born in Philadelphia in 1858, he graduated with top honors in the class of 1881 at the University of Pennsylvania Medical School. He worked at Jefferson Medical College as clinical professor of ophthalmology between 1892 and 1896; in 1896, he was made full professor. In 1901, he followed William Norris as professor at the University of Pennsylvania and worked there until his retirement in 1924. He was then appointed professor of ophthalmology in the graduate school of the University of Pennsylvania.

Dr. deSchweinitz was thoroughly devoted to the College of Physicians and served as its president between 1910 and 1912. He was also instrumental, with William Norris and Edward Jackson, in forming the Section of Ophthalmology in the College in 1893. His world renown in the field of ophthalmology became evident in 1923, when he was one of the first Americans invited to give the Bowman lecture.

T. B. Holloway and Francis Heed Adler

T. B. Holloway and Francis Heed Adler (Fig. 4-4) were originally attending surgeons at Wills Eye Hospital before becoming heads of the department of ophthalmology at the University of Pennsylva-

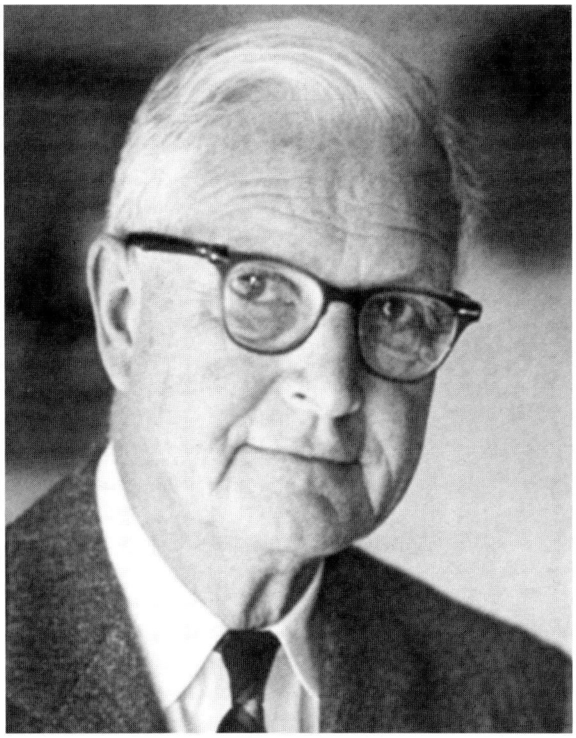

FIGURE 4-4
Francis Heed Adler.

nia. Holloway served from 1924 to 1936, and Adler from 1933 to 1960. Adler initiated the residency program at the University. His first resident, Harold G. Scheie, succeeded him as chairman.

Edward Jackson

Edward Jackson, an attending surgeon at the Wills Eye Hospital from 1890 to 1898, rose to national fame as an ophthalmologist, although most of this fame developed after he left Philadelphia for Denver, Colorado (Fig. 4-5). Nevertheless, Jackson did spend the first 44 years of his life in this area, and it was in the City of Brotherly Love that he first demonstrated his talents to the ophthalmic community.

Jackson was born in West Chester County and was a member of the Society of Friends. When he later moved to Denver, he became affiliated with the Unitarian Church, but in 1939 he renewed his membership in the Friends Meeting when he returned to Philadelphia.

A graduate of Union College with a degree in engineering, he immediately decided on a career in medicine rather than in engineering and entered the University of Pennsylvania, from which he graduated in 1878. His interest in ophthalmology resulted partly from an attack of diphtheria that left him with multiple paralyses, including a paralysis of accommodation. He read Donders' monumental work on refraction from cover to cover.

Jackson moved to Philadelphia, where he became associated with Drs. Harlan, Fox, Randall, Norris, Oliver and Risley. In 1888, he was made professor of ophthalmology at the Philadelphia Polyclinic School. He was instrumental in the formation of the section of ophthalmology at the College of Physicians and probably would have been content to remain in Philadelphia had his wife not developed tuberculosis in 1894. This precipitated his move to Denver with his wife, three sons, and two daughters. Despite the move, Mrs. Jackson died in 1896, and Jackson subsequently

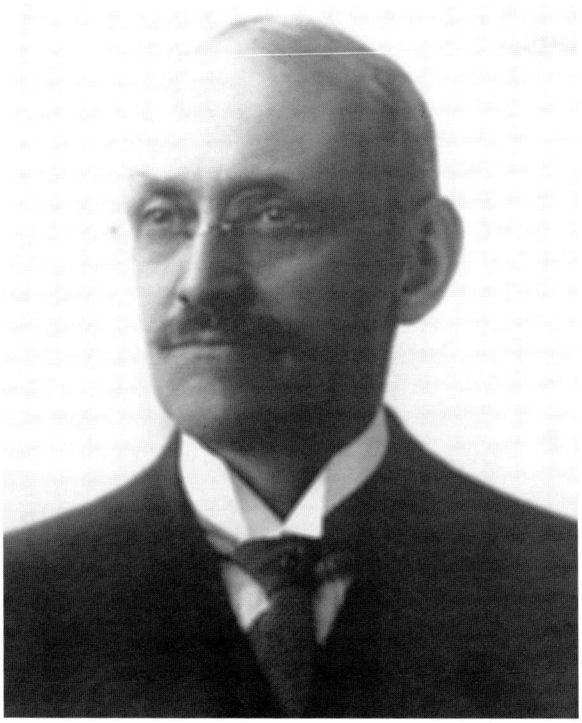

FIGURE 4-5
Edward Jackson's own ophthalmic problem, paralysis of his accommodation, inspired him to become an ophthalmologist and to establish two important institutions: the ophthalmology section at the College of Physicians and the American Academy of Ophthalmology and Otolaryngology.

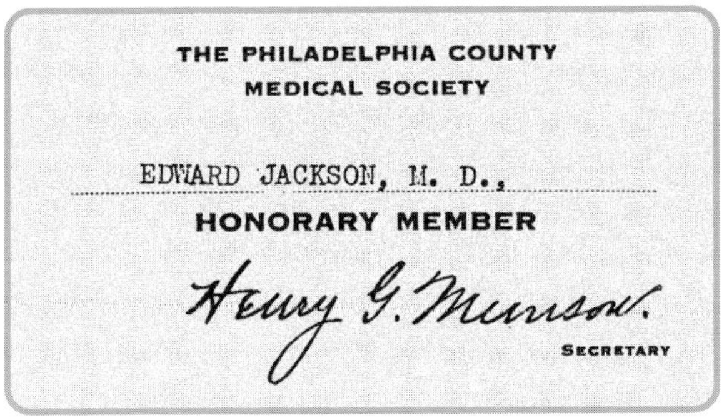

FIGURE 4-5A
Jackson's Philadelphia County Medical Society honorary membership card.

moved back to Philadelphia. However, he then became apprehensive that his children might have become infected with tuberculosis, so he once again returned to Denver.

While in Philadelphia, Jackson published 22 papers covering many subjects, but mainly refraction. One of his most notable contributions was the cross cylinder, which is still an essential instrument for the refractionist today.

The experience and satisfaction that came from his contributions to the organization of the section of ophthalmology of the College of Physicians inspired him to help in the formation of the American Academy of Ophthalmology and Otolaryngology. He is remembered for these efforts each year when the annual Jackson Memorial Lecture is given at the Academy meeting.

William Zentmayer

William Zentmayer was an extremely well liked and dedicated ophthalmologist. His father, Joseph, was an instrument worker and optician who invented and made many different types of micro-

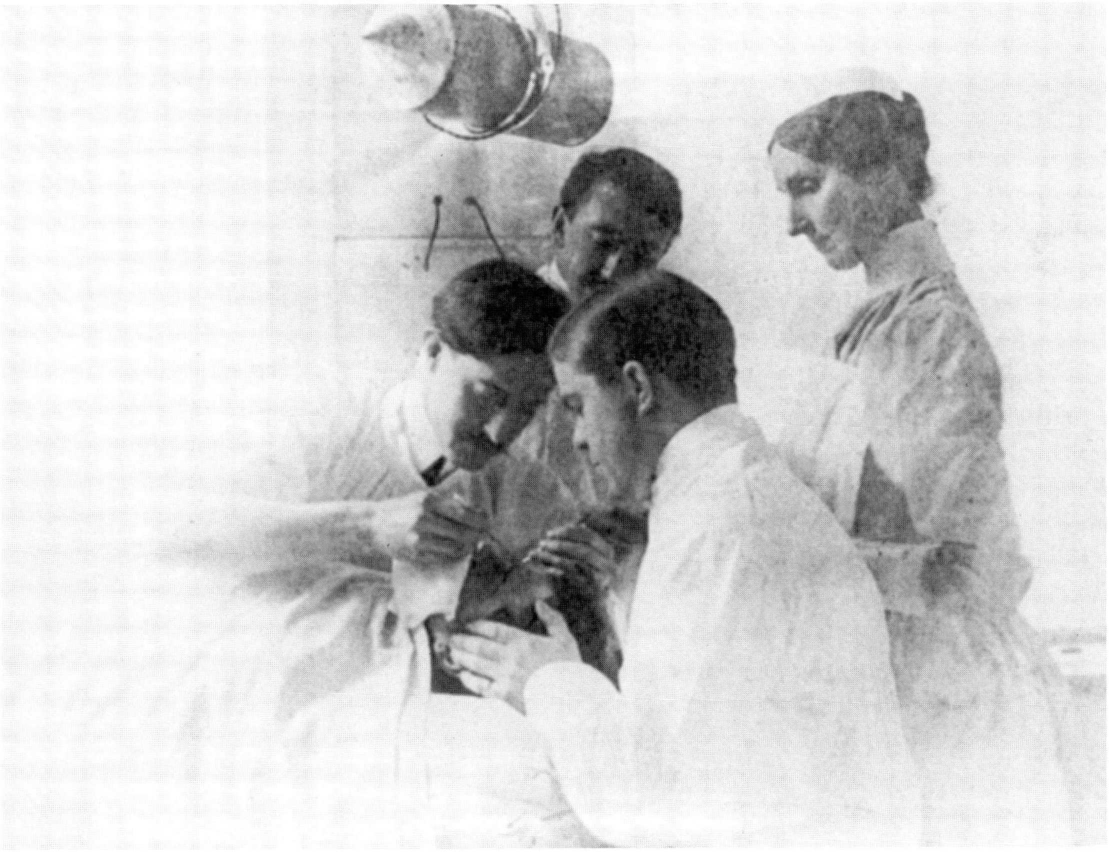

FIGURE 4-6
Homer Rhode, Harold Goldberg, Arthur Bedell, and Nurse Finley operating.

scopes and won several prizes both at home and abroad; he was also one of the first opticians to demand a prescription from the ophthalmologist before making spectacles.

Zentmayer graduated from the medical school of the University of Pennsylvania in 1887. In 1890, he was appointed assistant surgeon at the Wills Eye Hospital under the leadership of William Norris, and in 1901 he succeeded Norris as attending surgeon. He served in that position until 1928, when he retired at the age of 65.

Zentmayer was very active in the ophthalmic community. He was a fellow of the College of Physicians and served as chairman of the section of ophthalmology. In 1927, he served as president of the American Ophthalmological Society; he also served as chairman of the section of diseases of the eye, ear, nose, and throat of the State Medical Society.

An extremely knowledgeable and learned man, he was on the editorial board of the *Archives of Ophthalmology* and was editor of the *Transactions of the College of Physicians* from 1889 to 1920. He never married and truly devoted his life to the advancement of ophthalmology.

Arthur J. Bedell

Arthur J. Bedell was one of the most notable staff members who ever worked at Wills Eye Hospital (Figs. 4-6 and 4-7). One of the first ophthalmologists to realize the importance of fundus photographs, he amassed a collection of thousands of kodachrome pictures over the years and gave these to Wills.

He was a robust man and is known for his arguments with Freddie Verhoeff of Boston and his faithful attendance at the Wills conferences, to which he often traveled by bus from Albany, New York, even at the age of 90. With his death in 1972, Wills lost its oldest living ex-resident of the day. In many ways, his passing signified the end of an era.

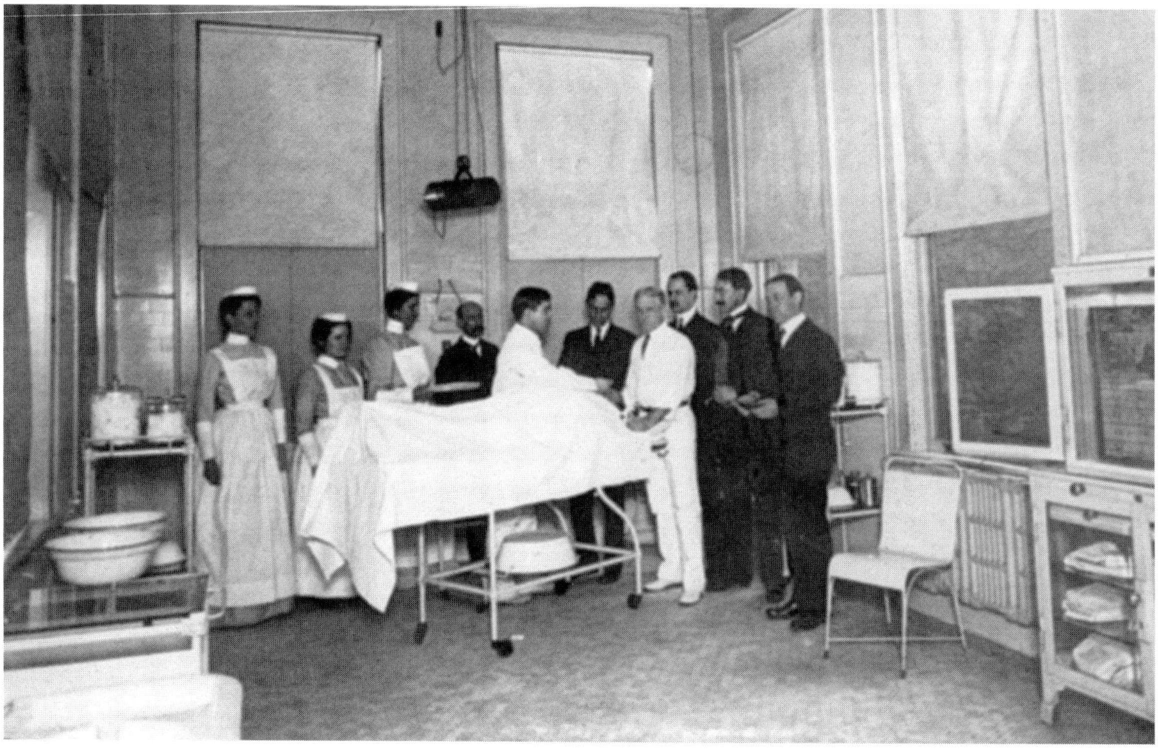

FIGURE 4-7
Operating room in the original Wills. A giant magnet hangs from the ceiling. Note the absence of surgical lights and surgical garb. A young Arthur Bedell stands near the patient's head.

Chapter 5

The Move to Spring Garden Street

Wills was growing fast and furiously when in 1873 there was an outbreak of contagious eye infection at the Wills Eye Hospital. Business came to an immediate halt, and a majority of the surgical staff refused to admit patients. About 44 fewer patients were admitted that year, and operations were postponed indefinitely. In the report for the year, the staff used this contagious outbreak to point to the need for better accommodations; in particular, they cited the fact that the infection was probably the result of poor ventilation and overcrowding in the wards. In addition, they said, the hospital had failed to keep pace with the increased population of the city; there had been no increase in the number of beds in the hospital since the structure was built 40 years earlier.

At that time, the population of Philadelphia was about 726,000, which was even larger than that of Berlin and Vienna, each of which had a population of about 600,000. However, both of these cities had 120 to 130 beds for eye patients, whereas Philadelphia could offer only 40 beds. Therefore, the committee agreed that two new wards should be built, and they sent out an appeal to the city's residents for funds.

The new wards opened on October 11, 1875.

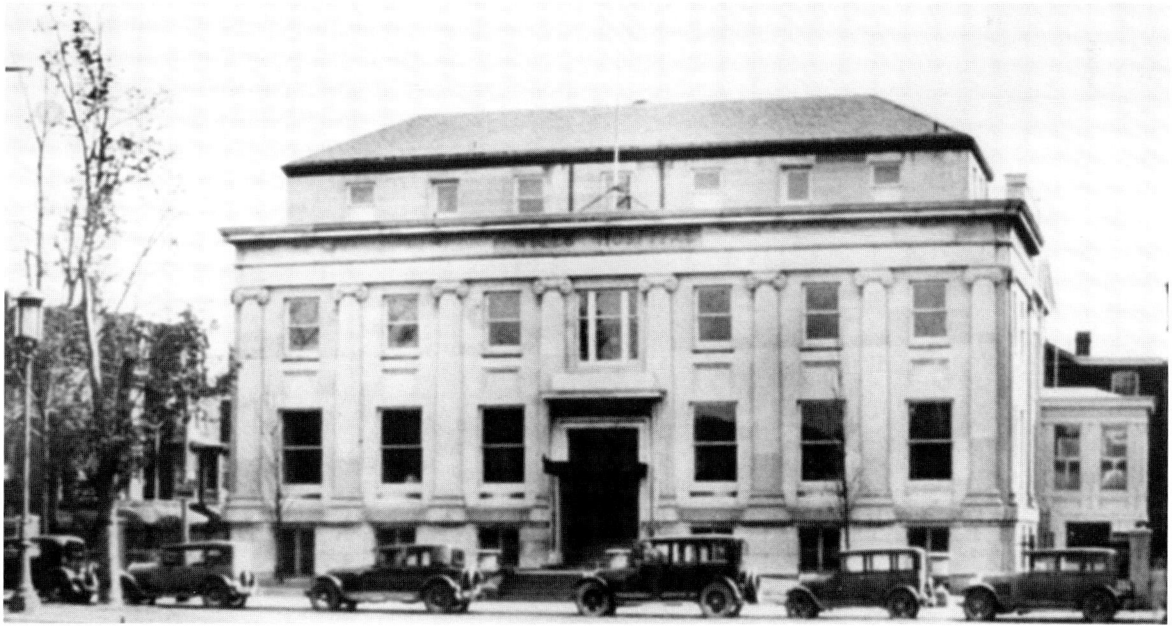

FIGURE 5-1
The original Wills after addition of a third floor. Cars of the period included a Packard (far left), Lincoln (fourth from left), and Erskine (fifth from left). The others could not be identified.

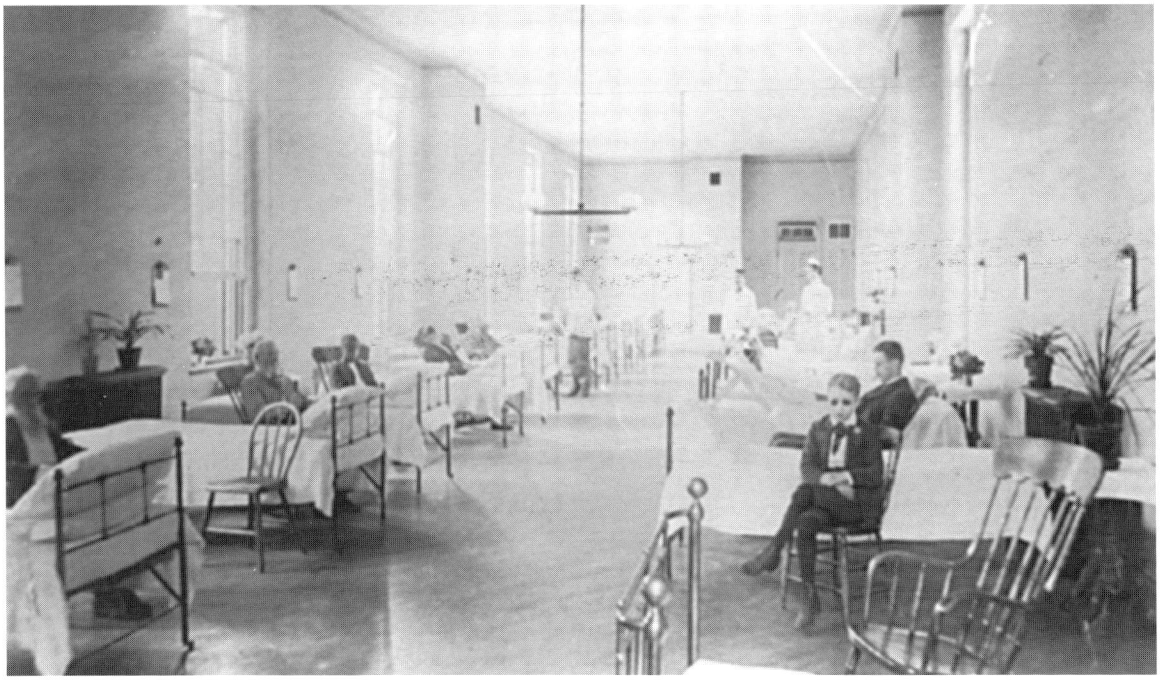

FIGURE 5-1A
Ward at the original Wills, c. 1900.

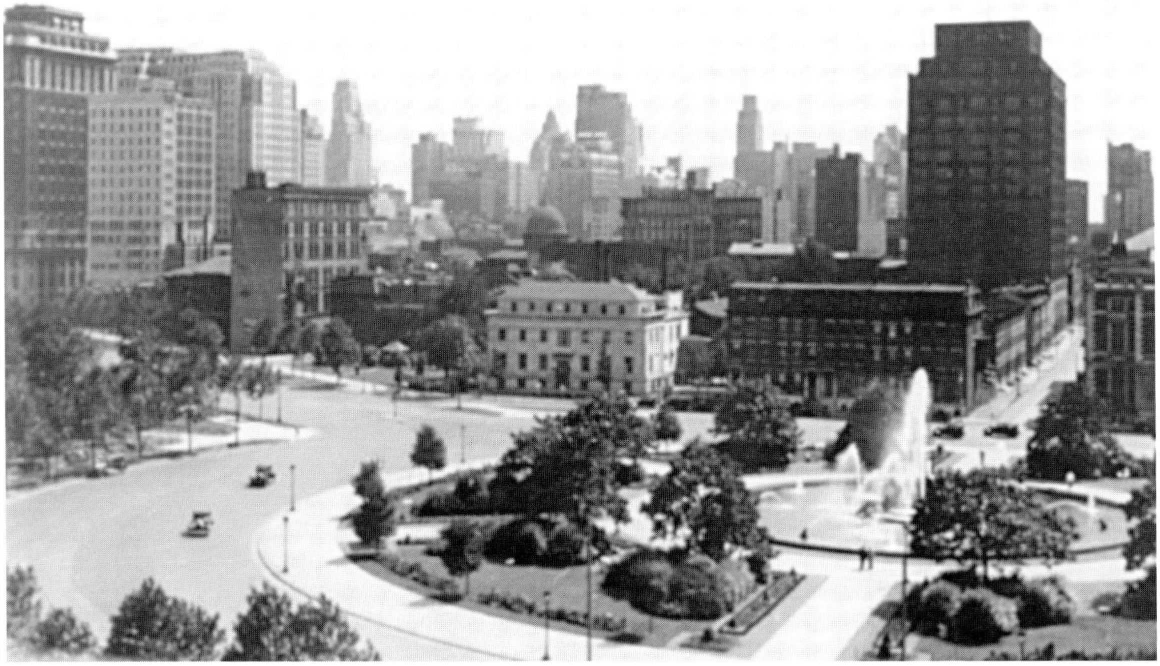

FIGURE 5-2
The Wills on Logan Square in 1931.

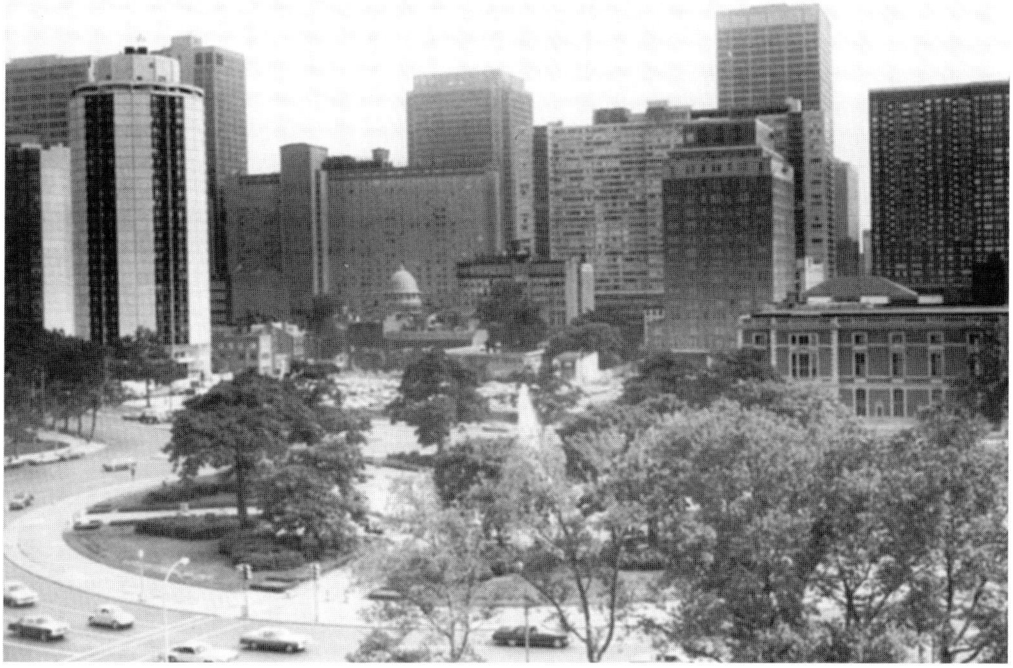

FIGURE 5-3
Logan Square as it appeared in 1980.

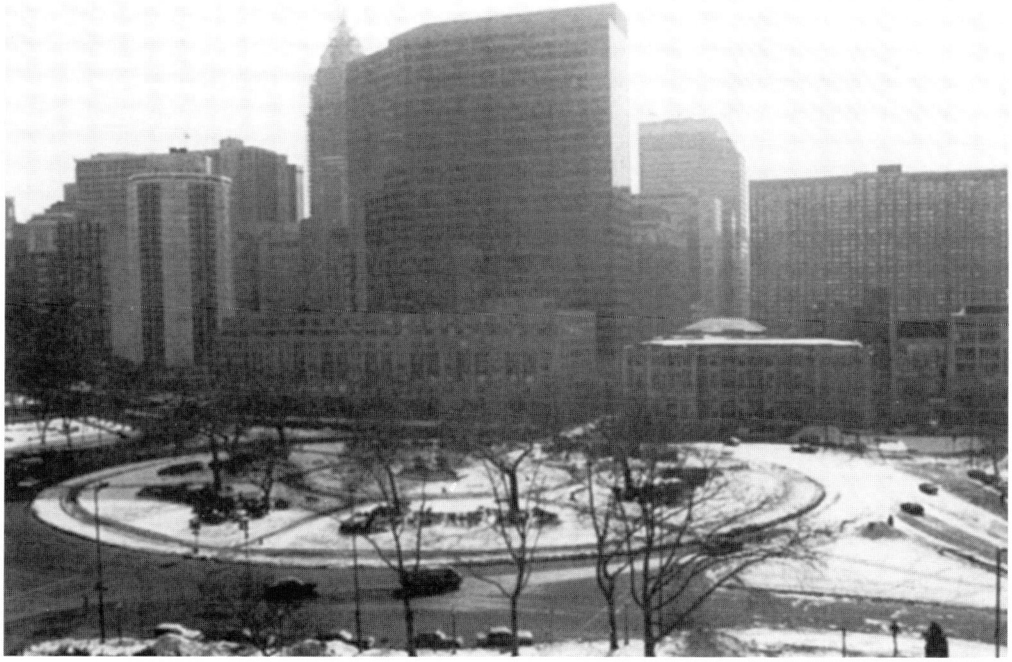

FIGURE 5-4
Logan Square, current site of the Four Seasons Hotel.

Each had a capacity of 20 beds. It took nearly 29 years, until 1908, for a third floor and basement to be completed (Figs. 5-1 through 5-4).

By 1923, a new era had begun. Mr. Stephen Wierzbicki was appointed superintendent of the hospital. He had previously been a warrant officer in the United States Navy, and he was very experienced in the administration of naval hospitals. The early 20th century brought more growth; in his report for 1928, Wierzbicki emphasized the marked increase in the number of patients admitted to the hospital compared with the number in former years. This was partly attributable to a reduction in the length of time patients stayed in the hospital; it dropped from 23 days in 1923 to 14 days in 1928 and to 12.06 days in 1930. Therefore, Wierzbicki concluded, a considerable amount of additional space was needed.

Plans were made for an entirely new Wills, and in June 1930 the property on Logan Square was sold to Mr. Cyrus H. K. Curtis for $1,100,000 (Fig. 5-5). It was understood that Mr. Curtis' purpose in acquiring the property was to erect a building in which musical programs could be held; unfortunately, this never came to pass. The old Wills Eye Hospital was used as a juvenile court from 1934 to 1938. It was not demolished until 1944. The permit for demolition was signed on December 30, 1943, at the request of Mary Curtis (Fig. 5-6). Today the site houses the Four Seasons Hotel.

In March 1931 the Board of Directors of City Trusts, after analyzing growth patterns in the city, acquired ground on the northwest corner of Sixteenth and Spring Garden Streets and planned to build a new hospital at a cost of $290,000 (Fig. 5-7). By the time the hospital was completed, however, it cost approximately $1,750,000. It was to be the largest hospital in the United States devoted to diseases of the eye.

The new site did not have the picturesque location of the old hospital, but it was felt to be con-

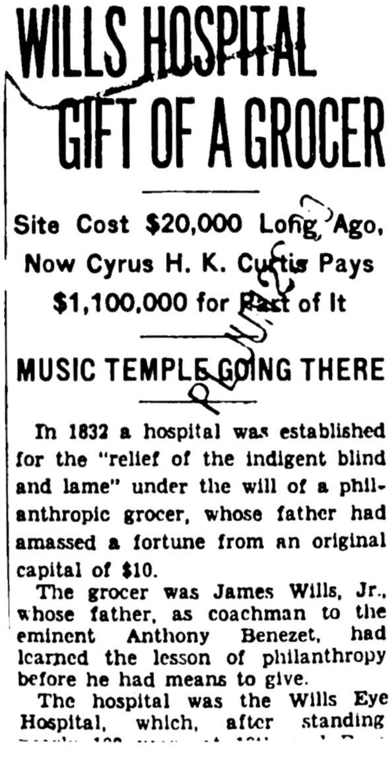

WILLS HOSPITAL GIFT OF A GROCER

Site Cost $20,000 Long Ago, Now Cyrus H. K. Curtis Pays $1,100,000 for Part of It

MUSIC TEMPLE GOING THERE

In 1832 a hospital was established for the "relief of the indigent blind and lame" under the will of a philanthropic grocer, whose father had amassed a fortune from an original capital of $10.

The grocer was James Wills, Jr., whose father, as coachman to the eminent Anthony Benezet, had learned the lesson of philanthropy before he had means to give.

The hospital was the Wills Eye Hospital, which, after standing

FIGURE 5-5
The sale of Wills to Cyrus Curtis.

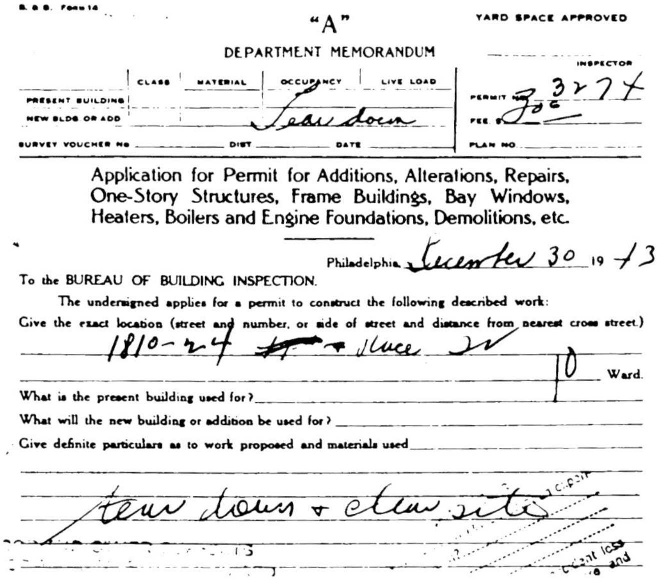

B. B. I. Form 14

"A"

DEPARTMENT MEMORANDUM

YARD SPACE APPROVED

INSPECTOR

	CLASS	MATERIAL	OCCUPANCY	LIVE LOAD
PRESENT BUILDING				
NEW BLDG OR ADD				

SURVEY VOUCHER No DIST DATE

PERMIT No

FEE $

PLAN NO

Application for Permit for Additions, Alterations, Repairs, One-Story Structures, Frame Buildings, Bay Windows, Heaters, Boilers and Engine Foundations, Demolitions, etc.

Philadelphia 30 19 43

To the BUREAU OF BUILDING INSPECTION.

The undersigned applies for a permit to construct the following described work:

Give the exact location (street and number, or side of street and distance from nearest cross street.)

10 Ward.

What is the present building used for?

What will the new building or addition be used for?

Give definite particulars as to work proposed and materials used

FIGURE 5-6
Mary Curtis signed the papers for the demolition of the Wills Hospital on Logan Square in 1943.

venient to both patients and staff because, at that time, Spring Garden Street was one of the most important thoroughfares of the city and Sixteenth Street was only two blocks from Broad Street. This made it accessible to traffic north, south, east, and west.

The lot was 197 feet by 170 feet, and was bordered on three sides by streets—Spring Garden Street on the south, Sixteenth Street on the east, and Brandywine Street on the north.

Mr. John Windrom, a well-known Philadelphia architect, was selected to design the new Wills Eye Hospital, which ultimately consisted of a basement, six floors, and a roof apartment for the superintendent (Fig. 5-8). John McShain constructed the 200-bed hospital, and it opened in November 1932 (Fig. 5-9).

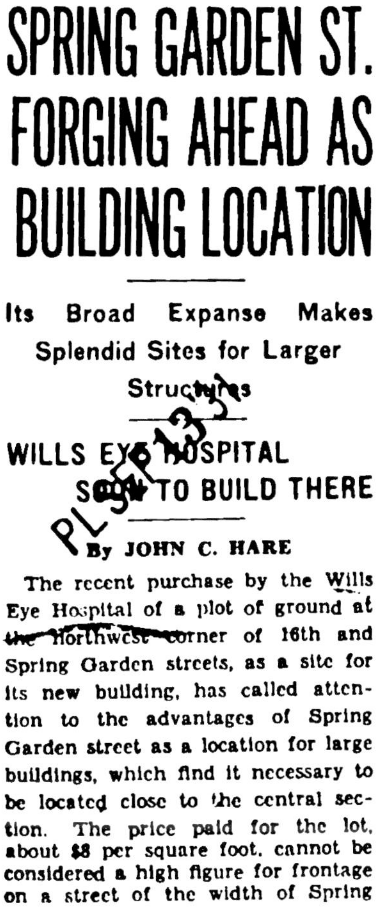

SPRING GARDEN ST. FORGING AHEAD AS BUILDING LOCATION

Its Broad Expanse Makes Splendid Sites for Larger Structures

WILLS EYE HOSPITAL SOON TO BUILD THERE

By JOHN C. HARE

The recent purchase by the Wills Eye Hospital of a plot of ground at the Northwest corner of 16th and Spring Garden streets, as a site for its new building, has called attention to the advantages of Spring Garden street as a location for large buildings, which find it necessary to be located close to the central section. The price paid for the lot, about $8 per square foot, cannot be considered a high figure for frontage on a street of the width of Spring

FIGURE 5-7
Plans to move to 16th and Spring Garden.

The roof apartment has an interesting story associated with it. Mr. Melvin Sutley, who succeeded Stephen Wierzbicki as superintendent of the hospital, held many séances in his apartment, particularly on Sunday nights. It was not uncommon for a resident on duty to see the best cuts of meats and freshest vegetables being transported upstairs for the séances. Mr. Sutley was so convinced of his ability to communicate with the dead that he often spoke of his late wife in the present tense. Once, when leaving for Japan on a trip, he spoke in the plural, stating that "we will visit Tokyo . . . " It was the day after his departure on this trip that a phone call came from his apartment. The caller obviously was in acute distress. When notified, the resident went to the emergency room to get a blood pressure cuff and stethoscope and asked one of the nurses working there to accompany him to Mr. Sutley's apartment. She was at first reluctant to go because of the "communications with the dead" that reportedly took place there but finally relented. A gentleman was found in the apartment with a perforated diverticulum; he identified himself as the medium who ran the séances. He was quickly transferred to Graduate Hospital, where, happily, he made a speedy recovery.

The operating rooms were on the fourth floor and were easily accessible from the elevators. At either end of the floor, there was an open surgical ward, so that guests arriving to visit relatives would walk through the operating suite. Not infrequently they peered through porthole windows in the operating room doors to catch a glimpse of the surgery taking place. Undoubtedly on more than one occasion someone looked in and, without realizing it, saw a relative or friend having a cataract removed.

This, fortunately, was remedied in the mid 1960s, when a new operating suite was constructed with all the latest equipment. It was isolated from the elevators, and unauthorized spectators were finally excluded from the surgical scene.

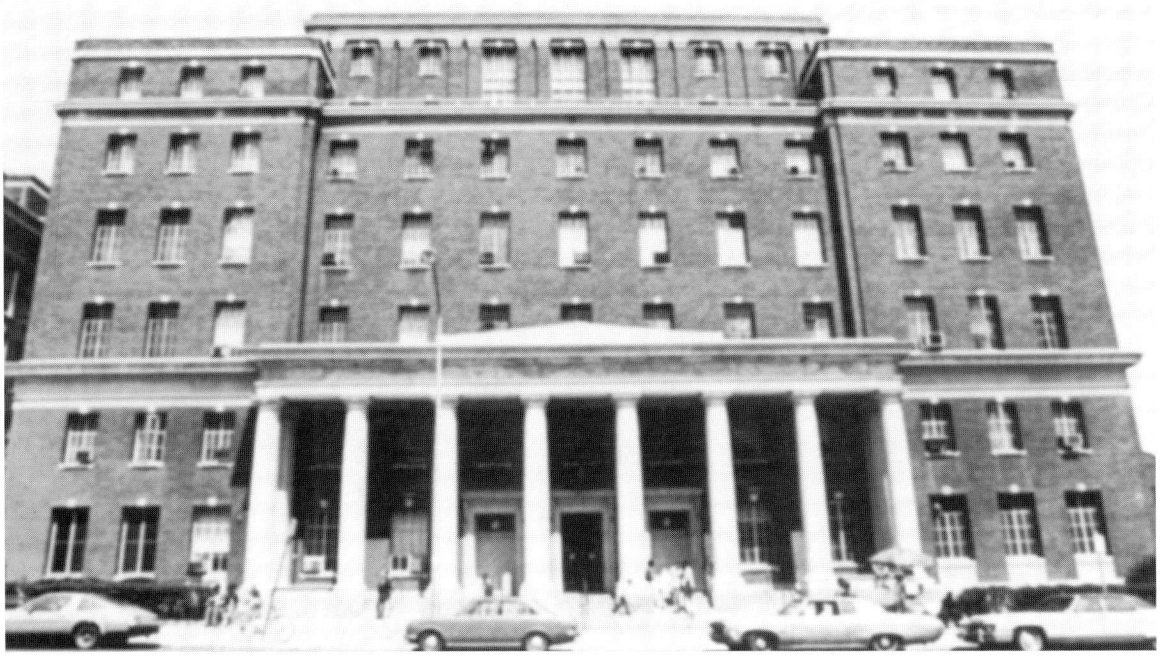

FIGURE 5-8
The Wills at 16th and Spring Garden Streets opened in November 1932.

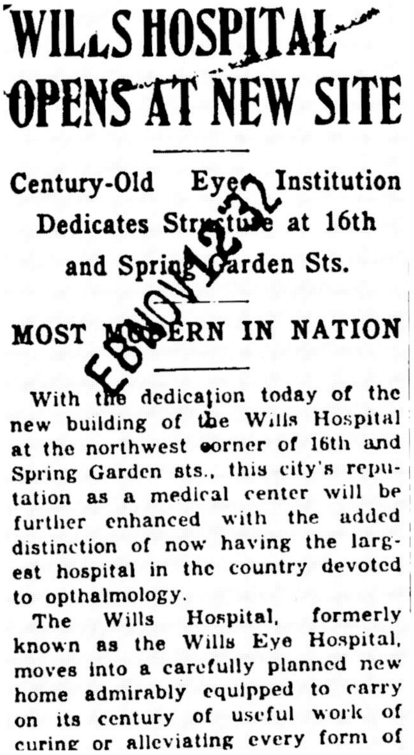

WILLS HOSPITAL OPENS AT NEW SITE

Century-Old Eye Institution Dedicates Structure at 16th and Spring Garden Sts.

MOST MODERN IN NATION

With the dedication today of the new building of the Wills Hospital at the northwest corner of 16th and Spring Garden sts., this city's reputation as a medical center will be further enhanced with the added distinction of now having the largest hospital in the country devoted to opthalmology.

The Wills Hospital, formerly known as the Wills Eye Hospital, moves into a carefully planned new home admirably equipped to carry on its century of useful work of curing or alleviating every form of

FIGURE 5-9
Dedication of Wills Hospital
at 16th and Spring Garden Streets.

Chapter 6

Cataract Surgery at Wills

The Wills Eye Hospital has always been known for its cataract surgery and for the training in cataract surgery that its resident surgeons receive. The evolution of the cataract operation as practiced in the United States may be traced by examining the contributions Wills Eye staff members made to the cataract technique. Littel, Hays, Agnew, and Norris all described procedures that were popular at their time, and each recorded his opinions of the early methods.

When the hospital was first founded, three ways of operating were in vogue: couching, keratonyxis (or breaking up of the lens), and extraction. Various modifications have since been made to these three methods.

Couching, or depression, was the operation of the earliest surgeons and until the beginning of the 18th century was the only procedure practiced. It consisted of simply displacing the lens below the level of the pupil. It was easy to do and often gave immediate, successful results.

Keratonyxis was performed by tearing the capsule and fragmenting the lens so that the lens substance might be exposed to the action of the aqueous and thus be gradually dissolved and absorbed. This procedure was very popular, and advances were made in this procedure well up to the end of the 1800s. In Wharton Jones's book (edited by Isaac Hays), the following opinion was given:

> *Considered as an operation, this is the most successful of all those of the cataract, both in performance and extent of injury necessarily inflicted upon the eye. . . . In the cases proper for the operation, the prognosis is good. . . . In general, it may be said that in children the absorption process proceeds more quickly than in adults.*

Littel also felt that this operation was particularly applicable for children. The instrument of choice was a needle, which in many cases, Littel pointed out, could not be well controlled by the surgeon, especially when it was introduced through the sclera, as it commonly was.

In 1745, Daviel revolutionized the operation for cataract by making an incision into the eyeball and removing the opaque lens from the eye. Some years later, Beer of Vienna modified Daviel's method and invented a triangular knife by means of which a sufficiently large section of the cornea could be made to allow removal of the lens from the eye. No iridectomy was done. Many cases were successful, but unfortunately many were lost to infection; this was thought to be because the incision lay anteriorly on the cornea. Therefore, for some years a more peripheral incision was made in the sclera, though the results obtained with this modification were not much better than those with the corneal incision.

Littel was not in favor of extraction and criticized it while still advocating couching. In any event, the procedure was adopted by most staff members after von Graefe made modifications in the method of extraction in 1862. The first improvement suggested by von Graefe was a linear incision, which did away with the gaping caused by the Beer incision. Von Graefe made his incision in the upper part of the cornea and combined it with an iridectomy, another modification. About the same time, Jacobson introduced a flap section in the sclera, also combining it with an iridectomy.

By this time, the complications of subacute inflammation with couching and excessive length of time for absorption with keratonyxis had been pointed out by Agnew. By 1890, Norris again emphasized the complications of discissions and absorption. Agnew practiced von Graefe's method from the very start and was impressed with his results. Excellent as von Graefe's results were, however, he further improved them a few years later by introducing the modified flap operations, which combined the advantages of the linear incision, by which he obtained a closed coaptation of the lips of the wound, with those of a scleral incision. A narrow or linear knife was soon almost universally employed.

Many modifications followed, including preliminary iridectomy, performed several weeks prior to lens extraction. The objections raised to this were a greater risk of infection with two operative procedures and the greater mental and physical strain experienced by the patient.

The methods of opening the capsule also differed, but the cystotome was preferred by most surgeons. Others tore off a bit of the capsule with forceps, while the more experienced and skillful operators incised the capsule with the tip of the cataract knife as the instrument was swept across the anterior section. Still others thought it was better to open the capsule and ripen the lens several days before completing the cataract operation. This approach, however, was never widely accepted.

From 1872 to 1891, about 1,428 cataract extractions were performed at Wills Eye Hospital. This represented 1.1 percent of the cases seen at the hospital. An interesting survey of cataract patients reported by Edward Jackson showed that 449 of 1,545 patients over the age of 50 were noted to have some lens opacities. Arranged in five-year periods, the percentages were as follows: 15 percent between ages 50 and 55, 16.1 percent between 55 and 60, 30.2 percent between 60 and 65. In a 10-year period, in patients between ages of 65 and 75, 77 percent were noted to have lens opacities.

Before the days of general anesthesia, even cocaine was not available. As a result, patients and surgeons had to make do as best as they could, the one enduring pain and the other trying to operate skillfully and swiftly. After general anesthetics were introduced in the 1840s, the question arose as to whether the relief from pain they afforded the patient combined with the opportunity given the surgeon to operate with greater precision and ease counterbalanced the evils of retching and vomiting that the anesthetic often produced. One must remember that no sutures were used at this time, so that the vomiting could be a considerable problem. Interestingly enough, Agnew felt that it was better not to use anesthetic because, he said, the operation was not painful and a few words of assurance from the surgeon could put a patient at ease. One must conclude from this that Agnew himself probably never had a cataract operation. Still, in an interesting survey conducted by Derby in Boston, 100 patients were operated on while under an anesthetic and eight eyes were lost. A second group of 100 patients were operated on without the advantage of an anesthetic and only one eye was lost. Once again, however, had sutures been used, the results certainly would have been different.

In 1881, antiseptics were introduced in ocular surgery, and aseptic precautions were observed. Still, antisepsis was not the great boon to ophthalmology that it was to general surgery. Many of us can still remember the barehanded ophthalmic surgeon (even in the 1950s and early 1960s) and the low incidence of infection in their operations.

In 1884, Carl Koller discovered cocaine. This was a big help to the ophthalmic surgeon, as was the later introduction of Novocain. With the advent of local anesthetics, the number of cataract operations increased markedly. In 1880, at the Wills Eye Hospital, 262 extractions were done; by 1920, there were over 600 extractions, and by 1930, over 1,000.

In 1921, Colonel Henry Smith, who had gained much experience performing cataract operations in India, visited the Wills Eye Hospital. An Irishman trained in Britain, Smith served for years in India as an officer in the British Medical Service. Although only a general medical officer in charge of the health in the Punjab, he developed a particular interest in diseases of the eye, especially cataract.

His operative skill was well known throughout India. He averaged 3,000 cataract operations each year. Since he could not speak the various dialects, he was unable to communicate with his patients; as a result, he devised an operation that could be performed without the patient's cooperation, and thus the intracapsular method of extraction was developed. By the time he retired in 1921, Colonel Smith had performed 50,000 cataract operations, mostly by the intracapsular method.

Actually, the intracapsular method did not originate with Colonel Smith, and he never claimed that it did. The first surgeons to practice this method of extraction were Richter and Beer and, later, the Pagenstechers of Germany, who obtained excellent results with it. The Pagenstechers maintained their clinic in Wiesbaden as late as 1959. Smith, however, modified the operation and had far greater experience with it than did anyone else.

He visited the Wills Eye Hospital on November 17, 1921, and operated on 18 senile cataracts. His results were followed up by Dr. William Zentmayer and showed a corrected vision of 6/6 in two cases, 6/9 and 6/12 in two cases, 6/15 in three cases, 6/20 in four cases, and 6/30 in two cases. In five cases, no follow-up was available. Vitreous loss and incarceration of the iris occurred in 38 percent of the patients, and in most there was residual haze.

Although Smith's results in this country were somewhat disastrous, it was the general opinion that he was operating at considerable disadvantage. His assistants were unknown to him and the surroundings were strange; also, large crowds watched him operate, which no doubt had an effect. Still, all those who witnessed his surgery admired his skill, poise, and command of the situation.

While operating in India for hours at a stretch, the Colonel had grown accustomed to smoking during the operation. He usually smoked cigars and lighted up before scrubbing. The cigar then remained in his mouth until the operation was almost completed. While smoking his customary cigar during surgery at Wills, one of the observers became concerned that the ash from the cigar would fall into the eye of the patient and actually felt compelled to draw attention to this. He said to Smith: "Pardon me, Colonel, but aren't you afraid that an ash from your cigar is going to fall into the patient's eye?" Smith replied quickly and with certainty: "It never has yet."

Although all admired the skill he demonstrated at Wills Eye Hospital, there were those who felt that he would be better named "Vitreous Smith" rather than "Indian Smith," the name that had been given to him because of his long service in the subcontinent.

Through the years, intracapsular cataract extraction became well accepted. However, innovations have evolved over the years, and Wills Eye Hospital has contributed to many. Probably one of the most significant contributions to cataract surgery was the use of the cryoprobe for extraction of the lens, a procedure devised by an ex-resident of the Wills Eye Hospital, Dr. Charles Kelman, who served his residency from 1958 to 1960.

Kelman also developed the technique of phacoemulsification, a method of fragmenting the lens with an ultrasonic tip. Thus, two significant innovations in cataract surgery are attributable to a Wills Eye Hospital ex-resident. The latter is currently state of the art.

Wills Eye Hospital also pioneered another popular modern addition to cataract surgery, the introduction of an intraocular lens into the eye to replace the removed cataractous one. Today posterior chamber implants are the procedure of choice, but initially they were quite controversial.

During the Battle of Britain in World War II, England survived, thanks to the Royal Air Force, to which Winston Churchill paid tribute when he said that never was "so much owed by so many to so few." It was during this time that a British ophthalmologist, Ridley, noted that when fragments of plastic material had been driven into the eye by an explosion or the impact of a bullet on the polymethyl methacrylate (Perspex) canopy of a fighter plane, tissue reaction was insignificant. The eye appeared to tolerate the plastic. As a result of this landmark observation, the first intraocular lens (IOL) became a reality in 1949. Ridley's work came to the attention of Dr. Warren Reese, an attending surgeon at Wills Eye, who began to correspond with Ridley. Ultimately, Dr. Reese performed 300 intraocular Ridley lenses between 1952 and 1956. This far exceeded the 77 that Ridley himself had inserted.

The first report by Reese on intraocular lenses concerned 20 cases. All had good results. Dr. Reese had wanted to perform his first Ridley implant without a crowd, so he inserted the first one four days before the annual clinical conference in 1952. Having performed one, he then did another during the Wills Eye Conference.

Reese performed the intraocular operation before he actually met Ridley, who lived in a cottage in Wiltshire, England. While driving in his car, Reese first glimpsed Ridley standing midstream in hip waders, intent upon fishing, and Dr. Reese was fond of recalling this memory, which marked the beginning of a long friendship. The two became very close and visited each other often.

As the only surgeon in the United States who had experience with Ridley's procedure, Dr. Reese discussed Ridley's first paper given at the Academy Meeting in Chicago. A short time later, under Reese's tutelage, Dr. Turgut Hamdi began inserting Ridley's implants and new implants as they were developed. Certainly until his death there was no one in the United States who had a longer follow-up of intraocular lenses than Dr. Hamdi.

Another close friend of Dr. Reese's was Cecil O'Brien. He was an excellent ophthalmologist, famous for his outspokenness as well as his intellect. He started his career at the Wills Eye Hospital, where he was a resident, but, restless for open spaces, he packed his bags and moved to the Midwest. There he became chairman of the University of Iowa Eye Department, where he subsequently taught Tom Duane, who afterward became an ophthalmologist-in-chief at Wills.

O'Brien used to teasingly accuse Reese of being afraid to visit him in the West for fear of being attacked by Indians. Reese denied the allegation and proved his fearlessness by arriving some months later on the train. To his surprise, O'Brien and his residents were waiting on the station platform dressed as Indians.

As already mentioned, O'Brien was a person who said what was on his mind. As a resident, he once watched Dr. William Zentmayer examine a young man. To relax the patient, Zentmayer asked what the young man did for a living. The answer was that he was a bricklayer. A few seconds later Zentmayer inquired again as to the patient's occupation, and the reply was again "bricklayer." Then as Zentmayer shifted to look in the second eye, he asked the same question a third time, but before he could finish, O'Brien said quietly from the doorway, "He's still a bricklayer, Doctor!"

Other cataract surgeons at Wills who were excellent technicians included Dr. Posey, who operated expeditiously, and Drs. William Zentmayer and Frank Parker, who are renowned for making cataract incisions and iridectomies at the same time with the von Graefe knife. More recently, Dr. Edmund Spaeth performed numerous cataract operations, as did Dr. James Shipman, both of whom developed national reputations as ophthalmic surgeons. Dr. Spaeth was also noted for his work in motility and for his abilities as a teacher.

In any discussion of cataract extraction, one cannot fail to mention the exceptional talent of P. Robb McDonald. His technical skill was matched by incomparable clinical judgment and an ability to keep pace with rapid changes in surgical technique. Because of his exceptional abilities, other cataract surgeons began to send their complications to him, and he became an authority in this field.

Today Wills Cataract Surgeons are among the best in the world, and they continue the legacy of those who preceded them.

Chapter 7

The Organization of Wills Eye Hospital

From the 1930s to the 1960s, Wills Eye Hospital was organized around several general eye services, each of which was headed by a chief. There were three clinic areas in the hospital, and each patient was examined by members of the staff as well as by one resident from each clinic. For example, the Tassman Service would see patients and operate on Monday and Thursday, the Leopold Service would see patients Tuesday and Friday, and the Spaeth Service would see patients on Wednesday and Saturday. After the external examination, patients were sent to a dark room for dilation and examination (usually with the direct ophthalmoscope) of the ocular fundus (Fig. 7-1). They later had to return on a different day for refraction.

Each service chief and his lieutenant were responsible for one of the clinic rooms and the surgery generated from the clinic two days each week. The result was that some of the staff would

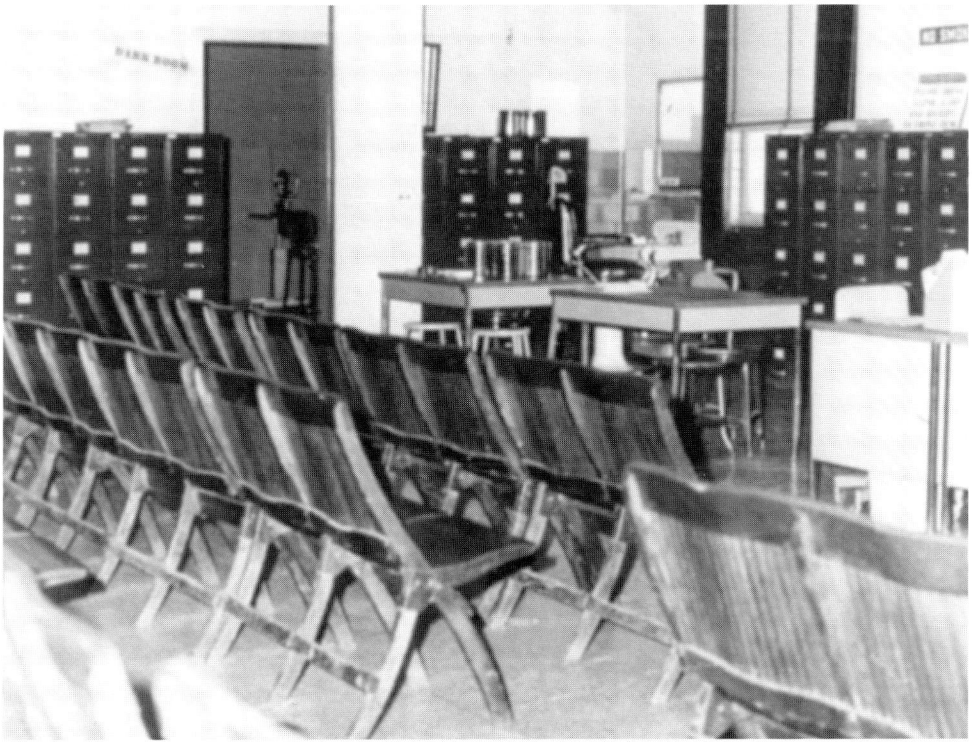

FIGURE 7-1
General receiving clinic, 16th and Spring Garden Streets, in the 1950s.

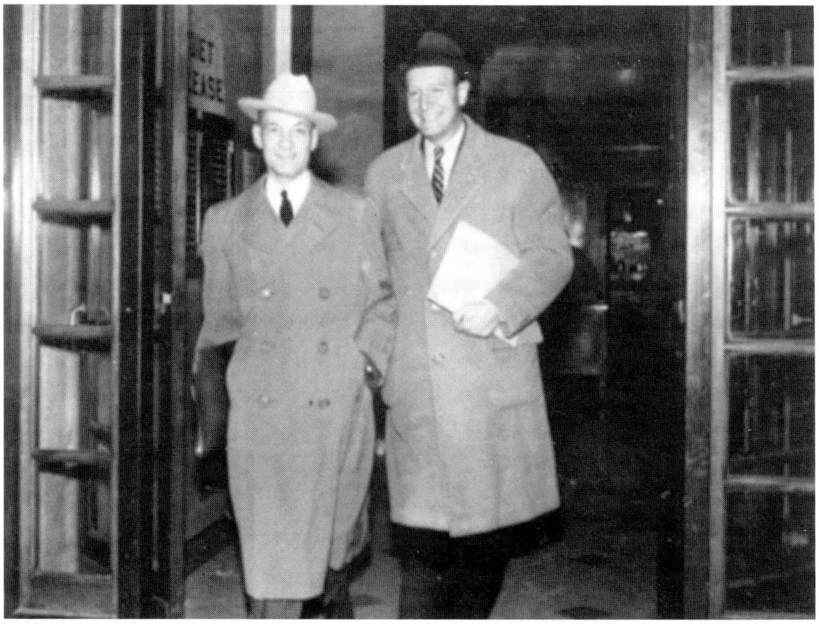

FIGURE 7-2
Jack Matthews and the late Irving Leopold leaving Wills Hospital.

be responsible for managing the clinics, while others would be in the operating room assisting residents with surgery. Each private physician would also operate on his private patients on those days.

By the late 1950s, one of the busiest chiefs was Irving Leopold (Fig. 7-2), who was instrumental in bringing about organizational changes. By this time, too, several offers came to Dr. Irving Leopold from other institutions. To counter these, the Board of City Trusts and the Board of Surgeons voted to make Leopold the overall chief with the idea of bringing together many of the potentially excellent functions and services at the Wills Hospital (Fig. 7-3). One of the first accomplishments of this new regime was to decrease the number of chiefs from nine to five. Instead of there being three services a day, each one performing twice a week, they were reduced to five, one for each of the working days of the week, and Saturdays became a teaching day, with use of the emergency room to handle the patients who could not come to the regular clinic during the week.

With Leopold as ophthalmologist-in-chief, specialty clinics in glaucoma, uveitis, and external disease were initiated. Pediatric ophthalmology, which was supported by a grant from the National Council to Combat Blindness, was successful from the start. Other subspecialty services were also introduced, and these are described in Chapter 9.

It also become apparent that it would be advisable for the Wills Hospital to have a medical school affiliation. Actually, Wills already had a loose connection with the University of Pennsylvania because Leopold was then professor and chairman of the Department of Ophthalmology in the Graduate School of Medicine at the University of Pennsylvania as well as head of Wills. The majority of the residents at that time were participating in the University formal course prior to coming to Wills as residents. Still, there were some ophthalmologists who felt that because the Wills Eye Hospital was not part of a

Dr. Leopold Gets Wills Eye Post

Dr. Irving H. Leopold, noted opthalmologist, has been appointed medical and research director of Wills Eye Hospital, it was announced Monday by Samuel H. Daroff, president of the Board of City Trusts, trustees of the hospital.

FIGURE 7-3
Irving Leopold becomes the first medical director and director of research. Note that ophthalmologist is misspelled.

university, it could not have a department quite as good as that found in a university. To make sure that Wills Eye Hospital was not losing stature and national and international prestige, the administration began looking for a firmer association with a medical school. Leopold organized a committee which approached the University of Pennsylvania Medical School, Thomas Jefferson, Temple, and Hahnemann. Each was asked to think about forming an association with the Wills Hospital. It took a number of years to resolve this situation. Ultimately, Leopold left for New York, and it had not yet been decided which institution would be associated with Wills. However, the groundwork was laid for the next chief, Arthur Keeney, and his group to consummate an affiliation.

Under the leadership of Arthur H. Keeney (Fig. 7-4), who was appointed in 1964, the inefficiency of seeing patients and having them come back later to the refraction clinic became apparent. Therefore, "one-stop" ophthalmic care developed. The clinic system was revamped, and better-equipped individual examining rooms were designed and built. This made for better patient/doctor relationships and more pleasant surroundings for the patients.

Keeney also carried on the quest for a university affiliation. This culminated in a marriage to Temple University, with the hope that a new Wills Hospital would be built at the North Broad Street Medical Complex. State funds never became available, however, and ultimately the association was dissolved.

Negotiations then began with the University of Pennsylvania and Jefferson. On July 20, 1972, Wills and Jefferson affiliated, and the 1980 hospital and a single residency program were fruits of that union.

In the 1950s and 1960s the chiefs were Drs. Wilfred Fry, Patrick J. Kennedy, Irving H. Leopold, P. Robb McDonald, Robert Mulberger, James Shipman, Edmund B. Spaeth, and Isaac Tassman. All contributed much to the modernization of Wills Eye Hospital.

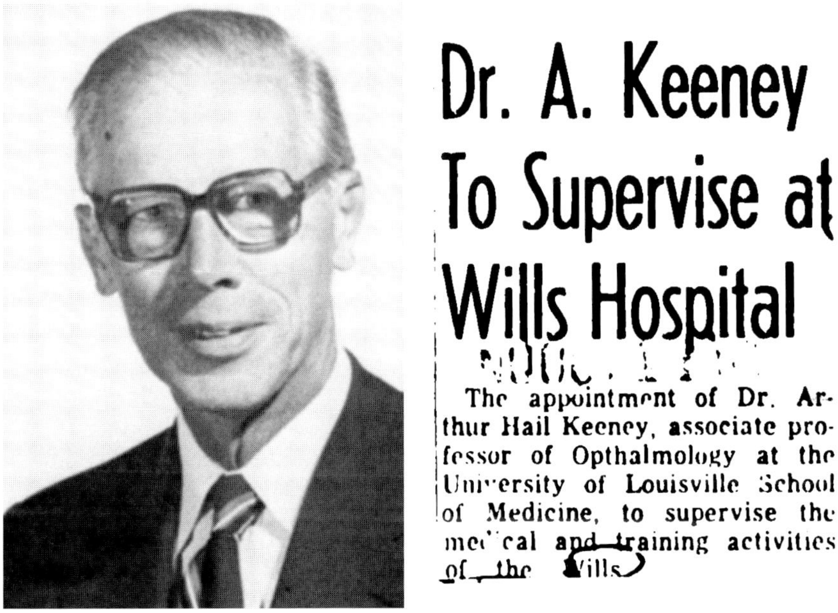

Dr. A. Keeney To Supervise at Wills Hospital

The appointment of Dr. Arthur Hail Keeney, associate professor of Opthalmology at the University of Louisville School of Medicine, to supervise the medical and training activities of the Wills

FIGURE 7-4
Arthur Keeney succeeds Irving Leopold as ophthalmologist-in-chief, November 1964. Ophthalmology is misspelled.

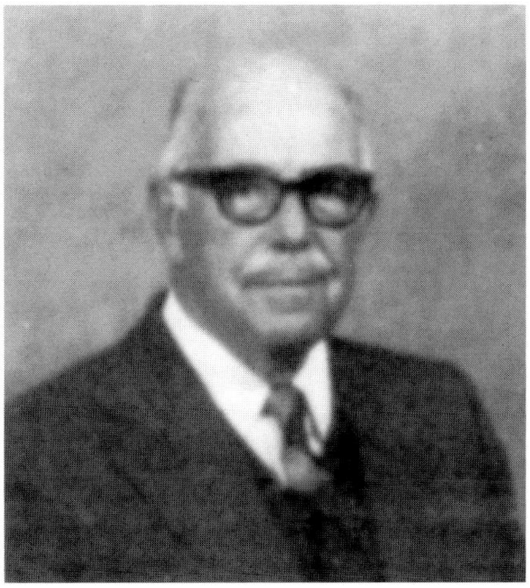

FIGURE 7-5
P. Robb McDonald

Known as "Mr. Wills," Shipman acquired a significant reputation for his skill as a surgeon. He was one of the first surgeons at Wills Eye Hospital to do corneal transplants with a two-blade knife and also did much to popularize the intrascapular cataract extraction in Philadelphia.

Shipman was also a local pioneer in retinal detachment surgery. Often after a person had a retinal detachment, the eye was lost. Bed rest was stressed for several weeks before and after surgery, and results were not what they are today. In his memory, there is a Shipman Memorial Fund, which is used to support a research retina fellowship.

P. Robb McDonald (Fig. 7-5) and Patrick Kennedy followed Shipman as pioneers in retinal detachment surgery. Quickly McDonald recognized the value of the work of Charles Schepens of Boston. Schepens developed and popularized the binocular indirect ophthalmoscope as a practical instrument to be worn on the head so that the surgeon could perform indirect ophthalmoscopy using scleral depression. This, as it turned out, was a major breakthrough in the cure of retinal detachment because the retina could now be adequately examined. Wills Eye Hospital thus became an early proponent of the new techniques of retinal detachment surgery, especially the use of a polyethylene tube to encircle the globe during retinal detachment surgery, This, however, was a rigid material that led to many cases of intrusion. As an alternative material, McDonald suggested to Schepens that he try silicone rubber instead, and this is still the material of choice today.

Two other chiefs active from the 1940s through the 1960s were E. B. Spaeth and I.S. Tassman. In addition to their contributions to Wills, both sired sons who have followed in their tradition at Wills: Philip G. Spaeth, George L. Spaeth, and William Tasman.

Edmund Spaeth was noted for his ophthalmic surgery, particularly in the fields of plastics and motility, and his textbook *Ophthalmic Surgery* was the classic of its day. Happily his son, George Spaeth, has continued publication of a surgical textbook entitled *Ophthalmic Surgery, Principles and Practice*.

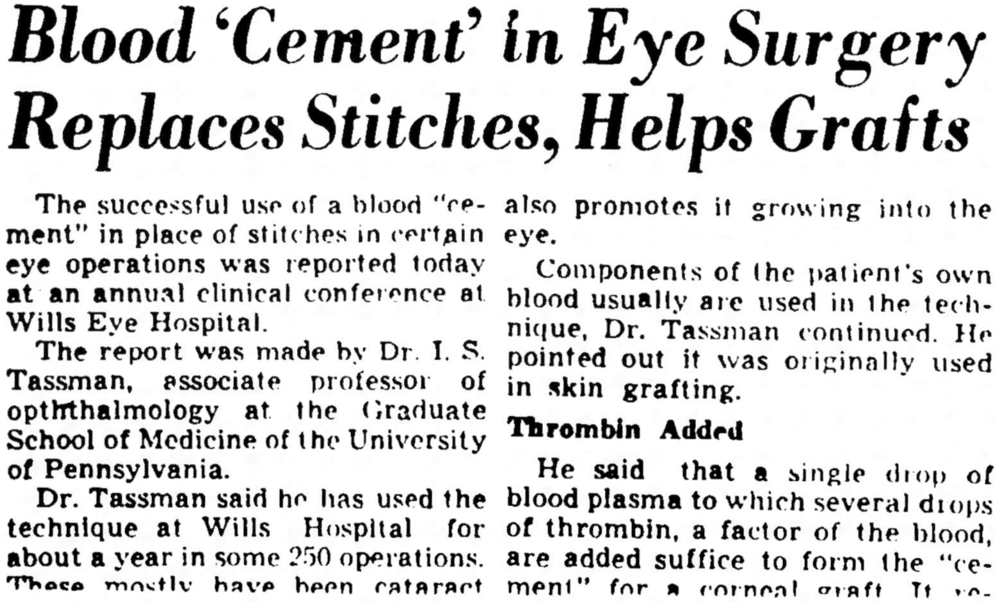

Blood 'Cement' in Eye Surgery Replaces Stitches, Helps Grafts

The successful use of a blood "cement" in place of stitches in certain eye operations was reported today at an annual clinical conference at Wills Eye Hospital.

The report was made by Dr. I. S. Tassman, associate professor of opththalmology at the Graduate School of Medicine of the University of Pennsylvania.

Dr. Tassman said he has used the technique at Wills Hospital for about a year in some 250 operations.

also promotes it growing into the eye.

Components of the patient's own blood usually are used in the technique, Dr. Tassman continued. He pointed out it was originally used in skin grafting.

Thrombin Added

He said that a single drop of blood plasma to which several drops of thrombin, a factor of the blood, are added suffice to form the "cement" for a corneal graft.

FIGURE 7-6

Description of the first physiologic glue.

Tassman was noted for his expertise in medical diseases affecting the eye and refraction and was the first chief of refraction at the Wills Eye Hospital. His book *Eye Manifestation of Internal Diseases* went through three editions and was a standard text of the day in Europe as well as the United States. He was also the first to devise a physiologic glue for corneal lacerations, which he first reported at the second annual Wills Eye Conference (Fig. 7-6), and he directed the Wills Eye Conference as chairman of the conference committee through the 1950s and into the 1960s.

Keeney's tenure lasted until 1972, when he was succeeded by Thomas D. Duane (see chapter 14). Duane retired in 1982. Robert D. Reinecke was recruited from Albany Medical College to become ophthalmologist-in-chief and professor and head of the department at Jefferson, a role he retained until he took over the Foerderer Research Department in 1985. William Tasman at that point became ophthalmologist-in-chief and department chairman for Jefferson (Fig. 7-7).

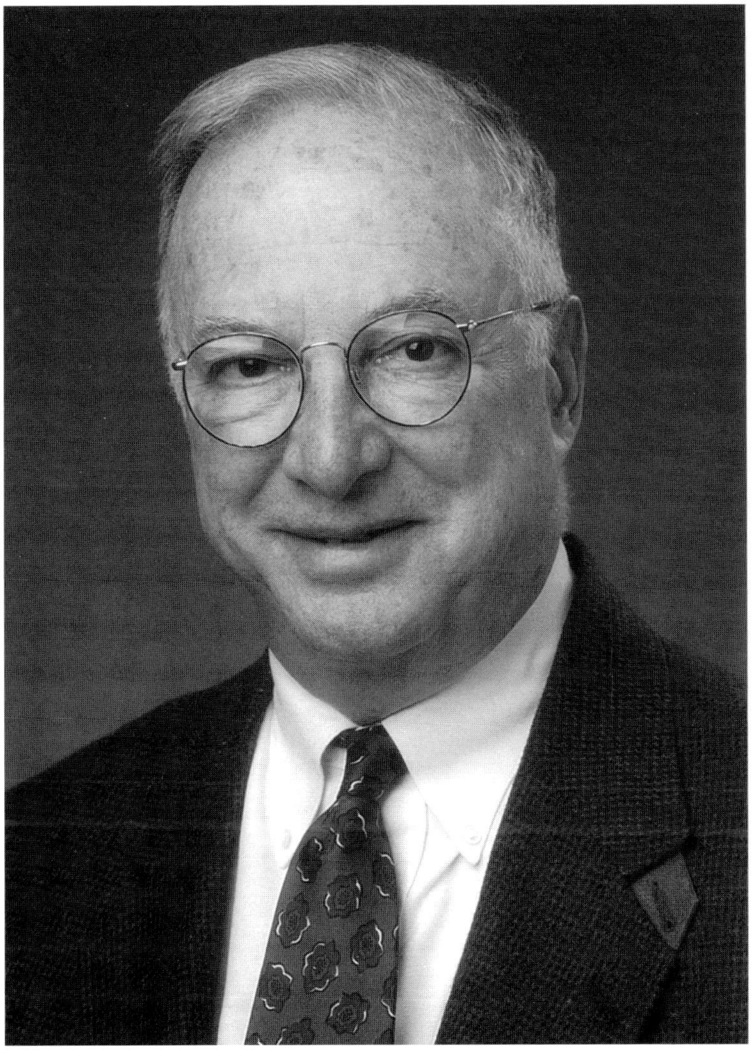

Figure 7-7
In 1985 Dr. William Tasman was appointed ophthalmologist-in-chief at Wills Eye Hospital and department chairman at Jefferson Medical College.

Chapter 8

The Residency Program

John Jeffers, M.D., Residency Program Director
Tara Uhler, M.D., Associate Residency Program Director

Wills Eye Hospital has always been actively involved in the teaching and training of ophthalmologists. As early as 1839, Isaac Parrish began a course of lectures in the hospital, which were continued until his death in 1852. Other members of the staff were also active in demonstrating cases to visiting physicians and students. By 1867, the Board passed a bylaw that lecturing and teaching should be continued.

During the period, it was the custom for students of the University of Pennsylvania and the Jefferson Medical School to attend clinics at Wills Eye Hospital, where their education in diseases of the eye were acquired. In Philadelphia, no regular courses of lectures on diseases of the eye were given in medical schools until 1870. That year, the department of ophthalmology was started at the University of Pennsylvania and was followed 24 years later by the department at the Jefferson Hospital. Although a chair of ophthalmology at Jefferson was not established until 1894, lectures had been given by Dr. Thompson for a number of years.

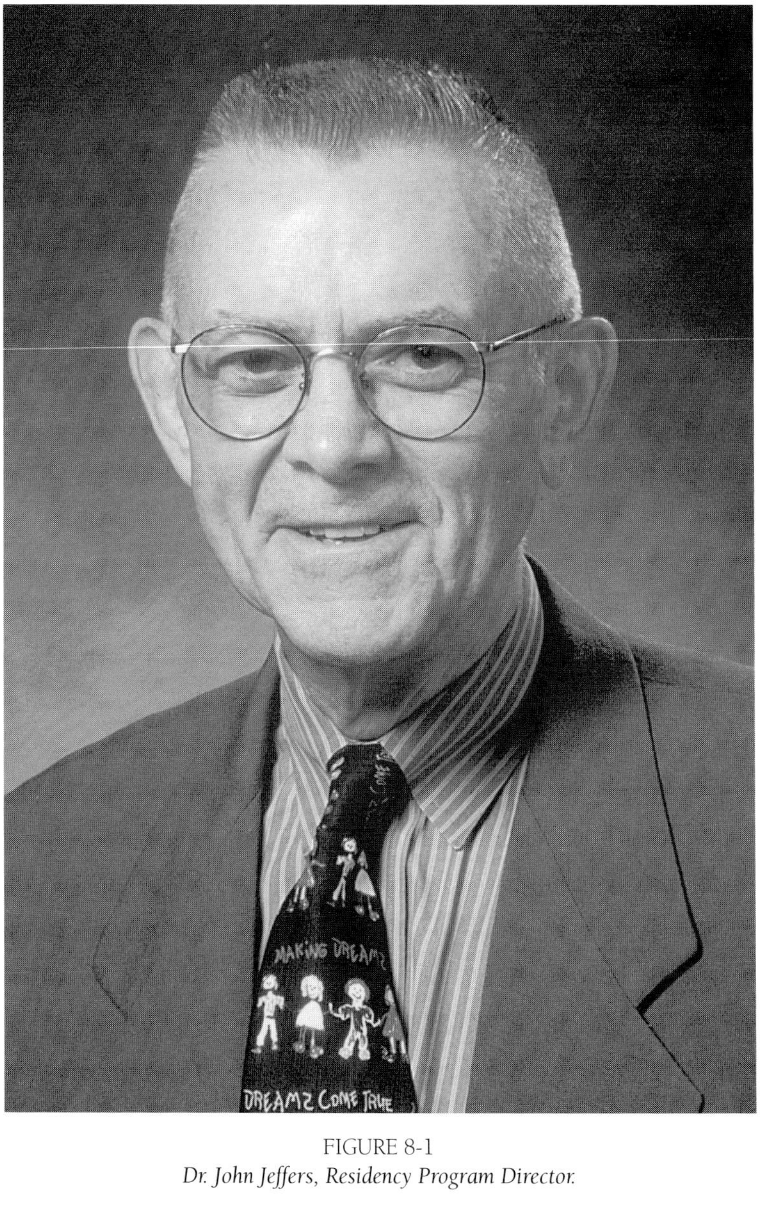

FIGURE 8-1
Dr. John Jeffers, Residency Program Director.

Advertisements in 1873 in the *American Journal of Medical Sciences* by Dr. Hall of the staff at Wills Eye Hospital and Drs. Levis and Dyer made known the fact that courses in ophthalmology were given at the Wills Eye Hospital. Dr. McClure, who initiated the lectures, had recently returned from studying abroad. His evening lectures at the Wills Eye Hospital illustrated various phases of the dioptric system of the eye, utilizing lantern slides that he had made himself. These lectures proved to be very popular, but their success created some jealousy among his peers.

It is difficult to pinpoint the exact time when official residency programs started at the Wills Eye Hospital, but the earliest listed ex-resident is John Neill in 1839. Certainly, the residency program was firmly in operation by the early 1900s.

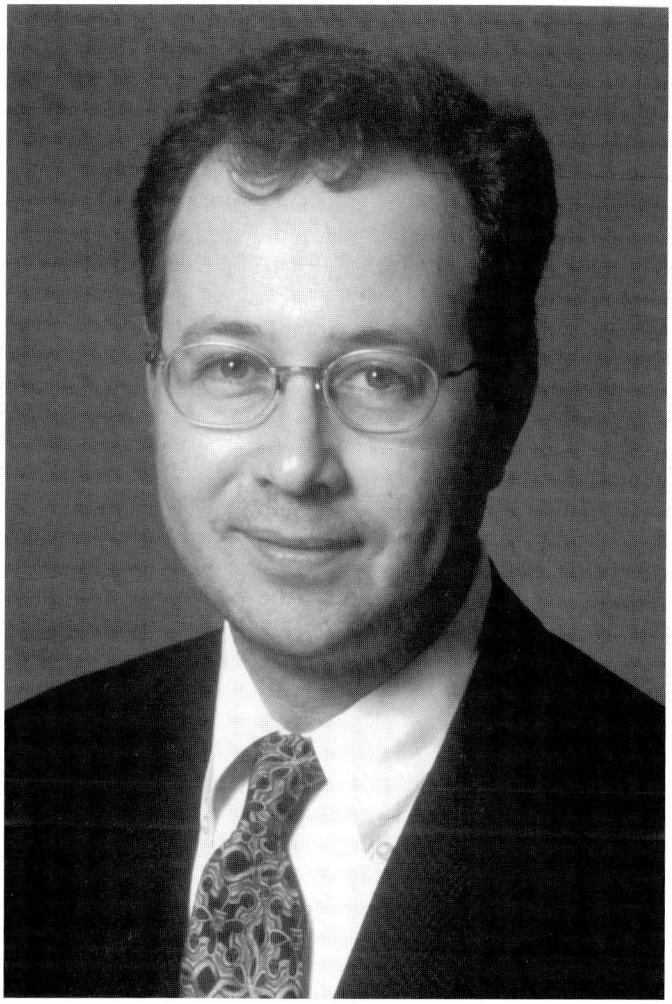

FIGURE 8-2
Dr. Marlon Maus, Co-Program Director (1997–2000).

The minutes of the Hospital meeting on November 4, 1912 reveal the emerging hierarchy of the hospital. The Board of Directors recommended that white uniforms be worn by the staff and that they should have the following insignia: surgeons, four one-half inch stripes on the sleeves: assistant surgeons, one one-half inch stripe and one one-fourth inch stripe; house surgeons, two one-fourth inch stripes; and clinical assistants, no stripe at all. They also recommended that a white apron be provided to cover the knees of the surgeons and assistant surgeons when they were treating cases in the clinic. A broad cape, which could be sterilized, was ordered for visitors in the operating rooms, and operating gowns were furnished for assistant surgeons and their assistants.

During the early 1900s, it was mandatory that the junior resident physicians and a junior nurse assist in operations and make visits in the ward as emergencies arose. As of 1911 and 1912, the resident physician served for one year, beginning January 1. During this period, there were two residents, a junior resident and a senior resident. However, by 1912, the workload was increasing at the hospital and a request for a third resident was made. It was also suggested that a committee consisting of three members of the staff be selected by the president of the staff to examine future applicants for the position of resident surgeon at the hospital. The committee was then to report to the Board of Surgeons "the general fitness of the gentlemen making application for the position."

Clinical training at the Wills Eye Hospital has always been excellent; its quality did not change through the transition of the move from Logan Square to Spring Garden Street. During this period, the number of residents gradually increased, as did the length of time served in the residency. From one year, it was increased to 18 months, and this was the requisite time until May 1947, when the committee on residents submitted a plan for increasing the resident service from 18 months to two years. This, they felt, would afford an additional two weeks on each service and would therefore upgrade the training.

The residency committee was given the responsibility of looking into the credentials of applicants for residency appointments. After an adequate number had been screened from the total number of applicants, a small number was selected and invited to appear before the Board of Attending Surgeons at their January meeting for further examination and recommendation to the Board of City Trusts for appointment as residents.

Many tales of these interviews have filtered down through the years. Applicants frequently stood around the perimeter of the boardroom, which at that time was on the Brandywine Street side of the first floor of the Spring Garden Street hospital; each wore a tag stating his or her name. There were at the time nine chiefs, and each of them moved around the room asking whatever question he desired of each applicant. There were no women chiefs at that time. Frequently this *modus operandi* of interviewing curdled the stomachs of even the most hearty.

One cannot forget, as well, how in the 1950s Dr. Wilfred Fry spent a good deal of his time selecting residents. Often he was seen interviewing candidates on the pew-type benches that were then present in the lobby. Usually two other members were on the committee with Dr. Fry. Two who served in that capacity were Drs. William Annesley and Philip Spaeth, but as the latter tell it, most of the decisions were actually made on the benches in the lobby, and their job was to ratify the selections.

During this period, residents entered every three months. This was a system with many hazards; the most significant of which was that if the resident three months ahead of you was a "turkey," your stay at Wills could be most unhappy. This system also allowed for each resident to eventually become the chief resident for the last three months of his (or her) tenure and was climaxed with farewell parties given by many of the staff men, including Drs. Shipman, Spaeth, Tassman and Kennedy.

The practice of taking on a new resident every three months was finally abolished in favor of having a class start each July 1. This process was in effect by the late 1950s and at the time seven residents were taken in each group, so that there were a total of 14 in the two-year class. By 1958, it was decided that one of the senior residents should be designated as the Chief Resident. The first to have this honor was Dr. Ralph Hamilton, who went on to practice in Memphis, Tennessee. He was succeeded by Dr. Jerome Montana in 1959. By 1982, because of the large number of residents (42), it was necessary to have two Co-Chief Residents.

Up until this time, it had been a prerequisite for a resident at Wills Eye Hospital to have a basic course in ophthalmology before entering the training program. Several courses were given, the most notable of which was at the graduate school of the University of Pennsylvania, headed successively by William Shoemaker, Edmund Spaeth and Irving Leopold. Many of the men who taught at the graduate school were members of the staff of Wills, as evidenced by Fig. 8-3, which shows the faculty at the graduate school of the University of Pennsylvania in 1937.

In 1965, the length of the residency increased to three years, and a new class of seven residents was selected. By then, too, Arthur H. Keeney had accepted the position of Ophthalmologist-In-Chief at Wills Eye, and under his guidance a basic science course given by staff members of the hospital was held on the premises. This course was much shorter than the nine-month course at the graduate school of the University of Pennsylvania, and covered only the most basic aspects of ophthalmology. Starting in the late 1970s a more formal three week Pre-Residency Course was given for the new first year residents. In addition to the Wills Eye Residents first year residents were invited from Temple University Hospital, Hahnemann Hospital, the Philadelphia School of Osteopathy, the University of South Carolina, Newark Eye and Ear Hospital and Tufts Medical College.

As of 2000 The University of South Carolina,

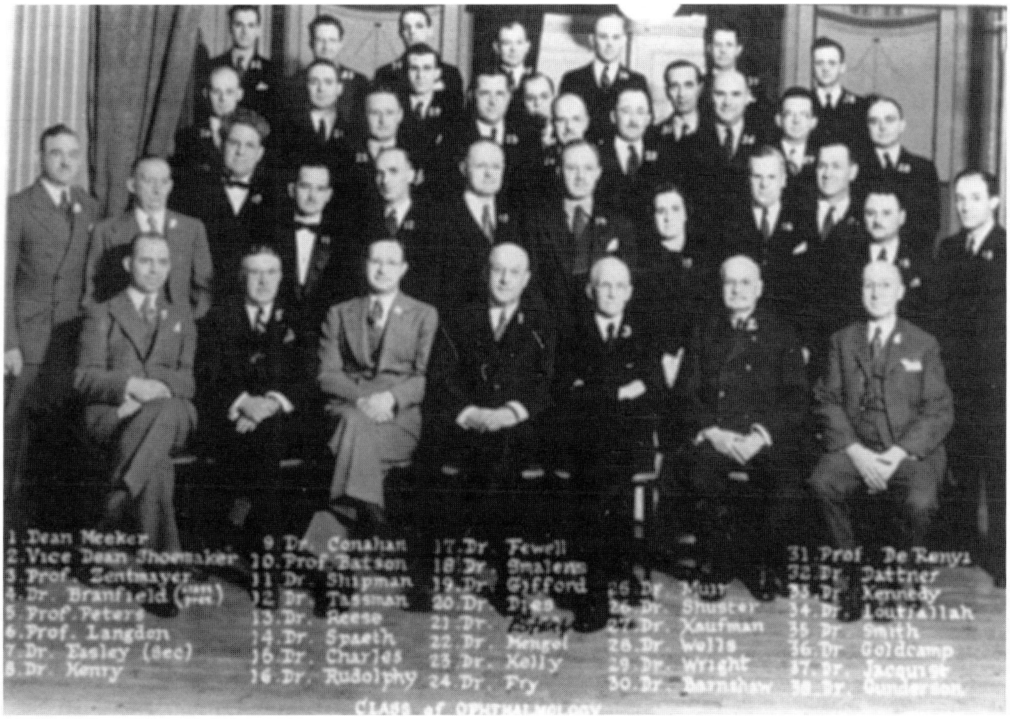

FIGURE 8-3
1937 faculty and class of ophthalmology. Graduate School of Medicine, University of Pennsylvania.

Newark, and Tufts established their own Pre-Residency Course. This year the Wills Class of 10 entering in 2002 for the Pre-Residency Course will be joined by first year residents from Temple University Hospital, Hahnemann Hospital and the Philadelphia School of Osteopathy.

Following the tenure of Dr. Keeney, the position of Ophthalmologist-In-Chief was filled by Thomas D. Duane, M.D., Robert D. Reinecke, M.D. and William Tasman, M.D. The changing times in medicine have required these physicians to lead Wills in the direction of appropriate modern teaching methods for residents to survive the health care environment following graduation.

When the residency increased from two to three years, some very well known Wills ex-residents were involved. The last two-year class included George Spaeth, Dick Green, Basil Manley, Donald Praeger, Horry H. Kerrison, Robert E. King and Ronald B. Vittone. The first three-year class, which included Peter Laibson, started just six weeks after the two-year class.

Members of the two-year class therefore considered themselves "sophomores" and immediately drew up a night-call schedule that totally victimized the incoming three-year freshman class. Needless to say, the latter would have none of it, and a more equitable arrangement was quickly worked out.

The number of residents gradually increased until it reached an all-time high of 42 in 1968. At that time Wills Eye Hospital became affiliated with Temple University Hospital with future plans to build a mega-health center which would include Temple University Hospital, St. Christopher's Hospital for Children and Wills Eye Hospital. Five residents had already been accepted into the Temple University Hospital program and with the affiliation, they joined the nine Wills Residents for a total number of 14 in the first year class. In the 1970s Wills severed its affiliation with Temple and joined forces with Jefferson Medical College.

Ultimately the Wills Program was gradually cut

back to 36 total House Staff. Because Wills has always been a leader in the field of ophthalmology training, it was felt that more severe cuts were necessary and therefore the class entering in 1994 was the last of 11 residents. The entering classes of 1995 and 1996 were reduced to ten each and the class entering in 1997 was reduced to eight residents. During the 1990s managed health care mandated that there be fewer specialists and more primary health care physicians trained.

The prestige of Wills has continued to grow, and the training program is one of the best in the country. This has been reflected in the huge number of applicants (approximately 500) and the high caliber of those applicants. The selection process uses the Ophthalmology Matching Program (OMP) that works to the advantage of both the candidate and the institution. Most important, however, it prevents the institution from trying to lure an exceptional candidate into its program before he/she has been interviewed elsewhere.

The process of reviewing some 450-500 applications is very work intensive for the dedicated members of the committee. All applications are reviewed by members of the committee to reduce the number to 70-80 applicants that are invited for interviews. All applications for residency positions come through the Central Application Service (CAS). The process for selecting residents is a result of a variety of opinions expressed by the 15 members and is extremely fair. Following the interviews, the rankings of the candidates are entered in the Ophthalmology Matching Program (OMC) and the applicants enter their rankings of the programs.

Over the years, the resident clinical experience has varied somewhat depending on the demands of ophthalmology. The first year resident spends most of the time learning aspects of general ophthalmology in the Cataract Primary Eye Care Service (CPEC) and Fight For Sight (FFS) with shorter rotations in some of the specialty services. They also spend a large portion of their time, both during the regular rotation and night and weekend call, in the very busy Emergency Room. Here they learn the various aspects of handling ophthalmic emergencies.

The first year residents also have an opportunity to take part in rotations on the Einstein and Cooper campuses along with contact lens fitting and low vision services at Wills Eye Hospital. These rotations were made possible July 1, 1999 when Cooper combined their residency with Wills and at the same time a rotation at Einstein was also agreed upon.

The second year training consists mainly of exposure to the specialty services, consultation service, pathology and an increased surgical experience during the Einstein rotation. The majority of time during a resident's third year is spent in the operating room learning the various modern techniques of ophthalmic surgery. They also have the opportunity to polish their ophthalmology skills with adults and children as well as the skills of the sub-specialty services.

Since 1998 four senior residents have had the opportunity to spend a three-month rotation in the Phoenix, Arizona Veterans Administration and County Hospitals. They share the residency tasks with a third year resident from the Mayo Ophthalmology Program. This rotation has served the residents well in that they get an increased number of surgical cases which does not subtract from the residents at the home base. They also have the opportunity to interact with a resident from another program.

From the early 1970s, the ever-changing cataract surgery technology has necessitated modifications of the teaching process. Up to that time intracapsular cataract extraction was performed with the correction of vision accomplished with a contact lens or "Coke bottle" spectacles. In the mid to late 1970s extracapsular cataract extraction by phacoemulsification was becoming popular. Insertion of a plastic intraocular lens (IOL) was coming into vogue. Now in the 21st century small incisions are used to insert foldable IOLs. The problem with the small incision, which requires no sutures, was that residents had to be taught suturing techniques. Special classes and wet lab practice were instrumental in addressing suturing by the time the third year resident had the opportunity to do corneal grafts.

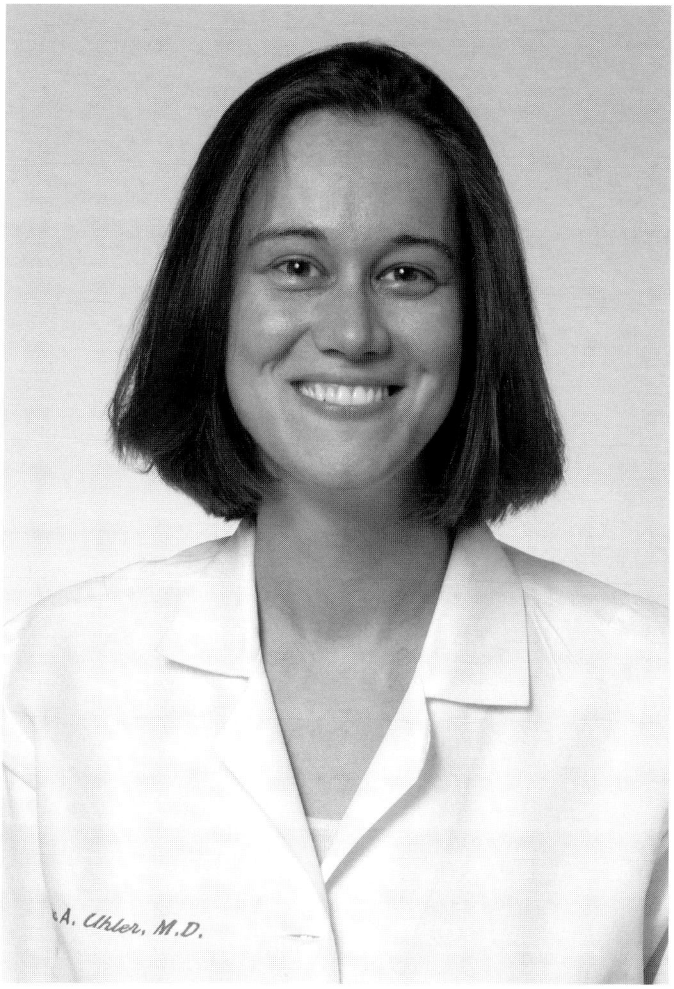

FIGURE 8-4
Dr. Tara Uhler was appointed Co-Residency Program Director in June 2002 succeeding Dr. Marlon Maus.

Also in the 1990s keratorefractive surgery evolved from radial keratotomy. As of the year 2000, a rotation was introduced to teach the art of keratorefractive surgery consisting of learning the basics and becoming certified in performing laser in situ keratomileusis (LASIK). In the year 2002, the residents will be introduced to the procedure known as laser in situ epithelial keratomileusis (LASEK). And now our residents are being introduced to operating in ambulatory surgery centers (ASCS).

An extensive didactic schedule, which includes morning core curriculum lectures, is ongoing. The lectures are preceded by sessions affectionately know as "eye-openers" beginning at 6:45 a.m., along with weekly Chiefs' Rounds when a resident from each year presents an interesting and often controversial ease. On a monthly basis a Visiting Professor, who is an expert in a particular specialty, is invited to participate in Grand Rounds.

Modern ophthalmology training requires the inclusion in the curriculum of business and coding lectures as well as evidence based medicine courses. An extensive ethics course is also a requirement for all residency training programs.

Each spring preceding the Ophthalmology Knowledge Assessment Program (OKAP) there is an extensive ophthalmology review course which all Wills Eye residents, residents from other city programs as well as Wills Eye fellows attend. Hands-on courses considered to be essential for the resident experience include the Introduction to Microsurgery Course for the new first year residents, the Cataract Extraction/Phaco Course for the second year residents, and the Laser Course and Orbital Dissection Course for all residents.

One of the most important aspects of the Wills Eye Hospital Training Program is the ongoing dedication and support of the ex-residents and fellows of the Wills Eye Society. The Society's financial support contributes to all aspects of resident training. The Wills Eye Annual Conference sponsored by the Society offers residents, fellows and staff the opportunity to present papers related to their research projects.

The Wills Eye Hospital residents also are actively involved in community services offering vision screening and examinations in Chinese and Hispanic communities and the underserved elementary and middle schools in Philadelphia and Chester county.

The Wills Eye Hospital Ophthalmology Training Program continues to produce a premium product, the Wills Resident, a well educated, well-rounded, caring resident physician dedicated to the best in patient care.

Chapter 9

Subspecialty Services and Fellowships

By the late 1950s, newer techniques in retinal detachment surgery were developed, mostly because of the ingenuity and perseverance of Dr. Charles Schepens in Boston. As mentioned earlier, his development of the binocular indirect ophthalmoscope as a practical instrument was a major breakthrough in the treatment of retinal detachment, one obtained against great odds and criticism. Ultimately, of course, his theories and preachings were proved correct. We at Wills were fortunate that Dr. P. Robb McDonald saw the wisdom of Dr. Schepen's teachings.

Under McDonald's direction, indirect ophthalmoscopy came into its own at Wills Eye, and one of the early proponents was his first retinal fellow, L. K. Sarin. He was preceded only by Dr. Leonard Apt who upon completion of his Wills residency was recruited by Irving Leopold to become a research fellow. By 1961, residents were learning the use of indirect ophthalmoscopy, and it became apparent that there were areas in ophthalmology that might be better handled by subspecialization. As a result, fellowship programs began to proliferate around the country, initially in retina, cornea, glaucoma, and oculoplastics. From this evolved the subspecialty or vertical service with its own director(s) and staff.

Accordingly, at Wills the subspecialty services of retina, cornea, glaucoma, pediatric ophthalmology, oculoplastics, oncology, and neuro-ophthalmology were initiated, and each of these now offers much-sought-after fellowships. Thus, the postgraduate experience at Wills Eye Hospital rivals resident training in quality. In all, there are 15 or more postgraduate fellows subspecializing each year.

In many ways it is flattering that Wills Eye attracts the good fellows that it does, because those who have completed their training in ophthalmology and seek further specialty training presumably look very critically at the program they choose.

Chapter 10

A Brief History of the Wills Eye Hospital Annual Conference

Robert B. Penne, M.D. and James Augsburger, M.D.

According to Annual Conference Program Notes and articles in the Wills Eye Hospital Society Newsletter by Dr. Jimmy Shipman (WEH '26), the principal guiding force behind the Wills Eye Hospital Society in its early years, and Dr. Jim Delaney (WEH '30), president of the Society in 1955-56 and a long-term member of its Executive Committee, the concept of an annual clinical conference of and by the alumni and staff of the Wills Hospital was initially suggested to the Medical Staff and the Board of Managers of the Wills Eye Hospital Society by two ex-residents, Dr. Edward C. Ellett (WEH 1892) of Memphis, TN, and Dr. Arthur J. Bedell (WEH '02) of Albany, NY, in about 1945. In 1947, two members of the medical staff, Dr. Carroll R. Mullen and Dr. Isaac S. Tassman (Fig. 10-2), were authorized by the Medical Staff and Society to plan the first such conference, and through their efforts the first Wills Eye Hospital Conference took place in Philadelphia in 1949.

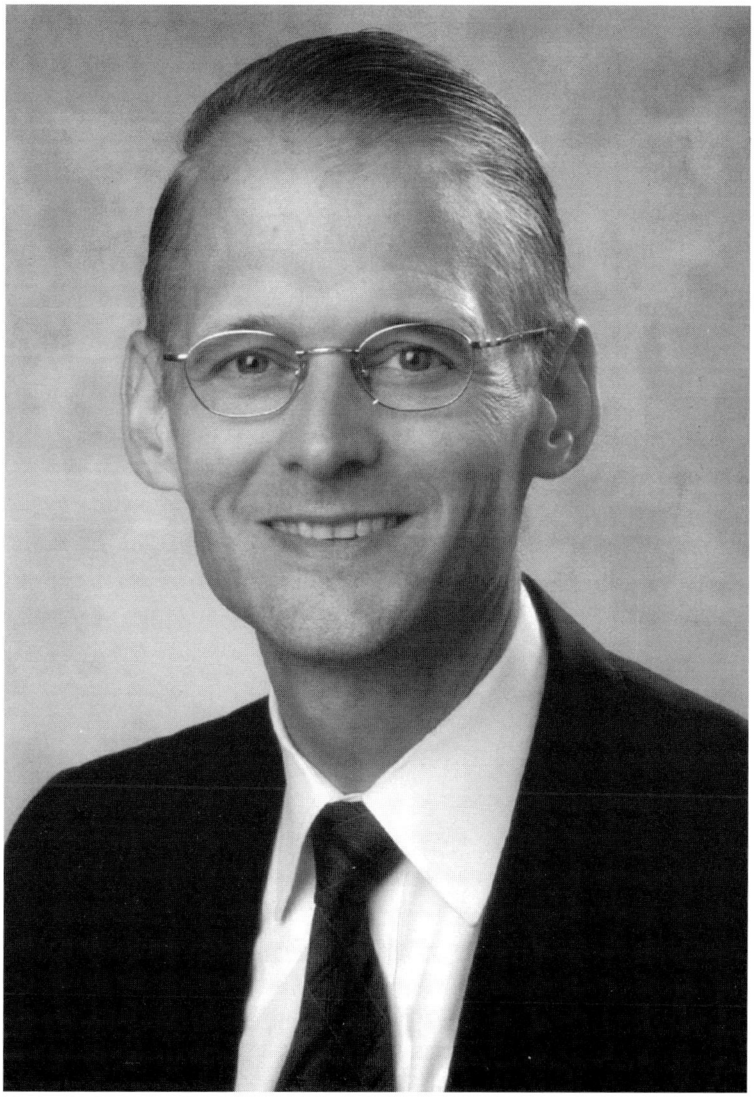

FIGURE 10-1
Robert B. Penne, M.D.

The First Conference

A program from that first conference in 1949 shows that it was a two-day meeting on May 6th and 7th (Fig. 10-3). The honor of delivering the first paper at the conference went to Dr. Bernard C. Gettes, who spoke on the subject "Dibutyline sulfate, a comparative study of its cycloplegic effects." Interestingly, there were only 13 papers (including the inaugural Bedell Lecture) presented during the conference, and those papers were all read by a Chief of Service, an Assistant Chief of Service, or an invited guest. The first conference attracted 226 ophthalmologists and was considered a great success.

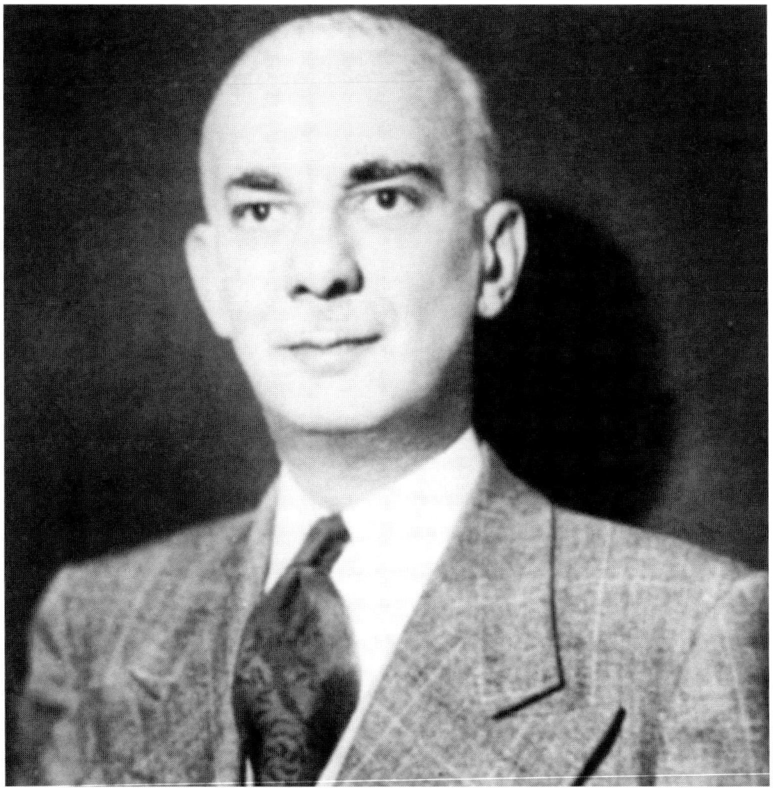

FIGURE 10-2
Dr. I.S. Tassman

The Early Years

The first through the 17th Annual Conferences took place at the old Wills Hospital at 16th and Spring Garden Streets. A major advance in the conference that cemented its national reputation was the introduction of live surgery demonstrations over closed circuit TV at the 3rd Annual Conference in 1951 (Fig. 10-4). Typically, eight to nine operative cases were performed by members of the medical staff and shown each afternoon. The TV monitors were set up in the lobby of the hospital, and the audience viewed the procedures there. Live TV surgery remained a highlight of each conference thereafter until 1969, when film and eventually videotape presentations finally supplanted it.

Maturation of the Conference

The venue for the Annual Conference was changed from the old Wills Eye Hospital to the Bellevue-Stratford Hotel in 1966, and the conference continued to be held at that hotel for the next 11 years. In 1977, after an outbreak of Legionnaires' Disease forced the abrupt closing of the Bellevue-Stratford Hotel, the conference was moved on rather short notice to the Philadelphia Sheraton. The next three years, from 1978 through 1980, the meeting was held at the City Line Marriott, and in 1981 it was held at the Franklin Plaza. The conference moved to the Adam's Mark Hotel in 1982 and has remained there to the present time.

Most of the early conferences were held in mid February, but the more recent conferences have been scheduled for mid March to mid April when the weather is likely to be better in Philadelphia. Attendance at the Annual Conference increased almost yearly during the early years until reaching a plateau at around 500-550 ophthalmologists in the mid 1960s through the late 1970s. At its peak in 1975, the conference registration exceeded 600 ophthalmologists. In recent years, approximately 300-350 ophthalmologists have attended the conference each year.

THE STAFF AND EX-RESIDENTS

OF

THE WILLS HOSPITAL

EXTEND TO YOU A CORDIAL INVITATION

TO PARTICIPATE IN

A CLINICAL CONFERENCE

AT THE HOSPITAL

16TH AND SPRING GARDEN STREETS

PHILADELPHIA

MAY 6 AND 7, 1949

FIGURE 10-3

Program from the first annual clinical conference.

Friday, May 6, 9:30 a.m.

DR. CARROLL R. MULLEN — *Presiding*

Dibutyline Sulfate, a Comparative Study of Its Cycloplegic Effects.
DR. BERNARD C. GETTES

Study of End Results of Glaucoma at the Wills Hospital.
DR. LOUIS LEHRFELD

Further Studies of the Chemical and Immunilogical Properties of Human Tears
DR. IRVING H. LEOPOLD

Diagnosis of Syphilitic Primary Optic Atrophy in the Pre-atrophic Stage
DR. JOSEPH V. KLAUDER *and* DR. GEORGE P. MEYER

Luncheon — 1:00 p.m.

Friday Afternoon, 2:00 p.m.

DR. WM. J. HARRISON — *Presiding*

A Follow-up Concerning Basket Implants
DR. WILFRED E. FRY

Experimental Studies with Physiologic Glue (Autogenous Plasma plus Thrombin) For Use in the Eyes
DR. ISAAC S. TASSMAN

Causes of Failure in the Surgical Treatment of Glaucoma
DR. JOHN S. McGAVIC

Some Practical Facts Regarding Retinal Surgery With a Report of Results in More Than Four Hundred Unselected and Consecutive Cases
DR. JAMES S. SHIPMAN

FIGURE 10-3 *(continued)*

Friday Evening, 8:15 p.m.

DR. WARREN S. REESE — *Presiding*

The Destruction of the Macula, Commonly Called Coloboma

DR. ARTHUR J. BEDELL

Saturday, May 7, 9:30 a.m.

DR. P. ROBB McDONALD — *Presiding*

Clinical Pathological Presentation

DR. JAMES H. PARKER

The Optics of Cylinder Magnification

DR. JOSEPH W. HALLETT

The Surgical Correction of Ptosis, Congenital and Acquired,
When Complicated by Other Oculomotor Situations.

DR. EDMUND B. SPAETH

Paper — Title to be announced

DR. CECIL O'BRIEN

Luncheon — 1:00 p.m.

Saturday Afternoon, 2:00 p.m.

OPERATIVE SURGERY

FIGURE 10-3 *(continued)*

Program Format Changes

As the years went by, the format of the conference gradually changed. Resident and ex-resident papers began to appear on the program after only the first couple of years, and papers by fellows and even medical students and non-ophthalmic physicians eventually followed. The length of the conference was increased from two to three days in 1959. In the interest of encouraging participation by as many people as were interested, the Program Committee gradually began to accept more and more abstracts for free papers each year. Since the total length of the conference was finite, this meant that the length of each presentation had to decrease. This policy ultimately resulted in a program that included 95 free papers (plus the special lectures, several symposia, and multiple workshops) in a single year (1988). Each of these papers was allotted seven minutes and each was presented in mind-numbing sequence, without any opportunity for questions or comments from moderators of the audience.

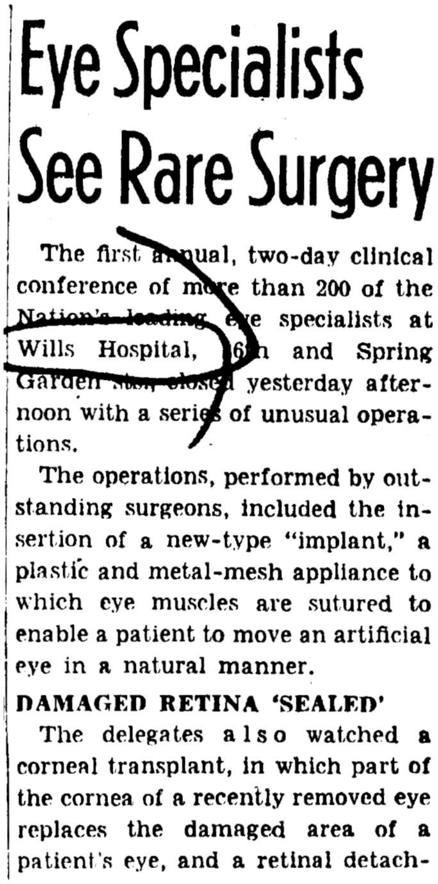

Eye Specialists See Rare Surgery

The first annual, two-day clinical conference of more than 200 of the Nation's leading eye specialists at Wills Hospital, 16th and Spring Garden Sts., closed yesterday afternoon with a series of unusual operations.

The operations, performed by outstanding surgeons, included the insertion of a new-type "implant," a plastic and metal-mesh appliance to which eye muscles are sutured to enable a patient to move an artificial eye in a natural manner.

DAMAGED RETINA 'SEALED'

The delegates also watched a corneal transplant, in which part of the cornea of a recently removed eye replaces the damaged area of a patient's eye, and a retinal detach-

FIGURE 10-4
Live surgery was a feature of the early conferences.

Workshops, which were in fact "Clinical Updates" like those currently being presented at Wills Eye Hospital on Saturday mornings throughout the year by members of the various Clinical Services, were introduced into the format of the conference in 1971. That year, a single workshop on retinal disease was presented by Drs. P. Robb McDonald, Bill Annesley, Bill Tasman, and Lov Sarin. This update must have been quite popular, because the number of updates presented at the conference increased to two in 1972, four in 1973, six in 1974, and eight in 1975. The peak number of workshops was attained in 1979, when 13 separate workshops were presented.

Saturday was changed to a subspecialty day presentation in 2000. At that meeting the retina service had a combined meeting honoring Dr. Bill Annesley. The format has continued with a refractive surgery meeting in 2001 and a glaucoma meeting in 2002.

Women at the Wills Conference

The first woman to speak at a Wills Eye Hospital Annual Conference appears to have been Dr. Georgianna Theobald, an invited guest speaker at the 10th Annual Conference in 1958. As far as I have been able to determine, the first woman to present a free paper at a Wills Conference was Dr. Ruth Fabritius, one of Dr. Irving Leopold's research assistants. She presented a paper entitled "Comparative study of anticoagulant therapy in occlusive vascular disease" at the 14th Annual Conference in 1962. The first woman resident to present a paper at the Wills Conference was Dr. Barbara Mitchell (WEH '67), who spoke on "Clinical use of the MacKay-Marge tonometer" at the 16th Annual Conference in 1964. The first woman staff member to speak at a Wills Conference appears to have been Dr. Anne Chan, who presented a paper on "A new miotic-mydriatic combination therapy of open angle glaucoma" in 1965. Dr. Marguerite McDonald was the first woman Leopold lecturer in 1999. Dr. Elisabeth Cohen was the first woman to receive the Silver Tray Award at the Conference in 2002.

Social Functions at the Annual Conference

Each of the six conferences included an "informal reception" (but no dinner or dinner-dance) for "Doctors and Wives." (Parenthetically, the Conference Programs continued to specify that these functions were for "Doctors and Wives" rather than "Registrants and Guests" through 1980!) The first five years of the conference, this reception was held at the Barclay Hotel. In 1954, the reception was held for the first time at the Union League. Starting with the 7th Annual Conference in 1955, the informal reception was expanded to include dinner. The first Conference Dinner-Dance took place in conjunction with the 14th Annual Conference in 1962 at the Union League. Beginning with the 18th Annual Conference in 1967, the conference included both a Dinner-Dance of the Wills Eye Hospital Society on Thursday evening and a Conference Dinner-Dance for all registrants and guests on Friday evening. This format remained essentially unchanged until 1990, when the Wills Eye Hospital Society's Dinner-Dance was moved to Friday and the Conference Dinner-Dance was discontinued as a regular feature and replaced with a cocktail reception on Thursday evening.

Joint Wills Annual Conference and PAO Annual Meeting

The Conference remained exclusively a Wills Eye Hospital Staff and Society function until 1991, when the first joint Wills Conference and Pennsylvania Academy of Ophthalmology (PAO) Annual Meeting was held. This year's 55th Annual Conference will mark the fifth joint conference with the PAO.

Ophthalmic Nursing at the Conference

The first Annual Clinical Conference for Nurses was held at the 33rd Annual Wills Eye Hospital Conference on April 24, 1981. Two years prior a similar "workshop" had first been introduced at the 31st Annual Wills Eye Hospital Conference. This was started since there was a need for education of ophthalmic nurses that was not being met. The Annual Clinical Conference for Nurses has continued as an annual part of the Wills Conference and has been very successful. The School Nurses' Ophthalmology Update was first held on Saturday, April 22, 1991, as part of the Annual Wills Eye Hospital Conference and was last held in 1999. Heather Boyd-Monk, SRN, BSN, CRNO has been program director of all these conferences. A stalwart member of the Wills family, Heather retired in 2002.

Ophthalmic Technicians at the Conference

The Ophthalmic Technicians' Program evolved from the Ophthalmic Nurses' Conference. As the educational needs of the ophthalmic nurses and technicians became different the need for a separate meeting was recognized. This was started as a workshop and then evolved into the current one-day meeting held at the Annual Wills Eye Hospital Conference each year.

Named Lectures and Symposia at Annual Conference

The Wills Eye Hospital Annual Conference has two named lectureships, the Arthur J. Bedell Lecture and the Irving H. Leopold Lecture, and one named symposium, the Bernard C. Gettes Symposium.

Arthur J. Bedell Lecture

The Bedell Lecture is named in honor of Dr. Arthur J. Bedell, a distinguished alumnus of the Wills Eye Hospital Residency Program (WEH '02) who went on to become Professor and Chairman of the Department of Ophthalmology at Albany Medical College. Dr. Bedell's chief ophthalmic interest was utilizing fundus photography as an aid in clinical diagnosis, patient management, and teaching. Over the course of his long lifetime, he amassed a collection of thousands of fundus photographs, many of which were included in his 1929 textbook entitled *Photographs of the Fundus Oculi*. Throughout his life, Dr. Bedell remained a loyal alumnus of Wills; he attended virtually every Wills Conference between 1949 and 1970. He died in Albany in 1973 at the age of 93 years.

TABLE 1. Arthur J. Bedell Lecturers at Wills Eye Hospital Annual Conference

YEAR	LECTURER	YEAR	LECTURER	YEAR	LECTURER
1949	Arthur J. Bedell	1967	Joaquin Barraquer	1985	Edward W. D. Norton
1950	Francis Heed Adler	1968	Gerd Meyer-Schwickerath	1986	John E. Wright
1951	Conrad Berens	1969	Harvey E. Thorpe	1987	H. Dunbar Hoskins
1952	Derrick T. Vail	1970	David G. Cogan	1988	Franz Fankhauser
1953	John H. Dunnington	1971	P. Robb McDonald	1989	W. Richard Green
1954	Daniel B. Kirby	1972	Lorenz E. Zimmerman	1990	Simmons Lessell
1955	Algernon B. Reese	1973	Harold G. Scheie	1991	Charles D. Kelman
1956	Albert D. Ruedemann	1974	John C. Mustarde	1992	Carl Kupfer
1957	John McLean	1975	Irving H. Leopold	1993	George W. Weinstein
1958	Paul Chandler	1976	David Shoch	1994	Thomas B. Hutchinson
1959	Brittain F. Payne	1977	Charles E. Iliff	1995	Robert Ritch
1960	Peter C. Kronfeld	1978	Frederick C. Blodi	1996	Alfred Sommer
1961	Michael J. Hogan	1979	Norman S. Jaffe	1997	Stanley Chang
1962	Frank Walsh	1980	Cornelius D. Binkhorst	1998	J. Donald Gass
1963	Hans Goldmann	1981	Stephen M. Drance	1999	Daniel Albert
1964	Edmund B. Spaeth	1982	J. Lawton Smith	2000	Richard Mills
1965	Donald J. Lyle	1983	G. Richard O'Connor	2001	Neil Miller
1966	A. Edward Maumenee	1984	Claes H. Dohlman	2002	Carmen Puliafito

The inaugural Bedell Lecture, which was given by Dr. Bedell, took place during the first Wills Conference at an evening session on Friday, May 6, 1949. Dr. Bedell's topic was "The Destruction of the Macula, Commonly Called Coloboma." In the years following that Conference, Dr. Bedell subsequently presented three more scientific free papers during Wills Conferences. The last one was in 1966 when he was 86. His topic for that last presentation was "How Fundus Photographs Prevent Enucleation."

The Bedell Lecturers have literally ranged from A (Adler) to Z (Zimmerman), and names on the list of Bedell Lecturers (Table 1) surely include many of the most distinguished and well-known ophthalmologists of the mid to late 20th century. The 54 Bedell Lecturers to date have chosen to speak on "glaucoma" eight times, "cataract or cataract surgery" seven times, "neuro-ophthalmology" six times, "oculoplastic surgery or orbital disease" five times, "tumors of the eye or orbit" four times, "cornea or anterior segment diseases other than cataract" three times, "retina" three times, and miscellaneous other subjects for the remaining 18 lectures.

There is an interesting paradox concerning the Bedell Lectureship. Although there have been 54 Bedell Lectures thus far, there have only been 53 Bedell Lecturers. How can this be? A possible explanation would be that a single individual presented more than one Bedell Lecture. Good guess, but that's not right. The true explanation lies in the fact that the individual scheduled to present the 6th Annual Bedell Lecture in 1954, Dr. Daniel Kirby of New York, died suddenly a short time before the conference. He had thoughtfully completed his lecture prior to his death, so an unspecified member of the medical staff was able to read his paper on "Various Means of Direct Separation of the Zonule in Extracapsular Cataract Surgery" to the audience at the conference.

Irving H. Leopold Lecture

The Leopold Lecture is named in honor of Dr. Irving H. Leopold, an Attending Surgeon at Wills Eye Hospital from 1952 through 1964, Director of the Wills Research Department from 1949 through 1964, and Ophthalmologist-in-Chief at Wills from

TABLE 2. Irving H. Leopold Lecturers at Wills Eye Hospital Annual Conference

YEAR	LECTURER	YEAR	LECTURER	YEAR	LECTURER
1987	Irving H. Leopold	1993	Richard K. Parrish, II	1999	Marguerite McDonald
1988	George Waring	1994	Jay Krachmer	2000	Robert Osher
1989	Richard L. Lindstrom	1995	Kenneth Abrams	2001	Gilbert Kliman
1990	Manus C. Kraff	1996	R. Doyle Stulting	2002	Douglas Koch
1991	Paul R. Lichter	1997	Norman Medow		
1992	Brian C. Leonard	1998	Richard Mackool		

1961 through 1964. Dr. Leopold passed away in 1993. The first Leopold Lecture was given in 1987 at the 39th Annual Conference. Dr. Leopold was the first lecturer, and he spoke on the rather unusual topic "Ocular Therapeutics through the Retrospectroscope." Most of the subsequent Leopold Lecturers (Table 2) have had some sort of prior affiliation with Wills, either as a resident, fellow, or member of the staff. Thus far, there have been sixteen Leopold Lectures given in conjunction with this conference.

Bernard C. Gettes Symposium

The Gettes Symposium is named in honor of Dr. Bernard C. Gettes, an Attending Surgeon at Wills (1967-73) who was President of the Medical Staff at the time of his death in 1973. The first Gettes Symposium was held at the 27th Annual Conference in 1975. The topic of that first symposium was "Ocular Therapy," moderated by Dr. Irving Leopold. Over the ensuing years, the topics of subsequent Gettes Symposia (Table 3) included Glaucoma, Cornea, Strabismus, Contact Lenses, Uveitis, Neuro-Ophthalmology, Cataract Surgery, and Tearing. Since 1991, the Gettes Symposium has been the "Cataract and IOL Surgery" symposium. This was moderated by Steve Lichtenstein (WEH '78) from 1991-2000 and is now rotated among members of the cataract service.

TABLE 3.
Bernard C. Gettes Symposia at Wills Eye Hospital Annual Conference

YEAR	TOPIC	MODERATOR
1975	Ocular Therapy	Irving H. Leopold, M.D.
1976	Tearing	Peter R. Laibson, M.D.
1978	Strabismus	Donelson R. Manley, M.D.
1979	Contact Lenses	Kenneth Michaile, M.D.
1980	Contact Lenses	Kenneth Michaile, M.D.
1981	Glaucoma	George L. Spaeth, M.D.
1982	Neuro-Ophthalmology	Norman J. Schatz, M.D.
1983	Uveitis	David H. Fischer, M.D.
1984	Cataract & IOL Surgery	Peter R. Laibson, M.D.
1985	Strabismus	Joseph H. Calhoun, M.D.
1986	Cataract & IOL Surgery	Stephen B. Lichtenstein, M.D.
1987	Glaucoma	George L. Spaeth, M.D.
1988	Cornea	Peter R. Laibson, M.D.
1991	Cataract & IOL Surgery	Stephen B. Lichtenstein, M.D.
1992	Cataract & IOL Surgery	Stephen B. Lichtenstein, M.D.
1993	Cataract & IOL Surgery	Stephen B. Lichtenstein, M.D.
1994	Cataract & IOL Surgery	Stephen B. Lichtenstein, M.D.
1995	Cataract & IOL Surgery	Stephen B. Lichtenstein, M.D.
1996	Cataract & IOL Surgery	Stephen B. Lichtenstein, M.D.
1997	Cataract & IOL Surgery	Stephen B. Lichtenstein, M.D.
1998	Cataract & IOL Surgery	Stephen B. Lichtenstein, M.D.
1999	Cataract & IOL Surgery	Stephen B. Lichtenstein, M.D.
2000	Cataract & IOL Surgery	Stephen B. Lichtenstein, M.D.
2001	Cataract & IOL Surgery	Richard Tipperman, M.D.
2002	Cataract & IOL Surgery	Mark H. Blecher, M.D.

"Wills Eye Hospital Heritage" Series of Presentations

There have certainly been many noteworthy and interesting presentations (and, to be fair, a generous number of lousy ones as well) given at the Annual Conference over the years. In my opinion,

TABLE 4. "Wills Eye Hospital Heritage" Presentations by Harold Barnshaw, M.D., at Wills Eye Hospital Annual Conference, 1967–1983

YEAR	TOPIC
1967	Edward Jackson, M.D. (AS 1890–1898)
1968	Samuel Doty Risley, M.D. (AS 1890–1917)
1969	S. Lewis Ziegler, M.D. (R 1887; AS 1904–1916)
1970	D. Hayes Agnew, M.D. (AS 1864–1869)
1971	William Zentmayer, M.D. (AS 1901–1928)
1972	Isaac Hays, M.D. (AS 1834–1854)
1973	William Fisher Norris, M.D. (AS 1872–1901)
1974	William Thompson, M.D. (AS 1872–1902)
1975	William Campbell Posey, M.D. (AS 1902–1919)
1976	Isaac Parrish, M.D. (AS 1834–1852)
1977	Leighton F. Appleman, M.D. (AS 1924–1939)
1978	Francis Heed Adler, M.D. (AS 1933–1937)
1979	James S. Shipman, M.D. (R 1926, AS 1939–1966)
1980	Edmund B. Spaeth, M.D. (AS 1939–1960)
1981	Warren S. Reese, M.D. (R 1917, AS 1939–1957)
1982	Isaac S. Tassman, M.D. (AS 1939–1960)
1983	George Fox, M.D. (AS 1834–1839)

AS = Attending Surgeon at Wills Hospital R = Resident Surgeon at Wills Hospital

TABLE 5. Silver Tray Award Recipients at Wills Eye Hospital Annual Conference

YEAR	RECIPIENT
1962	James S. Shipman, M.D. (R '26; AS '39–'66)
1963	James H. Delaney, M.D. (R '28)
1964	Edmund B. Spaeth, M.D. (AS '39–'60)
1965	Isaac S. Tassman*, M.D. (AS '39–'60)
1966	Wilfred E. Fry, M.D. (AS '43–'67)
1967	Warren S. Reese, M.D. (AS '39–'57)
1968	Patrick J. Kennedy*, M.D. (AS '53–'72)
1969	P. Robb McDonald, M.D. (R '36; AS '49–'71)
1970	Kelvin Kasper, M.D. (otolaryngologist)
1971	Harold D. Barnshaw,* M.D. (AS '66–'72)
1972	Albert F. Cleveland,* M.D. (R '46; AS '72–'76)
1973	James S. Jordan, M.D. (R '33)
1974	Curtis Pritchard (administrator)
1975	Robert Mulberger,* M.D. (AS '58–'81)
1976	Robert Shoemaker, M.D. (R '42)
1977	Arthur H. Keeney, M.D. (OIC '64–'72)
1978	Joseph Hallett, M.D. (AS '60–'78)
1979	Nathan Schleszinger, M.D. (neurologist)
1980	Robison Harley, M.D. (AS '67–'76)
1981	Thomas Duane, M.D. (OIC '72–'82)
1982	Oram R. Kline, Jr.,* M.D. (R '49; AS '72–'86)
1983	Owen Belmont,* M.D. (R '50; AS '79–'81)
1984	Philip G. Spaeth, M.D. (R '53; AS '73–'81)
1985	William H. Annesley, Jr., M.D. (R '51; AS '71–'93)
1986	Samuel Blank, M.D. (anesthesiologist)
1987	Malvin Dougherty, * M.D. (AS '79–'86)
1988	Joseph C. Flanagan, M.D. (R '67–; AS '81–)
1989	William Tasman, M.D. (R '61; AS '73–; OIC '85–)
1990	George L. Spaeth, M.D. (R '61; AS '73–)
1991	Hunter R. Stokes, M.D. (R '67)
1992	John Siliquini,* M.D. (AS '87–)
1993	William N. Offutt, IV, M.D. (R '72)
1994	Raymond Adams,* M.D. (R '64; AS '84–'00)
1995	Jack Jeffers, M.D. (R '71; AS '97–)
1996	Peter Laibson, M.D. (R '64; AS '73–)
1997	James Augsburger,* M.D. (AS '90–'99)
1998	Edward Jaeger, M.D. (AS '81–)
1999	William Benson, M.D. (AS '81–)
2000	Joseph Calhoun, M.D. (R '69; AS '78–)
2001	Robert C. Sergott, M.D. (R '79; AS '88–)
2002	Elisabeth J. Cohen, M.D. (R '79; AS '89–)

*Served as Chairman of the Annual Conference

AS = Attending Surgeon at Wills Hospital R = Resident Surgeon at Wills Hospital

TABLE 6. James S. Shipman Award Winners at Wills Eye Hospital Annual Conference*

YEAR	AWARD WINNER	YEAR	AWARD WINNER	YEAR	AWARD WINNER
1967	Kurt Gitter	1979	William G. Martin	1991	Richard Tipperman
1968	Ben Houser	1980	Stephen M. Felton	1992	Carl D. Regillo
1969	Donald Le Win	1981	Norman F. Woodhef	1993	John R. Tribble
1970	Jerry A. Shields	1982	Andrew W. Eller	1994	Ming X. Wang
1971	Jonathan D. Trobe	1983	Thaddeus S. Nowinski	1995	David Buerger
1972	George O. Waring	1984	Robert D. Lehman	1996	Jonathan S. Meyers
1973	Ido Egerer	1985	Gregory G. Tesluk	1997	Julian D. Perry
1974	John J. Purcell	1986	Carol L. Shields	1998	Brian P. Connolly
1975	John J. Purcell	1987	Eric P. Shakin	1999	Vincent Deramo
1976	Joseph B. Michelson	1988	Marc C. Cohen	2000	Anthony Aldave
1977	Ronald R. Reed	1989	Tamara R. Vrabec	2001	Rod Foroozan
1978	Robert C. Sergott	1990	Christopher J. Rapuano	2002	Brandon Busbee

the series of historical papers on the Wills Eye Hospital Heritage by Dr. Harold Barnshaw (Table 4) during the middle years of the conference remains a memorable highlight. Many of you undoubtedly recall some of those presentations. Starting at the 19th Annual Conference in 1967 with a presentation on Dr. Edward Jackson, "Barnie" (as he was known to his friends) presented a new vignette about a distinguished person in the Wills family every year for 17 consecutive years. His last presentation, in 1983, was on Dr. George Fox, one of the early attending surgeons at Wills.

Special Awards at the Annual Conference

There are three special awards presented each year at the Wills Eye Hospital Annual Conference. These awards include the Silver Tray Award, the Shipman Award, and the McDonald Award.

Silver Tray Award

A silver tray (Silver Tray Award) has been presented at the Annual Conference every year since 1962 to a member of the Wills family who has exhibited exceptional loyalty and service to the hospital, the residency or fellowship training programs, the Wills Eye Hospital Society, the Annual Conference Committee, or other areas in the field of Ophthalmology.

The recipients of this award (Table 5) include some of the best known and best loved members of the Wills family. Befitting his place in the history of the Wills Conference, Dr. Jimmy Shipman (see below) was the first person to be awarded the Silver Tray.

Shipman Award

The Shipman Award is named in honor of Dr. James S. Shipman, an Ex-Resident, an Attending Surgeon at Wills from 1939 through 1966, and one of the founding fathers of the Wills Eye Hospital Society. Dr. Shipman is generally credited with introducing Gonin's principles and techniques of retinal detachment surgery to Philadelphia and is therefore properly regarded as the father of modern retinal surgery at Wills. The Shipman Award has been presented yearly since 1967 to the resident-in-training who is judged to have presented the best scientific free paper (Table 6). Dr. Kurt Gitter (WEH '68) was the first Shipman Award winner for his paper entitled "A-scan Ultrasound in the Diagnosis of Unilateral Proptosis." Only one resident, Dr. John Purcell (WEH '75), has won the Shipman Award twice (in 1974 and 1975).

* *For up-to-date list see Appendix O*

TABLE 7. P. Robb McDonald Award Winners at Wills Eye Hospital Annual Conference*

YEAR	AWARD WINNER
1992	Andrew Michael
1993	Mary Ellen Cullom
1994	José Gomes
1995	Silvana Araujo
1996	Tarek Eid
1997	Richard Rodman
1998	Nathan Congdon
1999	Kenneth Kubis
2000	Helen Danesh-Meyer
2001	Beth Handwerger
2002	Mary Jude Cox

TABLE 8. Chairpersons of Wills Eye Hospital Annual Conference

CHAIRPERSON	YEARS	LENGTH OF SERVICE
Carroll R. Mullen	1949	1 year
Isaac S. Tassman	1950-1960	11 years
Carroll R. Mullen	1961	1 year
Patrick J. Kennedy	1962-1963	2 years
Harold Barnshaw	1964-1966	3 years
Albert Cleveland	1967-1969	3 years
Robert Mulberger	1970-1973	4 years
Gerard Shannon	1974-1976	3 years
Malvin Dougherty	1977	1 year
Oram Kline	1978-1980	3 years
John Siliquini	1981-1983	3 years
Raymond Adams	1984-1986	3 years
Owen Belmont	1987-1989	3 years
James Augsburger	1990-1994	5 years
Christopher Rapuano	1995-1999	5 years
Robert B. Penne	2000-	

McDonald Award

The McDonald Award is named in honor of Dr. P. Robb McDonald, an Attending Surgeon at Wills from 1949 through 1971, one of the last of the old-time Chiefs of Service at Wills, and the first Director of its Retina Service. The McDonald Award is given yearly at the Annual Conference to the clinical fellow-in-training who is judged to have presented the best scientific paper at the Annual Conference (Table 7). This award was first conferred in 1992.

Conference Chairpersons

In the 45-year history of the Wills Conference, there have been only 16 Conference Chairpersons (Table 8). Dr. Carroll Mullen, chairman for the first Annual Conference, was also chairman for the 13th Annual Conference in 1961. The individual who ran the conference for the longest period of time by far was Dr. Isaac Tassman, who was in charge for 11 consecutive years from 1950 through 1960. Dr. Christopher Rapuano and Dr. Jim Augsburger are second in line with five years of service (1994–1999 and 1990–1994), and Dr. Robert Mulberger was third in line with four years of service (1970–1973). Dr. Robert Penne (WEH '88) of the Oculoplastics Service has accepted the mantle of Conference Chairman from 2000 to present.

* *For up-to-date list see Appendix P*

Chapter 11

Development of Research

Research at Wills Eye was initiated almost single-handedly by Irving Leopold. A native of Philadelphia who trained with Francis Adler, he became involved with clinical warfare research during World War II. This led to his development of diisopropyl fluorophosphate or fluoropryl (DFP), which was first encountered and used in ophthalmology while being investigated as a chemical warfare agent. At that time, Leopold was working for the Office of Scientific Research and Development (OSRD), which had two major subdivisions: the Manhattan Project and the Committee on Medical Research (CMR). Leopold was on the OSRD and CMR, dealing with ocular gas casualties.

DFP was interesting because very small concentrations in vapor form produced marked miosis, lasting much longer than any miotic action previously observed in ophthalmology. Because of this unusual finding, at the end of the war the Chemical Warfare Service requested use of this agent in two ways: for study in patients with myasthenia gravis and to determine whether it could be used in the management of glaucoma. The hope was to reduce the frequency of instillation of drops required to maintain satisfactory intraocular pressure.

Considerable animal experimentation had already been done and had proved that this was an anticholinesterase agent. Experiments such as ciliary ganglionectomy and cervical sympathectomy were performed, and these established that this was a so-called irreversible anticholinesterase agent in the eye. With repeated instillation into rabbit eyes over a period of many months, no lens opacities could be demonstrated. Leopold also studied the ability of this agent, when topically applied to the eye, to inhibit human serum cholinesterase and set about trying the drug in various types of glaucoma. Response curves were established in rabbit eyes and normal human eyes, and the effectiveness of the drug in glaucoma was established.

The drug was tried in strabismus, and the results were published shortly after the war in the *Archives of Ophthalmology*. It was proved an effective agent for glaucoma cases that were not responding to pilocarpine or epinephrine.

DFP had one significant disadvantage in solution: it had to be made up in an anhydrous peanut oil, because it tended to very rapidly lose its potency in water. For this reason, after finding this drug and utilizing it for glaucoma, Leopold was on the constant lookout for an anticholinesterase agent that would be stable in water. One was called 217AO; the other, which did not penetrate into the central nervous system, was 217MI. 217MI, later known as phospholine iodide or echothiophate iodide, was selected for use in the eye because many researchers had discovered that DFP could penetrate into the central nervous system and on occasion produced bizarre dreams.

Phospholine iodide is stable in water for reasonable periods of time. Response curves were established, and it was tried in normal human eyes after studies in experimental eyes, where it was found to be effective. At no time was the development of lens opacities or retinal detachment in experimental animals demonstrated.

Human experience has shown a tendency for strong anticholinesterase agents, as well as all cholinergic agents, to produce lens opacities in glaucomatous eyes. Phospholine iodide was also found to be effective in esotropia and strabismus of the accommodative variety, but occasionally iris cysts developed.

When Leopold came to the Wills Hospital after World War II as an assistant in the Warren Reese Clinic, there was no experimental research going on. The Board of Surgeons and the Board of Trustees granted permission for him to set up some areas for research in basement rooms in which there were ventilation ducts. During that period a number of individuals worked in these facilities, including Robert Day, who is now in New York, and ex-resident Tom Dickinson. As research grants were obtained from NIH and other awarding groups, however, it became apparent that there was insufficient room to carry out the necessary work.

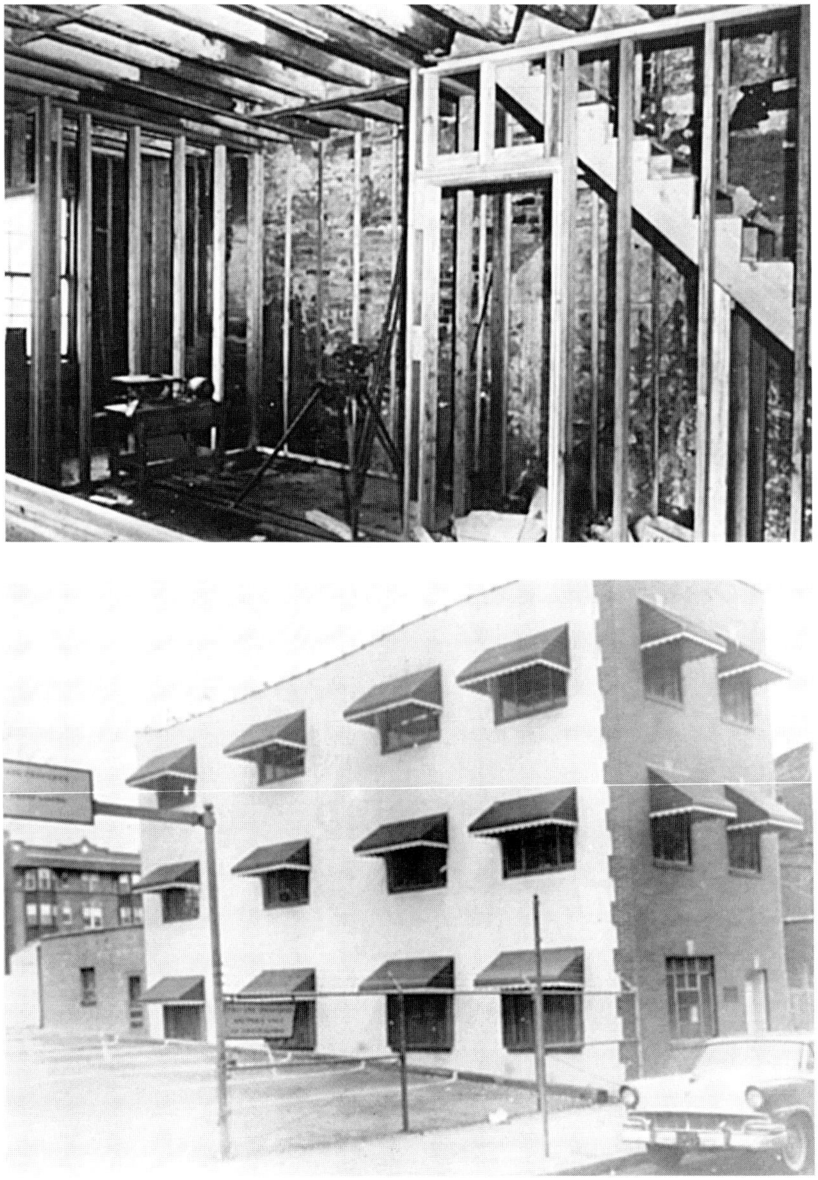

FIGURE 11-1
The first research building before, during, and after renovation.

As a result, the Board of City Trusts obtained a dilapidated building on Brandywine Street behind the hospital for approximately $3,000 (Fig. 11-1). (At that time, Mr. Ernest Trigg was the head of the Wills Committee of the Board of City Trusts.)

This building had to be refurbished, and the members of the staff of the Wills Hospital contributed toward its reconstruction. The funds raised at that time were $22,000. In addition, various philanthropic groups in the city purchased equipment and helped to refurbish the building and to set up a research laboratory. Some of the groups that contributed were the Lions and the Vida Lodge; many private patients of staff doctors also made contributions. Purchase of some of the equipment was supported by grants from NIH, the National Council to Combat Blindness, and the National Society for Prevention of Blindness.

The three floors were well equipped. The first floor included animal quarters in the rear, operating rooms, and an electron microscope on a firm base in the front. The second floor essentially housed microbiology and the third floor biochemistry. Individuals such as Dr. Virginia Weimer and Dr. Harry Green began to work in this department, along with a number of residents and research fellows, including Leonard Apt, Stanley Capper, a physiologist, H. Shapiro, Jim O'Rourke, George Spaeth, Arthur Calnan, and L. K. Sarin.

After this laboratory had been used for a reasonable period, it again became apparent that there was insufficient space, although the labs were doing creditable work that was calling attention to experimental studies at the Wills Eye Hospital.

Drs. Virginia Weimer and Harry Green were doing studies on corticosteroid penetration, lens metabolism, wound healing, and the factors that influence drug penetration. Harry Green and his staff were working on acetazolamide and its mechanism of action. Michael Kazurowski was beginning his anatomical studies. Frank Furguiele did a fellowship on antibiotic penetration, and Adolph Vogel started his oncologic drug toxicity and choroidal circulation studies. Enrique Wudka extended these and worked on scleral resections.

At this point, the Board of City Trusts was sufficiently impressed so that when the Ford Foundation funds were released to hospitals throughout the United States, the Board of City Trusts decided to use the funds for the construction of a new research laboratory.

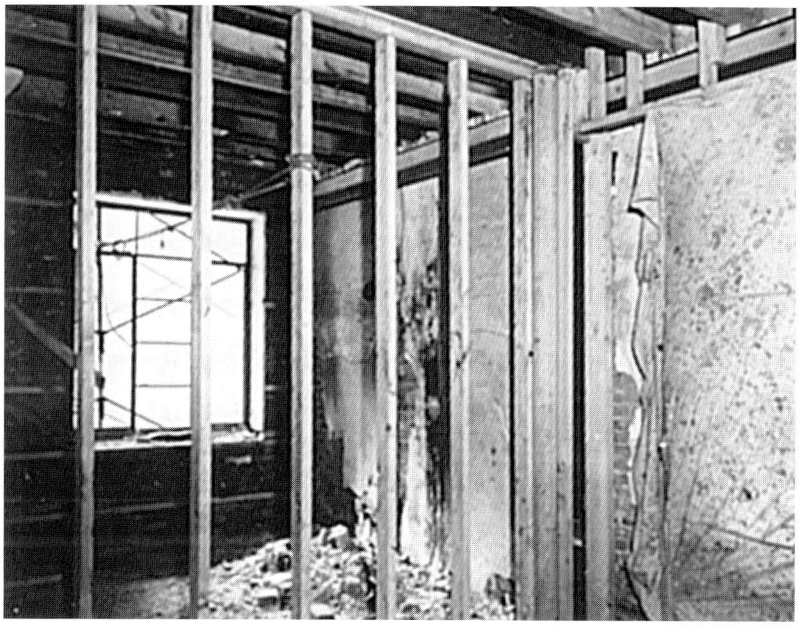

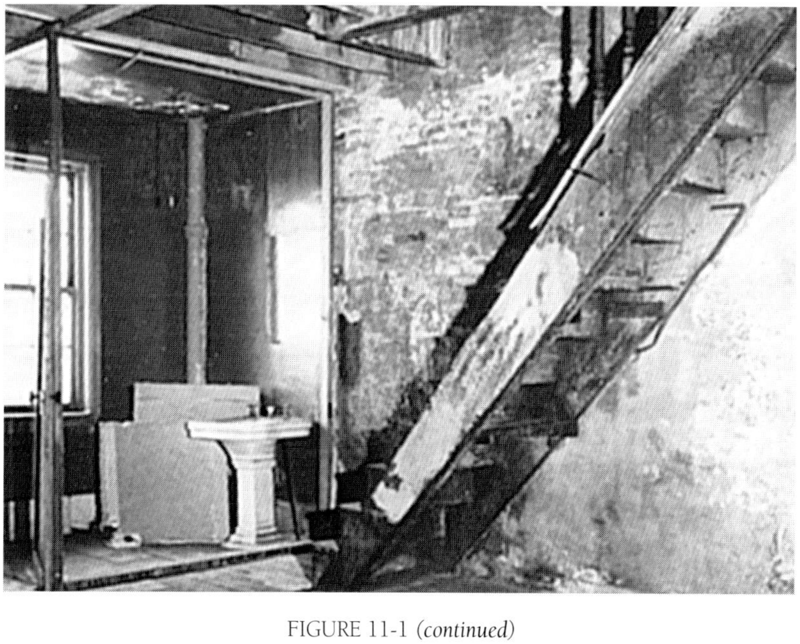

FIGURE 11-1 *(continued)*

With the architectural help of Vincent Kling, the new research laboratories were built; use of the initial research building also continued, because this space was still needed (Fig. 11-2).

By this time, Winston Barber and Ted Sery had joined the group, and the laboratory continued to be productive in many areas. Studies continued on penetration of antibiotics, corticosteroids, wound healing, herpes, and tumor growth. Additional hardworking research fellows included the late Florian Maylath, Fikret Mutlu, Satya Dev Paul, Paul Carmichael, and S. Kurose. Other contributors to this effort since its inception in 1949 have included Audrey Harris, D.Sc., Richard Peltz, Ph.D., Luke Huang, M.D., Rose Nagy, B.S., Michael Kaczurowski, M.D., the late Winston G. Barber, Ph.D., the late Ralph Pollikoff, Ph.D., and the late Norman T. Felberg, Ph.D.

Today Wills research includes NIH grants to study corneal diseases, glaucoma, immunology, intraocular tumors, and vitreoretinal diseases, in addition to continuation of basic research activities. As a result, Wills at present is in every sense of the word a tertiary eye care center. It is renowned for the diagnosis and management of

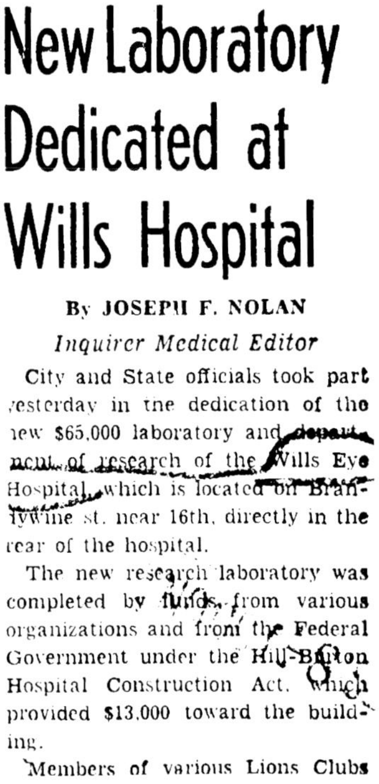

New Laboratory Dedicated at Wills Hospital

By JOSEPH F. NOLAN
Inquirer Medical Editor

City and State officials took part yesterday in the dedication of the new $65,000 laboratory and department of research of the Wills Eye Hospital, which is located on Brandywine st. near 16th, directly in the rear of the hospital.

The new research laboratory was completed by funds from various organizations and from the Federal Government under the Hill-Burton Hospital Construction Act, which provided $13,000 toward the building.

Members of various Lions Clubs

FIGURE 11-2
Dedication of a second research building.

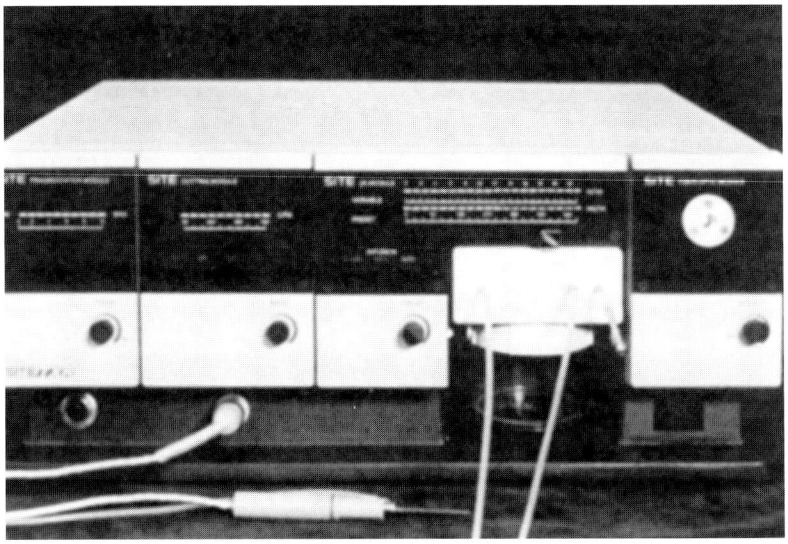

FIGURE 11-3
Suction infusion tissue extractor (SITE) for vitrectomy surgery.

ocular tumors and is credited with the development of the suction infusion tissue extractor (SITE) for vitreous surgery (Fig. 11-3). This instrument was developed by Dr. Jay Federman who previously served as director of research.

The Research Division of the Wills Eye Hospital continues to make innovative contributions to the understanding and treatment of eye diseases. An important addition to the staff in 1980 was Larry A. Donoso, M.D., Ph.D. (Fig. 11-4), a biochemist, ophthalmologist, and director of clinical retina research. Dr. Donoso has made advances in studies of retinal biochemistry and visual function.

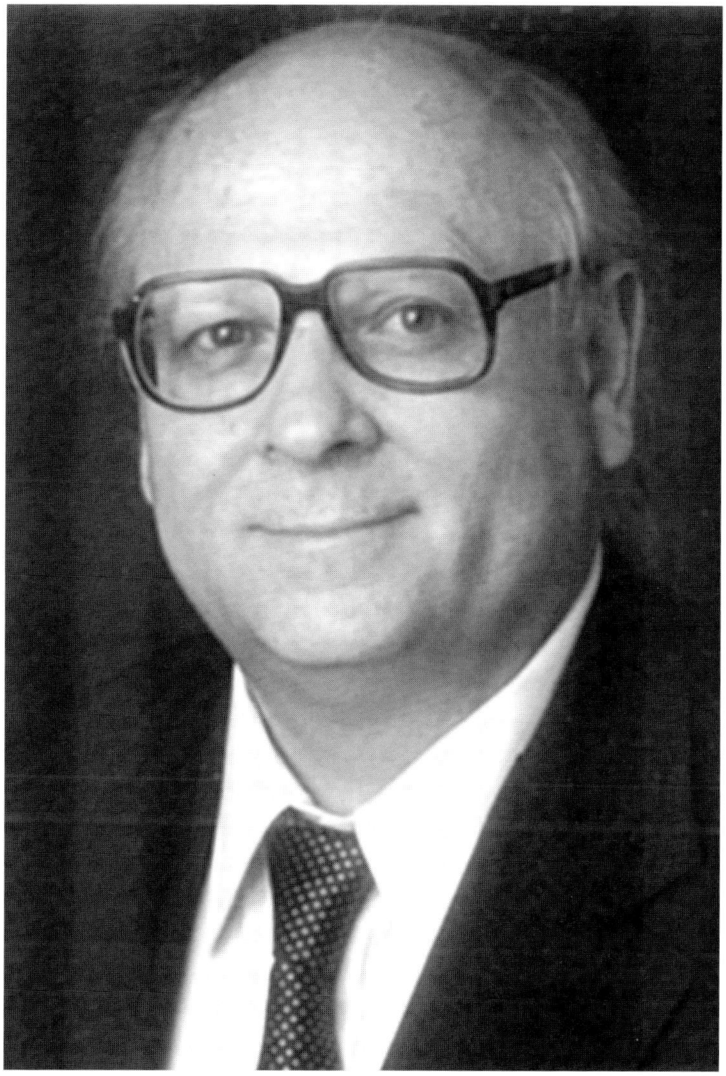

FIGURE 11-4
Dr. Larry Donoso

Of great importance to research at Wills was the establishment of an endowed chair—the first at Wills Eye Hospital and the first Chair of Ophthalmology at Jefferson. With an initial contribution in honor of former Ophthalmologist-in-Chief Thomas D. Duane as a start, over two million dollars was raised to fund the chair. Dr. Larry Donoso was named the first Thomas Duane Professor.

A generous bequest permitted establishment of the Henry and Corinne Bower Laboratory for macular degeneration within Wills Eye Hospital which is also directed by Dr. Donoso. In addition to supporting research related to macular degeneration, the endowment supports basic science research experience for clinicians. Tamara R. Vrabec, M.D. was named as the first Bower Research Fellow, followed by Ming Wang, M.D., Ph.D., Harminder S. Dua, M.D., Ph.D., Kang Zhang, M.D., Ph.D., Nina Ahmad, Ph.D., and José Gomes, M.D. Kang Zhang, M.D., Ph.D. was awarded the first Bower cup for studies related to hereditary macular degeneration.

Nina Ahmad, Ph.D., is a valued addition to retina research at Wills. She is intimately involved with the genetics of Stickler's syndrome, and with co-workers at Jefferson was the first to identify collagen 2 as one of the gene mutations in this condition.

Chapter 12
Administration

Dynamic forces have been re-shaping the organization of healthcare delivery systems in the U.S. The 1970s saw greater federal regulation. The 1980's introduced Diagnosis Related Groups (DRGs). And the 1990s was the decade of managed care—extreme cost control and accelerated outpatientization. The dynamics of these changes have been especially powerful and threatening to acute specialty hospitals. Many eye hospitals collapsed or were absorbed by bigger systems. Wills opened a new 120-bed inpatient hospital in 1980; nonetheless, the institution was financially threadbare by the middle of the decade.

In 1985, with the new chief executive officer came an administrative planning process which simultaneously focused on three broad strategic initiatives: internal management—improving clinical quality and access, streamlining systems, and enhancing Wills' financial and information systems; program development—the integration

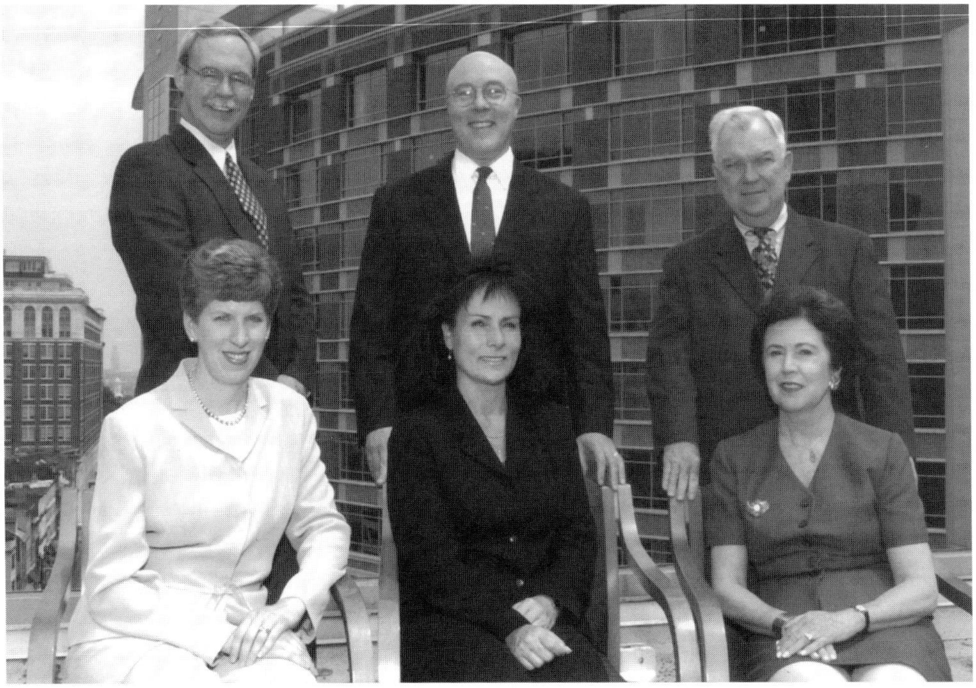

FIGURE 12-1
Front Row (from left ro right): Karla McCaney, Assistant Executive Director; Jeri Mogle, Chief Financial Officer; Lynn Gartland, Director for Institutional Advancement. Back Row (from left to right): Joseph Bilson, Managing Director of Wills Eye Hospital and President of the Wills Surgical Network; D. McWilliams Kessler, former Executive Director, and James J. Mulvihill, Current Executive Director of WIlls Eye Hospital.

of new clinical services; and endeavors in external relations—garnering congressional support and national leadership.

The advancing technology and tightening federal regulation of the 1980s moved much of traditionally inpatient ophthalmic surgery to outpatient settings. This rapid phenomenon created slack inpatient bed resources in the new Wills chassis. The Wills executive team, under the leadership of D. McWilliams Kessler, Executive Director & CEO, initiated plans to protect Wills, and begin the pre-positioning process for Wills' future. Through successful federal lobbying, Wills achieved favorable outpatient reimbursement to help in the transition years. Later Wills succeeded in obtaining special language to help support training costs in ambulatory surgery centers.

The 1990s was the decade of Wills' greatest clinical success, regional growth, and financial advancement. Introduced in 1990 in collaboration with Thomas Jefferson University, Wills Geriatric Psychiatry inpatient program gained national prominence within a few years. Next on the horizon, premiering one of the country's first few gamma knives and creating an instant success in 1995, was the Neurosensory program. Simultaneous with these diversification activities, ophthalmology kept growing at Wills and in another innovative way—through the creation and expansion of a three-state regional network of same day surgery facilities, the Wills Ambulatory Surgical Network.

As of this writing, the Surgical Network consists of 13 single- and multi-specialty facilities from one to five operating rooms. Since the opening of the first center in Cherry Hill, New Jersey in 1995 the surgical volume for the total Wills enterprise has grown from 8,000 cases annually to about 38,000; and tertiary referrals to the downtown facility have continued to grow.

The development, ownership and management skills gained during the building of the ASC network have been brought to bear in the creation of the new Wills Eye Hospital in 2002, thus completing the cycle of organizational expansion and re-integration.

The senior executive staff of Wills is comprised of the Executive Director and CEO, D. McWilliams Kessler; managing Director, James J. Mulvihill (Chief Operating Officer); Associate Executive Director, Joseph P. Bilson; Assistant Executive Director, Finance, Jeri Mogle (CFO); and Assistant Executive Director, Karla McCaney. Within the Wills Eye Surgical Network, Mr. Kessler served as Board Chairman and Mr. Bilson serves as President. The administrative team seeks its guidance through frequent consultation with the medical staff and Wills Society leadership, and is supervised by monthly Hospital Committee and Board of Directors of City Trusts meetings, as well as frequent conferencing with the Hospital Committee Chairman.

In June of 2002, Mr. Kessler departed to assume the position of President, Henry H. Kessler Foundation, New Jersey. Mr. Mulvihill was appointed as the new Executive Director.

Mission Statement

Wills Eye Hospital, through its dedication to the preservation and restoration of vision, serves as a comprehensive center of ophthalmology and other specialized services. Wills is committed to excellence in the provision of patient care to all those in need, to support of its medical staff, to education of healthcare professionals and the community, and to participation in medical research.

Wills Eye Hospital will fulfill the mission by operating as an independent not-for-profit hospital with a sound financial base.

Vision Statement

Wills seeks to remain the preeminent center for excellence in ophthalmology by creating a continuum of care accessible and responsive to the needs of the community. Additionally, Wills seeks to expand its services and become known as a center of excellence in other select medical and surgical programs.

Chapter 13

Wills Eye Hospital: 9th & Walnut to 840 Walnut

As surgical techniques grew more complex, it became apparent to officials of Wills Eye Hospital that it would be prudent for their hospital to be affiliated with a medical school. Each could then share the other's facilities, as well as their expertise. Therefore, on July 20, 1972, an agreement was signed between the Board of City Trusts and Thomas Jefferson University for such a merger.

This merger, however, did not change the fact that both institutions were separate and independent. It did mean that the new Wills Eye Hospital would be located near its partner school in an up-to-date modern facility. Therefore, the site on the southwest corner of 9th and Walnut Streets was selected (Fig. 13-1).

It is quite clear that the new hospital could not have been accomplished without the support of the Board of Directors of City Trusts and the even-handed leadership of the then ophthalmologist-in-chief, Thomas Duane (Fig.13-2). Working

Work slated on new home for Wills Eye Hospital

By Robert Fensterer
Inquirer Staff Writer

The Philadelphia hospital with a reputation as a world leader in eye treatment is moving to a larger building.

Wills Eye Hospital, located since 1932 in a six-story building at 16th and Spring Garden Streets, will break ground this winter for a $25 million building at Ninth and Walnut Streets, next to the Jefferson University campus. January 1980 is the target date for moving.

The City Planning Commission has approved the plans and the Hospitals Authority of Philadelphia has agreed to float a $22 million municipal bond issue.

The $3 million difference will be raised through contributions or by same number of beds as the old, as well as the same eye therapy equipment.

Staff doctors at Wills are pleased that they will be affiliated with the university next door.

"That means," said Dr. George L. Spaeth, head of the glaucoma clinic, "that when I examine a patient and find he has other ailments I will no longer have to send him all over town to other specialists. I will have all the specialists I need right here on the same campus."

A joint purchasing arrangement, Joseph said, will keep operating costs down.

The coming move reminded Dr. Spaeth of 1960, when he began his residency at Wills. Then, all patients were treated in three huge general clinics and all doctors saw all types of patients.

"It was fantastic training," he said. "But it was old-fashioned medicine. It hadn't changed since 1832."

That was the year that trustees of the James Wills estate interpreted the phrase in his will, "care for the indigent blind," to mean a hospital dedicated to the treatment of eye diseases.

A building on the southeast corner of Logan Square housed the hospital for exactly 100 years. In 1932, the Spring Garden building was opened.

FIGURE 13-1
Wills plans to move to 9th and Walnut Streets.

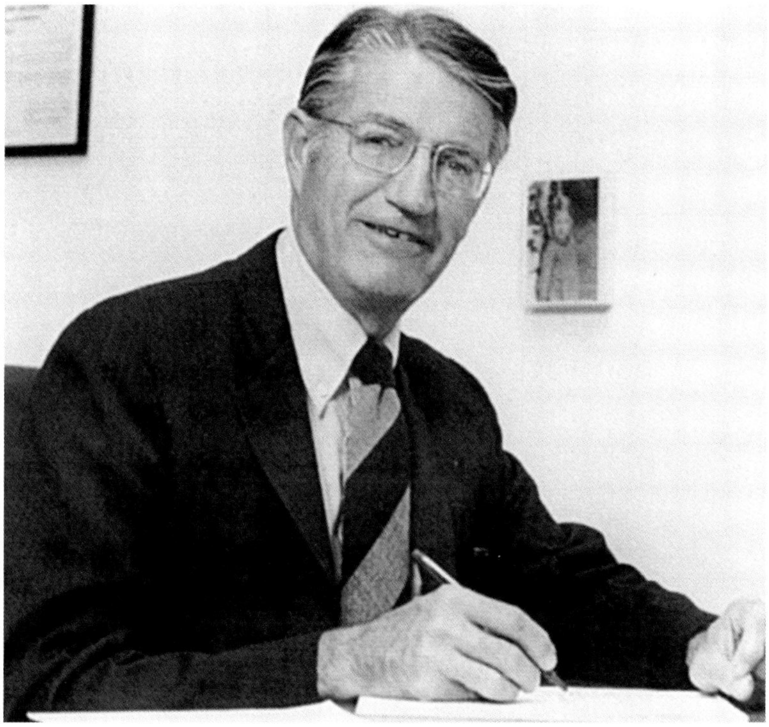

FIGURE 13-2
Ophthalmologist-in–chief Thomas D. Duane, 1972-1982.

with him and also sharing a major role in the accomplishment of our new facility was the administrator, Mr. David Joseph.

The new hospital was an eight-story building with 225,000 square feet of floor space (Fig. 13-3); this was considerably more than Spring Garden Street's 140,000 square feet. General ophthalmology continued and the same subspecialty clinics in retina, cornea, glaucoma, oculoplastics, neuro-ophthalmology, uveitis, oncology, and pediatric ophthalmology were available.

In addition to its own strong staff, Wills has supplied leaders to other institutions in this country and abroad, something discussed later in this chapter. One of its most illustrious alumni who is deserving of special recognition, however, is William R. Green, professor of ophthalmology and associate professor of pathology at the Johns Hopkins School of Medicine and director of the Eye Pathology Laboratory at the Wilmer Institute. His contributions to ophthalmology are legendary.

The Wills staff has depth in every department and is clinically and academically oriented. Members on all services have international reputations in their particular specialty. Many have authored or edited significant books, not the least of which is Duane's *Textbook of Ophthalmology*, a loose-leaf textbook of general ophthalmology available today, and kept current by Dr. Edward Jaeger. They serve on important committees, as officers in national societies, on the Academy Board, as Directors of the American Board of Ophthalmology, and on the editorial boards of important journals. Indeed, for 168 years Wills has been in the forefront of ophthalmology.

Changing Times

Even in 1985, it was apparent that the five-year-old facility would not be suitable for the times that were coming. That year heralded a new concept—diagnosis-related groups (DRGs)—which defined the number of days a patient could be hospitalized for an illness. Thus, if a condition was allotted four days of hospitalization and the patient was discharged in two days, it was possible for the hospital to make money. On the other hand, if the patient's hospital stay went beyond the designated four days, financial losses could be substantial.

The introduction of DRGs was the first harbinger that ophthalmology was becoming an outpatient specialty. As more and more eye cases were being managed without hospital stays, hospital services offered at Wills were broadened with the addition of geriatric psychiatry and, later, neurosurgery. Both of these initiatives were productive, and although they required an initial $20 million investment, the income generated amounted to a return of $30 million. Unfortunately, now other specialties are also doing more outpatient surgery, and reimbursements for geriatric psychiatry have plummeted.

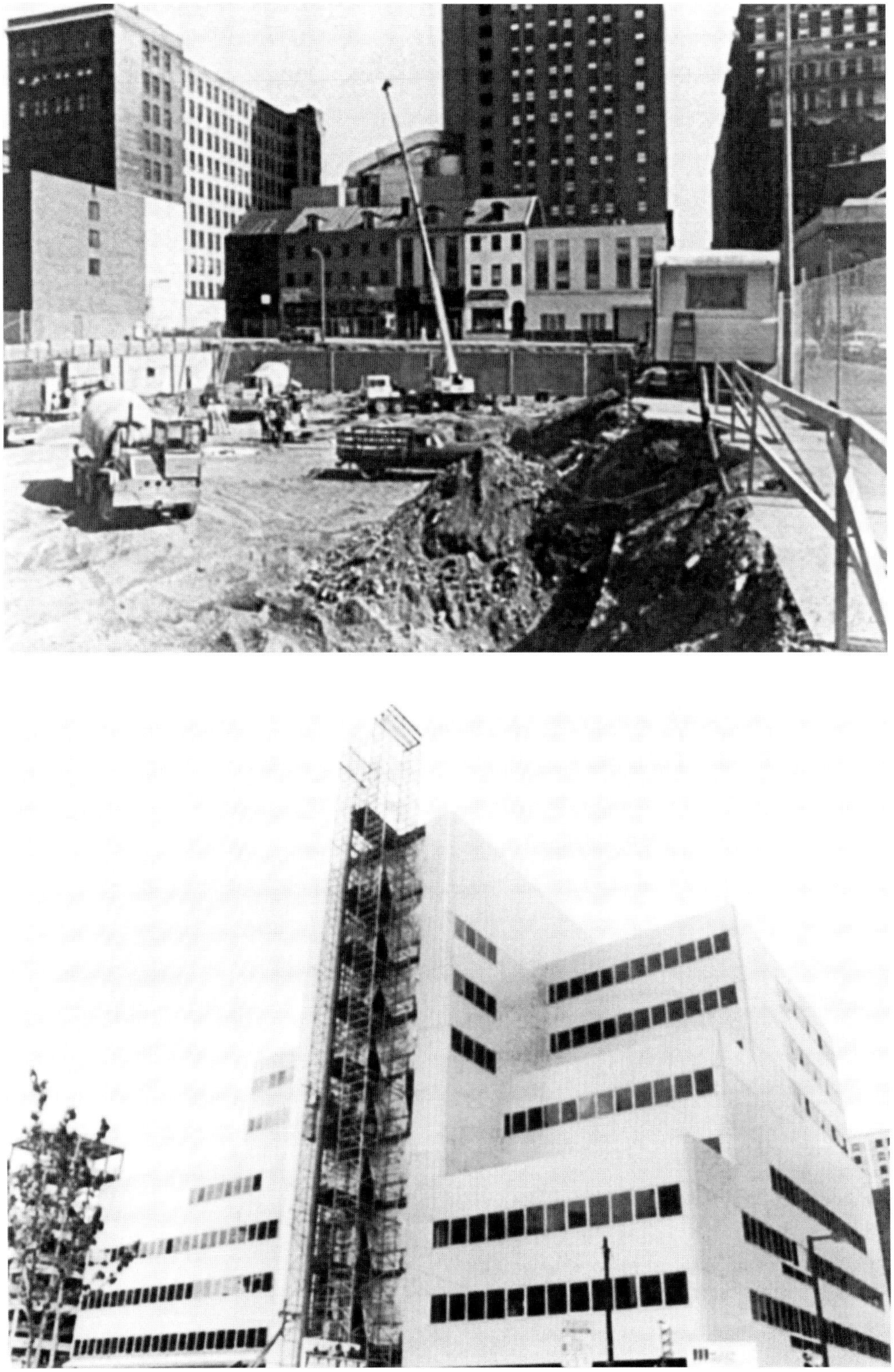

FIGURE 13-3
From a hole in the ground to near completion.

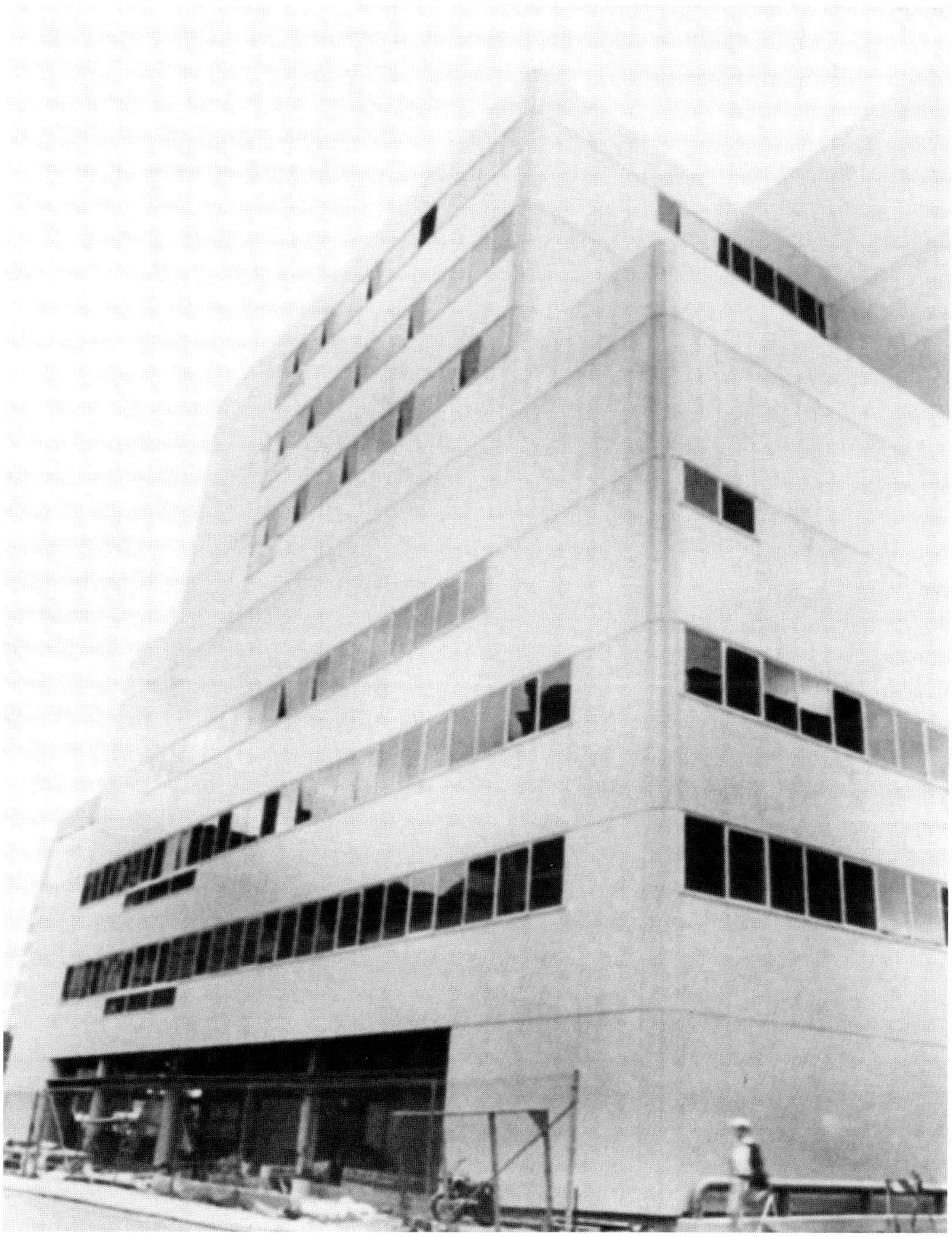

FIGURE 13-3 *(continued)*

Meanwhile, hospital administration spearheaded a network of ambulatory surgicenters around the Delaware Valley, and Wills gained valuable experience in community-based, same-day surgery centers, probably more than just about any other group.

The Old Facility

Initially, the 1980 facility was to be housed in Jefferson University's new Gibbon Building, slated to be constructed at the same time. Wills would have a Tenth Street entrance between Walnut and Chestnut Streets, and a high-speed elevator would take passengers to the tenth or eleventh floor, where the Wills condo would be located. This plan was endorsed by Donald Rubel, Chairman of the Board of Directors of City Trusts, and Mr. William Cairo, head of the Hospital Committee. However, the plan was vigorously opposed by the medical staff, who felt that Wills should be a freestanding hospital. Various meetings were held—including one on a Palm Sunday afternoon, led by Dr. Hunter Stokes, who had come up from South Carolina, and another at the Philadelphia Cricket Club—and the plan was finally scrapped. Subsequently, an attempt was made to obtain land within the Jefferson University campus to build a freestanding hospital.

Prior to this point, Wills had been affiliated with Temple University, which had promised to build a new Wills Eye Hospital with state funds. This never came to pass, and Wills and Temple separated. Wills affiliated with Thomas Jefferson University in 1972, at which time Tom Duane became Ophthalmologist-in-Chief. Plans for the Wills facility evolved under the guidance of Dr. Duane and David Joseph, CEO of the hospital. Redevelopment authority land was obtained, and the hospital was built.

At that time, the southeast corner of Ninth and Walnut Streets was a parking lot. Subsequently, of course, Walnut Park Towers was constructed, and fortunately, its foundation allowed for the construction of additional stories later.

The New Facility

Since July 1, 2002, the newest Wills Eye hospital, a state of the art facility, has been our residence. The celebration on November 1 and 2 includes scientific sessions and a special convocation by Thomas Jefferson University at which honorary degrees will be awarded to noted artist Andrew Wyeth and Professor Alan Bird of Moorfields Eye Hospital in London. Tony Auth, the Pulitzer Prize-winning political cartoonist for the *Philadelphia Inquirer*, is the guest speaker at the banquet. He will show many of his political cartoons and then review the mail that they generated.

The new hospital is located on the seventh through the 15th floors. The lobby entrance is on the ground floor on Walnut Street, and four high-speed elevators carry passengers to the upper floors, where various services are located: Cataract and Primary Eye Care, Cornea, Glaucoma, Neuro-ophthalmology, Oculoplastics, Oncology, Pediatric Ophthalmology and Retina.

The seventh floor houses eight operating rooms. Three operating rooms will be retained at the old Wills facility, and the Emergency Room will also remain there, at least for the present. The eighth floor houses an auditorium and an outdoor terrace where receptions can be held in good weather. There was much debate as to whether seating in the auditorium should be fixed or movable, but in the final analysis it was decided that movable chairs would make the room more functional. Also on the eighth floor are a classroom that seats about 40 people, the medical library, the residents lounge, the wet lab, and a meditation room (Fig. 13.4).

There was much discussion about the location of the new hospital. The biggest problem in Center City is parking, and some favored relocating to South Philadelphia near Veterans Stadium, where parking is plentiful. However, this move would have isolated Wills from the academic scene, and in the final analysis it was decided to purchase the air rights over Walnut Towers and build there.

In many ways, the new facility will present additional challenges. For example, for the first time, residents will be trained in a surgicenter environment, which in many ways simulates the real world that they will encounter when they enter practice.

A Firm Training Ground

Clearly, Wills' strength has always been its clinical training, and Wills consistently ranks high in surveys year after year. This reputation stems from a long tradition. The Wills residency was established in 1839. As one looks back over the years, it is probably fair to assume that Wills has trained more ophthalmologists than any other institution in the United States. When Wills opened its doors in 1834, it was the first hospital devoted exclusively to eye disease.

The first fellows at Wills Eye Hospital were Dr. Leonard Apt, who worked under Dr. Leopold, and Lov Sarin, who spent time with P. Robb McDonald and then specialized in retina. Since then, the training of fellows has mushroomed. In the late 1950s it became apparent that many subspecialties would become independent in that physicians became devoted exclusively to a particular part of the eye. Today we have fellowships in cornea, glaucoma, neuro-ophthalmology, oculoplastics, oncology, pediatric ophthalmology, and retina. Wills is fortunate to be able to attract the top candidates for both resident training and fellowship training.

Wills has always been a major contributor to the literature in the field of clinical ophthalmology but less so in basic research. Now that we have a new facility, the hope is that we can capitalize on our clinical expertise to develop epidemiologic and outcomes studies under the direction of a clinical research director with expertise in those fields.

As mentioned earlier, few people realize that Wills has served as a very firm training ground for academicians around the country. *Excluding ophthalmologists at Wills*, many alumni hold significant academic posts in the United States and even around the world. While it is dangerous to list these individuals for fear of leaving someone out, we attempt to do so here because it will be somewhat of a revelation to ophthalmologists who are not familiar with Wills' contribution to academic ophthalmology, something of which we are very proud.

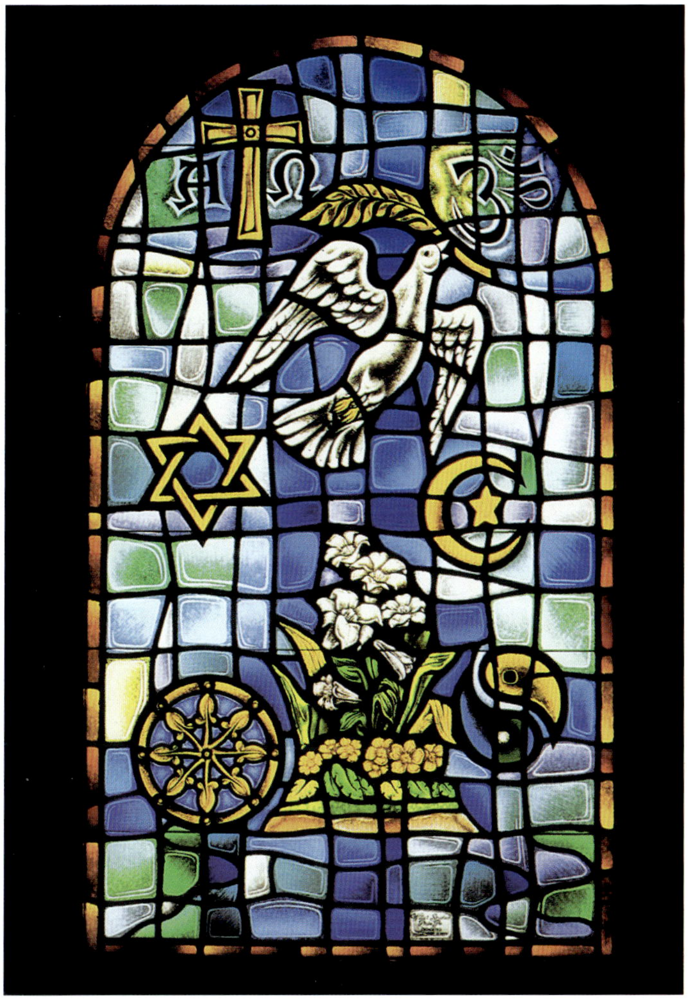

FIGURE 13-4
The meditation room and its stained glass window dedicated to Mr. Alfred Stern whose life was saved by Wills physician, Dr. Sidney Tyson, when he administered CPR to Mr. Stern, was moved across the street to the 8th floor of the new hospital.

Academic Positions Held by Former Residents and Fellows of Wills Eye Hospital*

Tony Aldave, M.D
Cornea
Jules Stein Eye Institute
UCLA
Los Angeles, CA

Leonard Apt, M.D.
Pediatric Ophthalmology
Jules Stein Eye Institute
UCLA
Los Angeles, CA

Geoffrey Broocker, M.D.
Program Director
Department of Ophthalmology
Emory
Atlanta, GA

Mary Lou Collins, M.D.
Residency Program Director
GBMC-Wilmer
Pediatric Ophthalmology
Greater Baltimore Eye
Baltimore, MD

Jay Duker, M.D.
Vitreoretinal Service
Chairman
Department of Ophthalmology
Tufts New England Eye Center
Boston, MA

Robert Folberg, M.D.
Chairman of Pathology
(Dr. Folberg is in
Ophthalmology & Pathology)
University of Illinois
Chicago, IL

Steven Gedde, M.D.
Program Director
Glaucoma
Bascom Palmer Eye Institute
Miami, FL

Cono Grasso, M.D.
Chairman
Department of Ophthalmology
St. Vincent's Catholic Medical Center
Brooklyn and Queens Region
New York, NY

William Richard Green, M.D.
Professor of Ophthalmology –
Pathology
Wilmer Eye Institute
Baltimore, MD

James Handa, M.D.
Vitreoretinal Service
Chairman
Wilmer Eye Institute
Baltimore, MD

William Harbour, M.D.
Oncology
Washington University
St. Louis, MO

Roscoe Kennedy, M.D.**
Chairman of Ophthalmoogy
Cleveland Clinic
Cleveland, OH

Stephanie J. Marioneaux, M.D.
Assistant Professor
Department of Ophthalmology
Eastern Virginia Medical School

C.S. O'Brien, M.D.**
Chairman of Ophthalmology
University of Iowa
Iowa City, IA

William Offutt, M.D.
Oculoplastics
University of Kentucky
Lexington, KY

Richard Parrish, M.D.
Glaucoma
Professor and former Chairman
Bascom Palmer Eye Institute
Miami, FL

Julian Perry, M.D.
Oculoplastics
Cole Eye Institute at the
Cleveland Clinic
Cleveland, OH

Michael Repka, M.D.
Professor of Pediatric
and Neuro-Ophthalmology
Wilmer Eye Institute
Baltimore, MD

Madison Slusher, M.D.
Chairman
Department of Ophthalmology
Wake Forest
Winston Salem, NC

Jonathan Trobe, M.D.
Neuro-Ophthalmology
Professor, University of Michigan
Ann Arbor, MI

Ming Wang, M.D.
Lasik and Cornea
Formerly Vanderbilt University

George Waring, M.D.
Professor of Ophthalmology
Emory University School of Medicine
Atlanta, GA

* *See Appendix H for updated list*
** Deceased

Glaucoma Fellows

Myung Douk Ahn, M.D.
Associate Professor
Department of Ophthalmology
Kangnam St. Mary's Hospital
Seoul Korea

Nursen Ariturk, M.D.
Assistant Professor
Ondokuzmayis Universitesi
Tip Fakültesi
Samsun, Turkey

Ioannis M. Aslanides, M.D., PhD
Assistant Professor
Vardinoyannion Eye Institute
of Crete
University of Crete
Heraklion, Greece

Augusto Azuara-Blanco, M.D., PhD
Honorary Clinical Senior Lecturer
University of Aberdeen
Aberdeen, UK

Stephen Best, M.D.
Clinical Lecturer
Discipline of Ophthalmology
University of Auckland, New Zealand

Janet Betchkal, M.D.
Professor and Chairman
Dept. of Ophthalmology
U. Hospital of Jacksonville
Jacksonville, FL

J. Brent Bond, M.D.
Assistant Professor
Wake Forest University
Winston-Salem, NC

James Brandt, M.D.
Associate Professor
Director, Glaucoma Service
University of California – Davis

Louis B. Cantor, M.D.
Associate Professor
Director, Glaucoma Service
Indiana University
Indianapolis, IN

Joseph Caprioli, M.D.
Professor of Ophthalmology
Jules Stein Eye Institute
University of California
Los Angeles, CA

Neil T. Choplin, M.D.
Associate Clinical Professor
University Service
Bethesda, MD

Nathan G. Congdon, M.D., MPH
Assistant Professor
Wilmer Institute
Baltimore, MD

Vital Costa, M.D.
Assistant Professor
Department of Ophthalmology
University Campinas
Sao Paulo, Brazil

Tasos Costarides, M.D.
Assistant Professor
Department of Ophthalmology
Emory University School of Medicine
Atlanta, GA

Helen Danesh-Meyer, M.D.
Discipline of Ophthalmology
The University of Auckland
Auckland, New Zealand

Richard Daniel, M.D.
President
Christian Medical College
and Hospital
Ludhiana, Punjab, India

Tarek El-Mohammady Eid, M.D.
El-Maghraby Eye & Ear Hospital
Jeddah, Saudi Arabia

Fathi El Sayyad, M.D.
El Maghraby Eye Hospital
Jeddah, Saudi Arabia

Robert M. Feldman, M.D.
Assistant Clinical Professor
Dept of Ophthalmology
University of Texas at Houston
Houston, TX

Ronald L. Fellman, M.D.
Associate Clinical Professor
University of Texas – Southwestern
Dallas, TX

Sai Gandham, M.D.
Director, Glaucoma Service
Assistant Professor of Ophthalmology
Albany Medical College
Albany, NY

Kevin Greenidge, M.D.
Professor and Chairman
Ophthalmology Dept
SUNY Health Science Center
Brooklyn, NY

Ronald L. Gross, M.D.
Professor and Director of Glaucoma
Baylor College of Medicine
Houston, TX

Paul Harasymowicz, M.D.
Department of Ophthalmology
University of Montreal
Montreal, Quebec, Canada

Roger Hitchings
Professor of Glaucoma and Allied Studies
Institute of Ophthalmology
Moorfields Eye Hospital
London, England

Lawrence M. Hurvitz, M.D.
Associate Clinical Professor
University of South Florida
Sarasota, FL

Yo-Quin Jiang, M.D.
Associate Professor
Department of Ophthalmology
Hunan Medical University
Chang-sha, China

Lawrence Jindra, M.D.
Clinical Assistant Professor
SUNY Stony Brook
Stony Brook, NY

Leslie Jones, M.D.
Assistant Professor
Department of Ophthalmology
Director of Glaucoma Services
Howard University College of Medicine
Washington, DC

Anup Khatana, M.D.
Cincinnati Eye Institute
Cincinnati, OH

Dr.med. Ines Lanzl
Augenklinik und Poliklinik
Klinikum rechts der Isar der Technischen Universität München
München, Germany

Martha Leen, M.D.
Clinical Assistant Professor
University of Washington
Poulsbo, WA

Ordan J. Lehmann
Lecturer
Department of Molecular Genetics
Institute of Ophthalmology
London, England

Mark Lesk, M.D.
Assistant Clinical Professor
Ophthalmology Department
University of Montreal
Montreal, Quebec, Canada

Suzanne Li, M.D.
Assistant Clinical Professor
California Pacific Medical Center
San Francisco, CA

James A. McAllister, FRCS
Associate
Moorfields Eye Hospital
London, England

Andrew J. Michael, M.D.
Assistant Clinical Professor
Department of Ophthalmology
Medical College of Virginia
Richmond, VA

Clive Migdal
Senior Lecturer
University of London
London, England

Erkan Mutlukan, M.D., PhD
Assistant Professor of Surgery
University of Massachusetts at Lowell
Lowell, MA

Dan A. Nichols, M.D.
Clinical Assistant Professor
University of Minnesota
St. Paul, MN

Y. Grace Oh, M.D.
Assistant Professor
University of Southern California
Doheny Eye Institute
Los Angeles, CA

Silvia Orengo-Nania, M.D.
Assistant Professor
Baylor College of Medicine
Department of Ophthalmology
Houston, TX

Fred Orlando, M.D.
Assistant Clinical Professor
Department of Ophthalmology
University of Massachusetts – Amherst
Amherst, MA

Richard Parrish, M.D.
Professor and former Chairman
University of Miami – Bascom Palmer Eye Institute
Miami, FL

Alfred "Fritz" Paul, M.D.
Clinical Faculty
Brown University Medical School
Providence, RI

Tom Samuelson, M.D.
Associate Clinical Professor
University of Minnesota
Minneapolis, MN

Mark B. Sherwood, M.D.
Professor and Chair
Department of Ophthalmology
University of Florida at Gainesville
Gainesville, FL

Robb Shrader, M.D.
Assistant Clinical Professor
University of Louisville
Louisville, KY

Steven Simmons, M.D.
Assistant Professor
Department of Ophthalmology
Albany Medical College
Albany, NY

Priv. Doz. Dr. Detlev Spiegel
Klinik und Poliklinik für Augenheilkunde der Universitäts Regensburg
Regensburg, Germany

Richard Starita, M.D.
Assistant Clinical Professor
Texas – Southwestern
Dallas, TX

Michael Stiles, M.D
Assistant Clinical Professor
University of Kansas at Kansas City
Kansas City, MO

Scott Stoller, M.D.
Clinical Instructor
University of Illinois – Urbana
Urbana, IL

Chryssa Terzidou, M.D.
Clinical Assistant Professor
Aristotle University
Thessalonika, Greece

Patrick Tiedeken, M.D.
Assistant Clinical Professor
Vanderbilt University
Nashville, TN

Carlo Traverso, M.D.
Professor and Chair
University Eye Clinic
Genoa, Italy

Shigeo Tsukahara, M.D.
Professor and Chair
Yamanashi Medical University
Department of Ophthalmology
Yamanashi, Japan

Stephen Wahl, M.D.
Assistant Clinical Professor
University of South Florida
Sarasota, FL

Rohit Varma, M.D.
Assistant Professor
University of Southern California
Doheny Eye Institute
Los Angeles, CA

William R. Whalen, M.D.
Assistant Clinical Professor
University of Colorado
Denver, CO

Asher Weiner, M.D., PhD
Assistant Professor
Department of Ophthalmology
SUNY Down – State
Brooklyn, NY

Kun Jin Yang, M.D.
Associate Professor
Department of Ophthalmology
Chonnam University Medical School
Kwangju, Korea

Isam J. Zakhour, M.D.
Assistant Clinical Professor
Medical University of South Carolina
Florence, SC

Cornea Fellows

Charles Adams, M.D.
Clinical Assistant Professor
Ophthalmology
University of Florida
Jacksonville, FL

James Allen, M.D.
Clinical Associate Professor
University of Minnesota, St. Paul

Paulo T.S. Alvim, M.D.
Assistant Professor Ophthalmology
Pontifical Catholic University of
Sao Paulo, Brazil

Helia Angotti, M.D., PhD
Professor of Ophthalmology &
Chairperson
Department of Ophthalmology
Faculdade de Medicina
do Triangulo Mineiro
Uberaba, Brazil

Peter Berkowitz, M.D.
Clinical Associate Professor
Ophthalmology
University of Pittsburgh

Christopher Blanton, M.D.
Clinical Assistant Professor of Surgery
Department of Ophthalmology
Loma Linda University
Medical Center
Loma Linda CA

Carol S. Clemons, M.D.
Associate Clinical Professor
Louisiana State University
Medical College
Shreveport, LA

Stephanie Croll, M.D.
Clinical Assistant Professor of
Ophthalmology
Storm Eye Institute, Medical
University of South Carolina
Savannah, GA

Robert Cykiert, M.D.
Clinical Associate Professor
Ophthalmology
NYU School of Medicine

M. Reza Dana, M.D.
Associate Professor of Ophthalmology
Harvard Medical School
Boston MA

Regis de Figueiredo, M.D.
Professor of Ophthalmology
Faculdade de Medicina
de Juazeiro do Norte
Ceara, Brazil

René Dinh, M.D.
Assistant Professor
Department of Ophthalmology
Université Laval
Quebec City, Quebec, Canada

Eric Donnenfeld, M.D.
Co-Chairman, Cornea &
External Disease
Manhattan Eye, Ear, Throat Hospital
Assistant Professor Ophthalmology
New York University Medical Center.

Harminder S. Dua, M.D.
Professor & Chairman
Department of Ophthalmology
University of Nottingham, UK

Richard Eiferman, M.D.
Clinical Professor of Ophthalmology
University of Louisville
Louisville, Kentucky

Michael Ference, III, M.D.
Associate Clinical Professor
University of Texas
Health Science Center
San Antonio, Texas

Todd Fladden, M.D.
Clinical Instructor in Ophthalmology
Northeast Ohio University
College of Medicine
Canton, Ohio

Matthew B. Goren, M.D.
Assistant Professor Clinical
Ophthalmology
Northwestern University
Medical School
Chicago, IL

Sanjeev Grewal, M.D.
Assistant Professor of Ophthalmology
University South Carolina
School of Medicine

Lewis Groden, M.D.
Associate Professor
Department of Ophthalmology
University of South Florida
Tampa, FL

Wee Jin Heng, M.D.
Head, Training & Education
The Eye Institute National
Healthcare Group
Singapore

Marc A. Honig, M.D.
Instructor, Wilmer
Ophthalmological Institute
Johns Hopkins University School of Medicine
Owings Mills MD

Jack Kabak, M.D.
Clinical Associate Professor
Ophthalmology
Stanford University Medical School
Palo Alto, CA

Terry Kim, M.D.
Assistant Professor of Ophthalmology
Duke, University
Atlanta, GA

Wilson Ko, M.D.
Instructor in Ophthalmology
New York Eye & Ear Infirmary
NYU Medical Center
New York, NY

Vera O. Kowal, M.D.
Clinical Assistant Professor, Department of Surgery
University of South Dakota School of Medicine
Rapid City, SD

Jay Krachmer, M.D.
Professor & Chairman
Department of Ophthalmology
University of Minnesota

Patricia Laughrea, M.D.
Professor de Clinique
Program Director Ophthalmology
Laval, University, Quebec Canada

Jy-Been Liang, M.D.
Clinical Assistant Professor
Taipei, Taiwan

Jodi Ian Luchs, M.D.
Assistant Clinical Professor of
Ophthalmology and Visual Sciences
Albert Einstein College of Medicine
Wantagh, NY

Stephanie J. Marioneaux, M.D.
Assistant Professor
Department of Ophthalmology
Eastern Virginia Medical School

Jose T. Oconer, M.D.
Manila, Philippines

Steve Poleski, M.D.
Assistant Professor
Department of Ophthalmology
University of Ottawa
Ottawa, Ontario

Noemi Lois Puente, M.D.
Clinical Senior Lecturer
University of Aberdeen, Scotland

Irving M. Raber, M.D.
Clinical Assistant Professor of Ophthalmology
Thomas Jefferson University School of Medicine
Philadelphia, PA

Jed Rabinovitch, M.D.
Chief Division Ophthalmology
Scarborough Hospital, Grace Division
Toronto

Rajesh Rajpal, M.D.
Clinical Assistant Professor Ophthalmology
George Washington University
Tysons Corner, VA

Richard C. Rodman, M.D.
Clinical Assistant Professor of Ophthalmology
Brown University School of Medicine
Lexington MA

Yaacov Rozenman, M.D.
Chairman, Department of Ophthalmology
Shaare Zedek Hospital
Jerusalem, Israel

Roy Rubinfeld, M.D.
Clinical Associate Professor
Department of Ophthalmology
Georgetown University Medical Center
Chevy Chase MD

Aisha Simjee, M.D.
Clinical Professor of Ophthalmology
University of California, Irvine
Orange County, CA

Raymond M. Stein, M.D.
Assistant Professor
University of Toronto
Co-Director
Bochner Eye Institute
Toronto, Canada

George W. Stubbs, M.D.
Associate Clinical Professor Surgery
Medical College of Pennsylvania
Philadelphia, PA

Emanuel Tanne, M.D.
Clinical Assistant Professor of Ophthalmology
Casey Eye Institute
Oregon Health & Science University
Portland, Oregon

David Varssano, M.D.
Clinical Instructor
Tel Aviv, Israel

George Waring, M.D.
Professor of Ophthalmology
Emory University
School of Medicine
Atlanta, GA

Wendell E. Willis, M.D.
Associate Professor of
Ophthalmology
Queens University
Deputy Head of Ophthalmology
Kingston, Ontario

William Yeakley, M.D.
Associate Professor of Clinical
Ophthalmology
Northeastern Ohio University
College of Medicine
Senior Clinical Instructor in
Ophthalmology
Case Western Reserve University
School of Medicine
Akron, Ohio

Oncology Ex-Fellows

J. Fernando Arevalo, M.D.
Diretor, Retina and Vitreous Service
Clinica Oftalmologica Centro Caracas
Caracas, Venezuela

Cynthia Carvalho, M.D.

An Ning Chao, M.D.
Chang Gung Memorial Hospital
at Taipei

Patrick De Potter, M.D.
Professor of Ophthalmology
and Chairman
Cliniques Universitaires St-Luc
Brussels, Belgium

Chaim Edelstein, M.D., FRCSC
Assistant Professor, McGill University
Department of Ophthalmology
Division of Orbital and Ophthalmic
Plastic and Reconstructive Surgery
and Ocular Oncology

Michael E. Giblin, MB, BS,
Visiting Medical Officer
Sydney Eye Hospital
Sydney, Australia

Kaan Gunduz, M.D.
Associate Professor of Ophthalomogy
Oncology Service
Department of Ophthalmology
Ankara University Medical School
Ankara, Turkey

Santosh Honavar, M.D.
Associate Professor
Ocular Oncology, Ophthalmic Plastic
Surgery, and Orbital Diseases
LV Prasad Eye Institute
Hyderabad, India

Sundeep Kheterpal, M.D.
Prince Charles Eye Unit
King Edward VII Hospital
Windsor, England

Hatem Krema, FRCS
Director, Ocular Oncology Service
Maghraby Eye Hospital
Cairo, Egypt

Prof. Dr. med. Wolfgang E. Lieb
Professor of Ophthalmology
Julius-maximilians University
Wuerzburg, Germany

Noemi Lois, M.D.
Consultant Ophthalmic Surgeon
Aberdeen Royal Infirmary
University of Aberdeen
Scotland, UK

John V. Mercado, M.D.
Clinical Associate Professor
Philippine General Hospital
Manila, Philippines

William F. Mieler, M.D.
Professor of Ophthalmology
Baylor College of Medicine
Houston, TX

Masood Naseripour, M.D.
Retina Specialist & Ocular Oncologist
Associate Professor
Ophthalmology
Rasool Akram Hospital
Iran University of Medical Sciences

Ihab Saad M Othman, MDFRCOphth
Consultant Ophthalmic Surgeon
Cairo University
Cairo, Egypt

Hugh Parsons, M.D.
Lecturer
University of British Columbia

Moel Perez, M.D.
Clinical Fellow, Ophthalmic Plastics
and Reconstructive Surgery
Medical College of Wisconsin
Milwaukee, Wisconsin

Paul Rundle, FRCOphth
Consultant Ocular Oncologist
Ophthalmology
Royal Hallamshire Hospital
Sheffield, UK

Arun Singh, M.D., FRCS
Department of Ophthalmology
Royal Hallamshire Hsopital
United Kingdom

Chenet Suvarnamani, M.D.
Bangkok, Thailand

Neuro-Ophthalmology Fellows

1980
Susan Benes, M.D.
Associate Clinical Professor
Ohio State University
Columbus, OH

1982
Roy W. Beck, M.D.
Clinical Professor
University of Southern Florida
Tampa, FL

1987
Susan Ksiazek, M.D.
Associate Clinical Professor
Indiana University
Indianapolis, IN

1990
William Cantore, M.D.
Associate Professor
Penn State University
Hershey, PA

1993
Edsel Ing, M.D.
Assistant Professor
Kresge Eye Institute
Wayne State University
Detroit, MI

1993
David Weinberg, M.D.
Assistant Professor
University of Vermont
Burlington, VT

1998
Helen V. Danesh-Meyer, FRACO
University of Auckland
Auckland, New Zealand

2001
Rod Foroozan, M.D.
Instructor
Baylor University
Waco, TX

Pediatric Ophthalmology Fellows

Maher F.D. Attia, M.D.
Quebec, Canada

David W. Day, M.D.
Arkansas Children's Hospital
Department of Ophthalmology
Little Rock, AR

Brian J. Forbes, M.D.
Children's Hospital of Philadelphia
Philadelphia, PA

Kammi B. Gunton, M.D.
St. Christopher's Hospital
for Children
Philadelphia, PA

Linda K. Nakanishi, M.D.
David Grant USAF Medical Center
Travis AFB, CA

Hulya Orer, M.D.
Ankara, Turkey

Retina Fellows

Emad Abboud, M.D.
Asst. Medical Director
Chief of the Vitreoretinal Division
King Khalid Eye Hospital
Saudi Arabia

James Augsburger, M.D.
Professor and Chairman
of Ophthalmology
University of Cincinnati

James Bolling, M.D.
Associate Professor
Mayo Graduate School of Medicine
Chair of Ophthalmology
Mayo Clinic Jacksonville

Gordon Byrnes, M.D.
Associate Professor & Director
of Retina Service
Uniformed Services
University of Health Sciences
Bethesda, MD

Alan Cruess, M.D.
Professor and Head
Department of Ophthalmology
Queen's University
Medical Director
Hotel Dieu Hospital
Kingston, Ontario

Jay Duker, M.D.
Professor and Chairman
of Ophthalmology
Tufts University New England
Eye Center
Boston, MA

Craig Greven, M.D.
Professor of Ophthalmology
Bowman Gray School of Medicine
Wake Forest
Winston Salem, NC

Brian Leonard, M.D.
Professor and ex-Chairman of
Ophthalmology
University of Ottawa
Former Director
General University
of Ottawa Eye Institute
Ottawa, Canada

William Phillips, M.D.
Director of Retinal Fellowship
Program
Washington Hospital Center
Assistant Professor
Howard University and
George Washington University
Washington, DC

Hermann Schubert, M.D.
Professor of Clinical Ophthalmology
Columbia University
New York, NY

Andrew Schachat, M.D.
Professor of Ophthalmology
Director of Retinovascular Service
Wilmer Institute
Johns Hopkins
Baltimore, MD

Sanjay Sharma, M.D.
Director
Cost-Effective Ocular Health
Policy Unit
Queen's University
Kingston, Ontario

Stephen Wong, M.D.
Director, Retina Service
Professor of Ophthalmology
Temple University School of Medicine
Philadelphia, PA

Myron Yanoff, M.D.
Professor and Chairman of
Ophthalmology
Hahnemann and MCP
Drexel University
Philadelphia, PA

Chapter 14

The Cataract & Primary Eye Care Service

Robert S. Bailey, Jr., M.D., Chief of Service

The Cataract & Primary Eye Care Service of CPEC is the largest service in the Wills Eye Hospital. Indeed, prior to the development of the vertical services it was the only service. Approximately 100 physicians serve on the CPEC staff. Most are on the active teaching staff interacting with residents in the clinic and operating room.

CPEC functions as the medical nucleus of the hospital. Most patients entering what was formerly the Wills Clinic system are examined here first and triaged to the various vertical services when necessary.

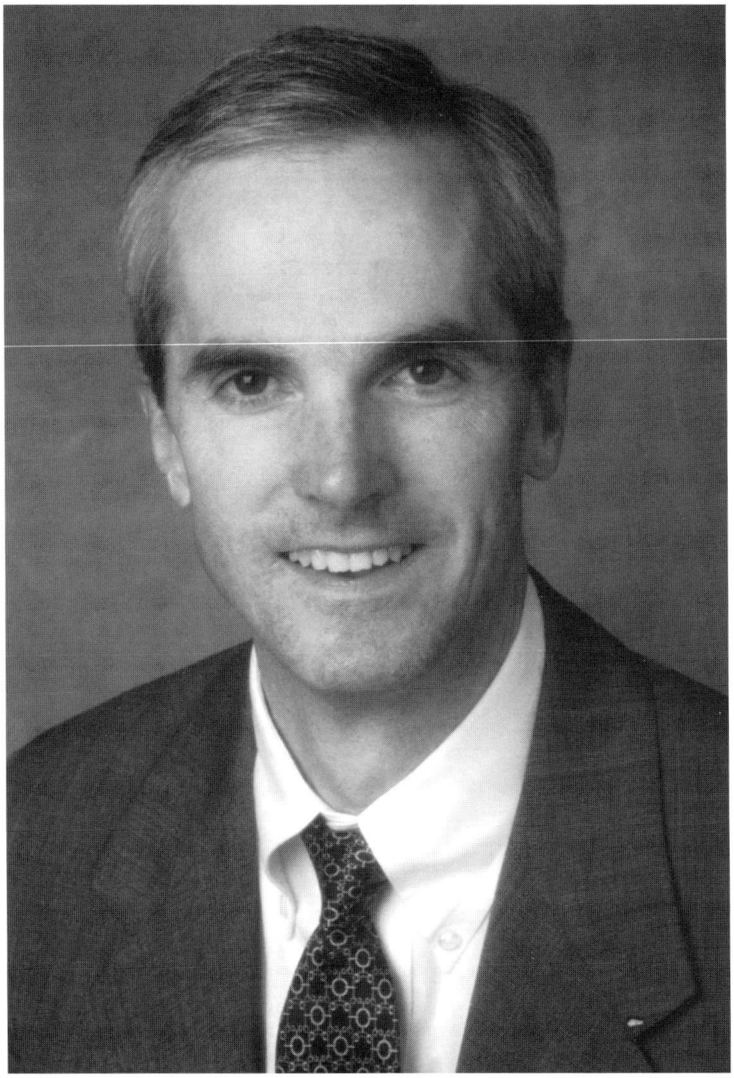

FIGURE 14-1
Robert S. Bailey, Jr., M.D.

The Original Service

The era of the Spring Garden Street Wills Eye Hospital (1950–1979) found the general ophthalmology clinic(s) on the first floor of the hospital. Ancillary clinics were located around the balcony, overlooking the hospital lobby. Some of them were the slit-lamp clinic (George Dublin), visual fields clinic (various attendings), refraction clinic (I.S. Tassman, Bernard Gettes; later, Owen Belmont) and orthoptics clinic (William Krewson), neuro-ophthalmology, dermatology and syphilology, ENT and dental. The last four clinics were staffed by non-ophthalmologists.

Five general ophthalmology clinics operated Monday through Friday (Saturdays were discontinued by 1960), between 2:00 P.M. and 4:00 P.M. A separate Chief of Service was responsible for each day of the week. The clinic was divided into three rooms (called clinic I, clinic II, clinic III). The Chief of Service appointed directors for each clinic and staff ophthalmologists. The physical dimensions of each clinic were similar with a large waiting room, long tables at the front of the room, a barbershop chair for tonometry and a dark room for slit-lamp and fundus examinations. All established ("old") service patients were examined by the attendings seated at the tables. The residents examined "new" clinic arrivals, performed Schiotz tonometry and examined dilated ("new" and "old") patients in the dark room with the attendings.

Service patients were assigned to a specific day/clinic, whether they came for a routine eye examination or an ocular emergency. For example, if a patient registered on a Thursday, he or she was enrolled with the Thursday clinic and given a color-coded clinic card. This handwritten card contained the clinic name, the patient's name and a clinic record number, in English or native language (such as German) (Fig. 14-2).

The service chief supervised most resident surgery. However, the attending staff was expected to be available and private surgery was also performed on the assigned clinic-surgery day. Service surgical emergencies operated on a Tuesday were assigned to the Thursday clinic for post-operative care. When a clinic visit was required sooner than one week, the patient was examined in the emergency room.

Some Friday service chiefs were James S. Shipman followed by Harold Barnshaw and lastly Oram R. Kline, Jr. Oram Kline served as Chief of the General Ophthalmology service from 1977 to 1987. Other chiefs were Wilfred E. Fry, R. Robb McDonald, Irving Leopold, Patrick Kennedy, William Krewson, J.W. Hallett, Al Cleveland, Philip Spaeth, Bernard Gettes and others.

Cataract & Primary Eye Care Service

In 1987 Raymond E. Adams was appointed Chief of the General Ophthalmology Service. One of his first acts was to rename the service the Cataract & Primary Eye Care Service, or CPEC. This change was to better define the purpose and role of the service. Daniel M. Kane, M.D. served as co-director of the service during the time Dr. Adams served as director.

In 1990, Dr. Adams performed a live cataract surgery broadcast at Wills on Channel 12, the local Public Broadcasting Systems Network. This telecast continues to be rerun even today, and has been seen by literally hundreds of thousands of people.

In 1992 CPEC purchased and donated a Visx excimer laser to the hospital. This laser was initially used for investigational work for the removal of scars, called photo-therapeutic-keratoplasty (PTK) and the correction of myopia, called photo-refractive-keratoplasty (PRK). Later it was used for LASIK.

In 2001 Robert S. Bailey, Jr., M.D. was named Director of the Cataract & Primary Eye Care Service.

The Service Today

Today, CPEC continues to be the largest service at Wills Eye Hospital in terms of:

a. Active staff volunteer ophthalmologists number more than 80 board-certified ophthalmologists
b. Affiliate staff non-volunteer ophthalmologists, primarily active in the Wills network of outpatient surgical centers in the surrounding tri-state area, number more than 50 members
c. Including the surgery centers, geographic distribution of the staff covers a radius of more than 100 miles around the Wills Eye Hospital

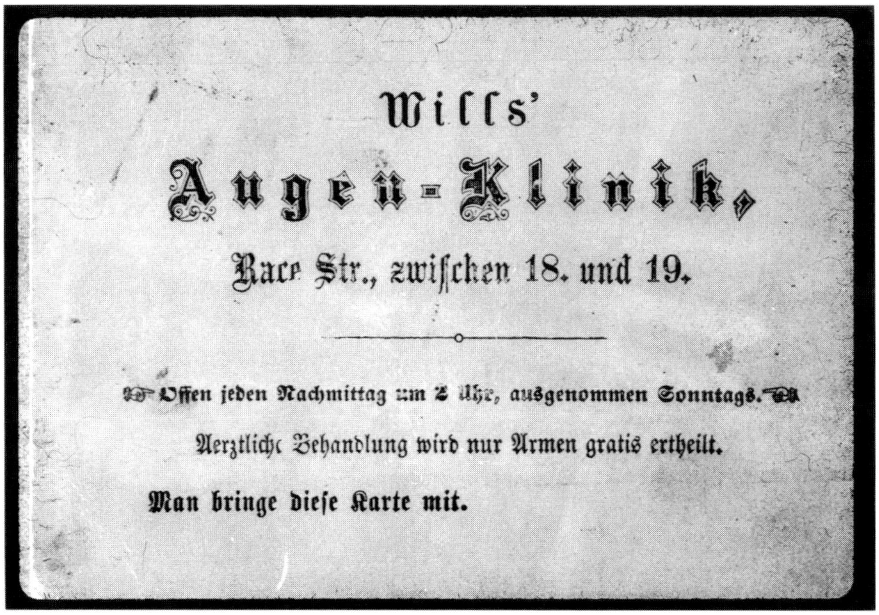

Wills'

Augen-Klinik,

Race Str., zwischen 18. und 19.

Offen jeden Nachmittag um 2 Uhr, ausgenommen Sonntags.

Aerztliche Behandlung wird nur Armen gratis ertheilt.

Man bringe diese Karte mit.

FIGURE 14-2

In the late 1800s and first part of the 20th century clinic cards were also printed in foreign languages because of the waves of immigration from Europe to the United States.

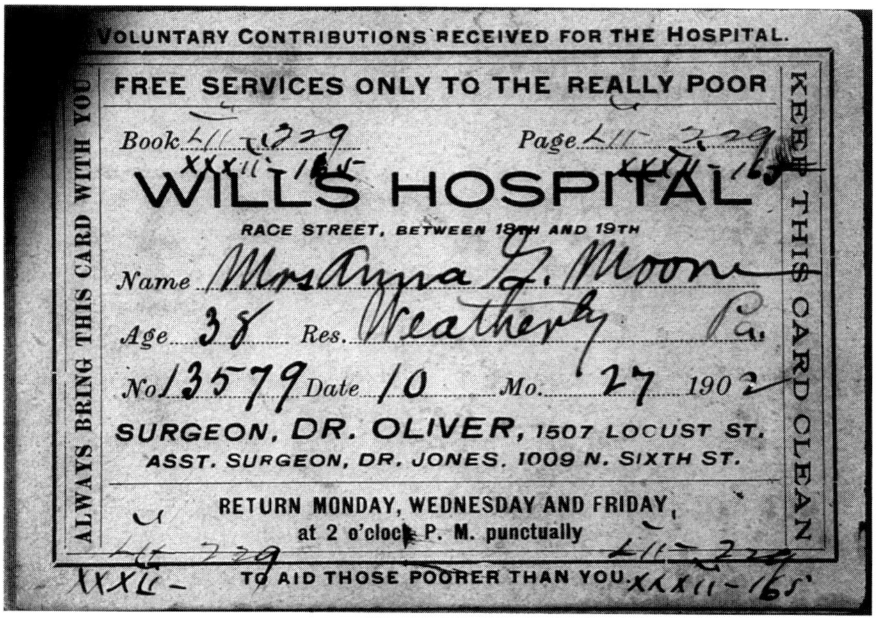

VOLUNTARY CONTRIBUTIONS RECEIVED FOR THE HOSPITAL.

ALWAYS BRING THIS CARD WITH YOU

KEEP THIS CARD CLEAN

FREE SERVICES ONLY TO THE REALLY POOR

Book 411–329 Page 411–329

XXXII–165 XXXII–165

WILLS HOSPITAL

RACE STREET, BETWEEN 18TH AND 19TH

Name Mrs Anna L. Moore

Age 38 Res. Weatherly Pa.

No 13579 Date 10 Mo. 27 1902

SURGEON, DR. OLIVER, 1507 LOCUST ST.

ASST. SURGEON, DR. JONES, 1009 N. SIXTH ST.

RETURN MONDAY, WEDNESDAY AND FRIDAY, at 2 o'clock P. M. punctually

411–329 411–329

XXXII– TO AID THOSE POORER THAN YOU. XXXII–165

FIGURE 14-3

A 1902 clinic card for Dr. Oliver's service.

d. Outpatient clinic visits per year number over 18,000
e. Private and service surgery performed
f. Residents on duty and clinic rotations
g. Operates 40+ hours per week

The majority of surgery performed by CPEC involves the removal of cataracts. Each resident performs over 100 cases during the three-year residency. Residents utilize phacoemulsification with intraocular lens implantation in 98 percent of cases. Planned extracapsular cataract extractions with intraocular lens implantation constitute the remainder.

An elected Board of Directors oversees the operation of the service and reports to the hospital executive committee and members of the CPEC staff. The Board members are Mark Blecher, M.D., medical director, who is responsible for clinic operations, Robert Lehman, M.D., who plans and reviews educational aspects of the service, Sydney Tyson, M.D., the financial officer, Marc Garden, M.D., who is responsible for legal issues, and Joanna Fisher, M.D., who oversees quality assurance. The CPEC staff is active on many hospital committees and has three representatives on the hospital executive committee.

All CPEC staff members are active in private practices throughout the greater Delaware Valley. Many are staff members in Wills Eye Surgical centers. Besides resident training, members participate in the resident phacoemulsification and microsurgery course, grand rounds, family practitioner ophthalmic updates, the Ex-Resident Annual Clinical Conference, and national ophthalmic meetings.

In summary, CPEC is a large and diverse collection of dedicated ophthalmologists who contribute to the education, strength and reputation of Wills Eye Hospital.

Chapter 15

The Retina Service

William E. Benson, M.D.

Early History

The Wills Eye Hospital Retina Service, one of the world's most outstanding retina services, was founded 42 years ago. However, our story really began 151 years ago, when, in 1851, von Helmholtz invented the ophthalmoscope. Shortly thereafter, von Graefe and von Arlt reported the first accurate clinical descriptions of retinal detachment. Although numerous clinicians found breaks in the detached retina, nearly 70 years passed without any successful treatment, until Jules Gonin, the father of retinal surgery, recognized cause and effect and, in 1919, actually repaired a detached retina by closing the retinal breaks. It took him ten years to convince the world that his operation could actually cure retinal detachment. For his great contribution to the fight against blindness, Gonin was considered for the Nobel Prize in Medicine, but he died before a final decision was made.

It took several more years for Gonin's innovation to be put into practice in Philadelphia. The first detachment operations were done at Wills Eye Hospital in the 1930s by Dr. James S. Shipman (Fig. 15-2). Two of his early students, Drs. Patrick J. Kennedy and P. Robb McDonald, went on to become leaders in the field following World War II. Many eyes were cured even though direct ophthalmoscopy was all that was available to find and localize the breaks. Photocoagulation and cryotherapy had not yet been invented, so the breaks were treated with diathermy. In the 1950s Dr. Charles L. Schepens, at the Massachusetts Eye

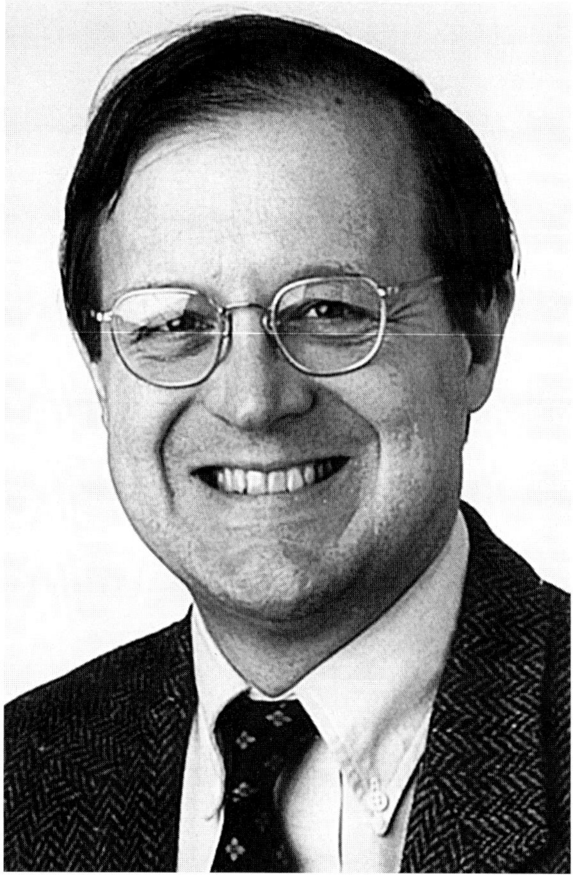

FIGURE 15-1
Dr. William E. Benson, the current Director of the Retina Service.

and Ear Infirmary in Boston, demonstrated that indirect ophthalmoscopy was superior to direct ophthalmoscopy in finding retinal breaks. This innovation, combined with scleral buckling procedures, increased the success rate from 50 to 90

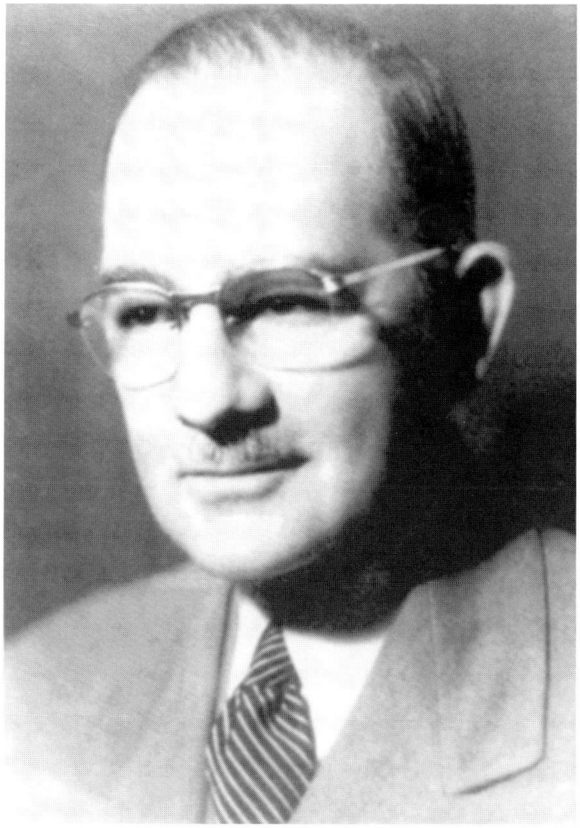

FIGURE 15-2
Dr. James S. Shipman, the father of retinal detachment surgery at Wills.

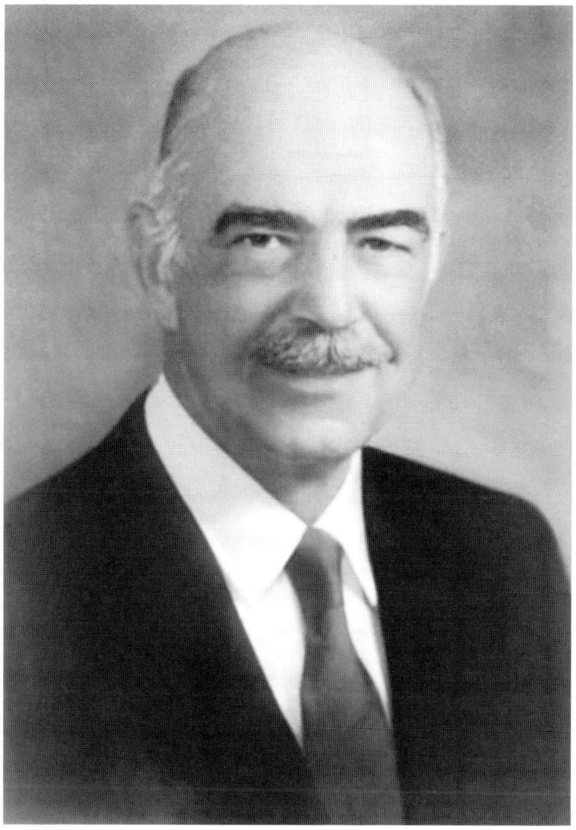

FIGURE 15-3
Dr. P. Robb McDonald, the first Director of the Retina Service.

percent. Gone were the days of prolonged pre- and postoperative bed rest with sandbags to prevent head movements. Instead, patients were mobilized the next day. Because of Dr. McDonald's close personal association with Dr. Schepens these advances were promptly brought to Wills.

Also in the 1950s, Professor Gerd-Meyer-Schwickerath in Bonn, Germany revolutionized the management of retinovascular diseases, intraocular tumors, and retinal detachment with his invention of the xenon arc photocoagulator. Between 1957 and 1959 he trained Dr. William Tasman (Fig. 15-4), who was serving with the U.S. Air Force in Germany, in the use of his new instrument. In 1960 Dr. William H. Annesley, Jr. (Fig. 15-5) traveled to Bonn, where he, too, became proficient in using the photocoagulator. He was the first to use it at Wills and later was instrumental in bringing the argon, krypton, and dye lasers to Wills.

For about 125 years after its founding, Wills had no subspecialists. During the era of nine service chiefs most of the staff performed all types of surgery including retinal detachment surgery. In 1957, however, Dr. Kennedy took the first steps toward the creation of vertical services at Wills. He assigned certain individuals to do oculoplastics, others to cornea, and a third contingent to retina. Dr. McDonald's service soon followed suit. In 1960 the Board of City Trusts recognized the changing times and certified the Retina Service as the first vertical service at Wills. The original members were the first Director, Dr. McDonald, Dr. Annesley and Dr. Charles J. Rife. Dr. Shipman (for whom the service was renamed in 1969) was

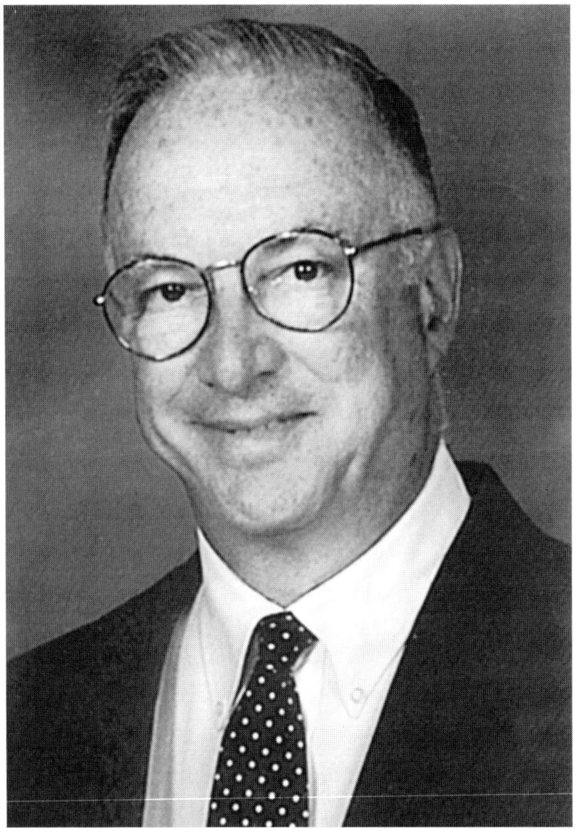

FIGURE 15-4
Dr. William Tasman, former co-Director of the Retina Service and current Ophthalmologist-in-Chief.

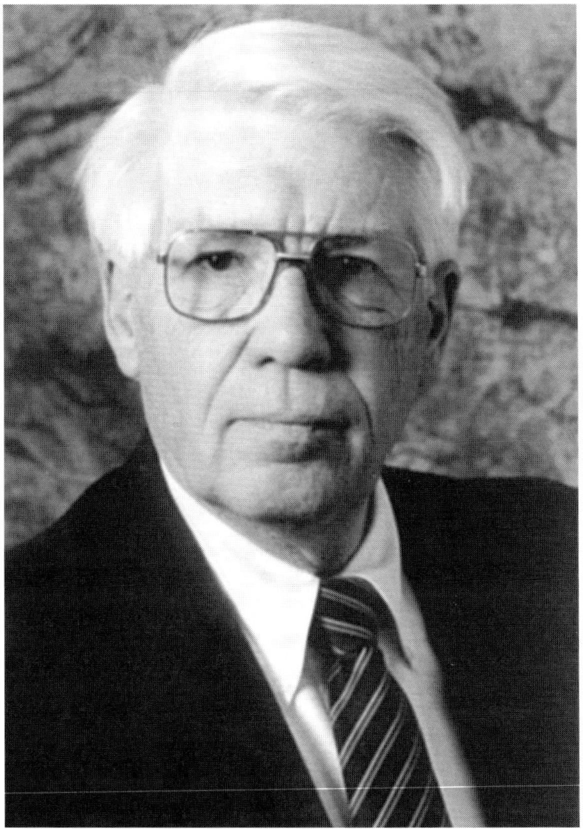

FIGURE 15-5
Dr. William H. Annesley, Jr., the second Director of the Retina Service.

Consultant. Within the next few years, the Retina Service was treating the majority of retinal detachment cases at Wills.

In 1962 Dr. Tasman completed a fellowship with Dr. Schepens and returned to Philadelphia to become the fourth member of the service. The fifth member of the service, Dr. Lov K. Sarin (Fig. 15-6) was also its first retinal fellow. Although he initially came to Wills to work in research under Dr. Irving Leopold, Wills' first ophthalmologist-in-chief, his interest and skill in the use of the indirect ophthalmoscope soon led him to become a leading retinal surgeon. In the mid-1960s Drs. Tasman and Sarin were named co-Directors of the service. Dr. McDonald continued as Director until 1970 when he moved his practice to Lankenau Hospital. Dr. Annesley succeeded him, serving as Director until 1992.

The 1970s

In 1970, Dr. Robert Machemer at the Bascom Palmer Eye Institute in Miami invented pars plana vitrectomy, which has saved the vision of many patients with diabetic retinopathy, complicated retinal detachments, and other conditions with opaque media. One of his early fellows was Dr. William E. Benson (Fig. 15-7), the current Director of the Wills Retina Service. Dr. Alfred C. Lucier, an excellent teacher who has taught scleral buckling procedures to many residents and fellows, joined the service in 1970. In 1971, Dr. Jay L. Federman, who has been the leader in bringing many new vitrectomy techniques to Wills, joined the service. He invented the SITE, an early improvement on Dr. Machemer's instrument. He later introduced the use of silicone oil and perfluorocarbon liquids to Wills.

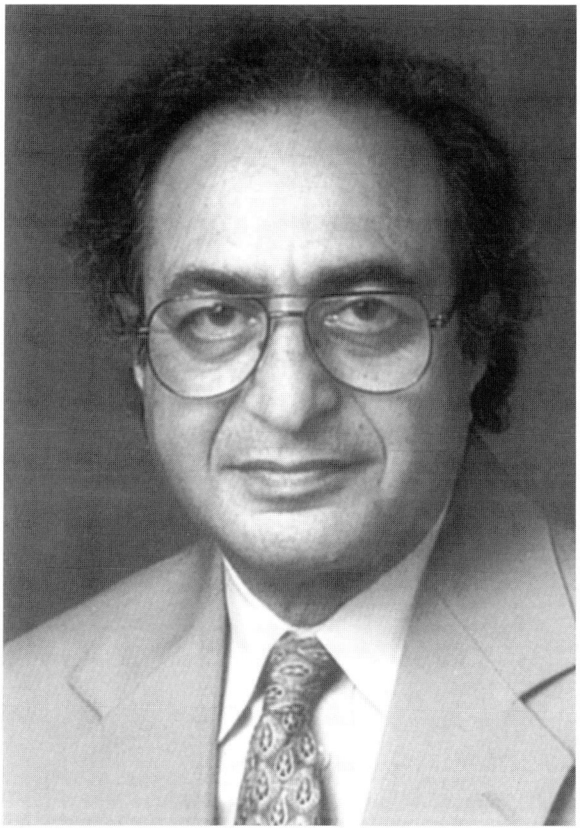

FIGURE 15-6
Dr. Lov K. Sarin, first fellow and current co-Director of the Retina Service.

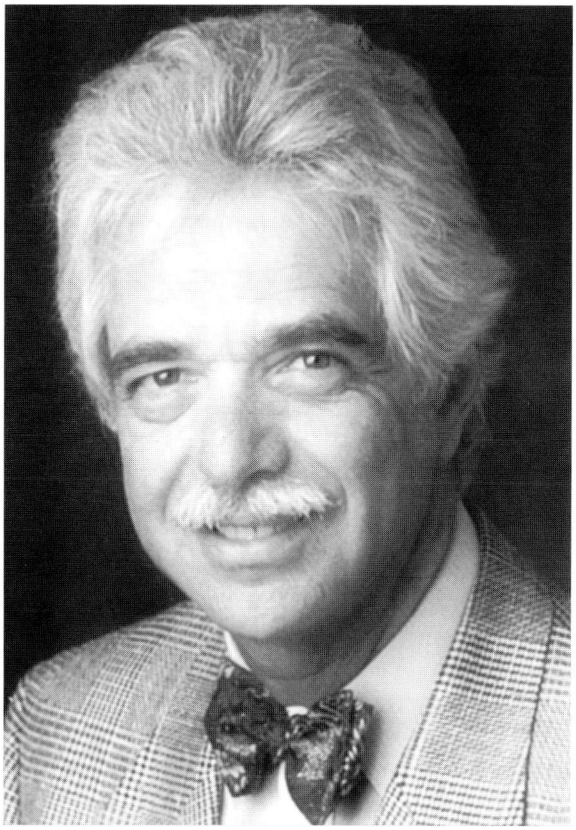

FIGURE 15-7
Dr. Jay L. Federman, current co-Director of the Retina Service.

In 1974, only 14 years after the "revolutionary" founding of the Retina Service itself, Dr. Annesley recognized that the continuing explosion of knowledge required further subspecialization. He created the Oncology Unit under the direction of Dr. Jerry A. Shields, an ex-resident and ex-retinal fellow. In 1978, it became a vertical service in its own right. The Oncology Service added ex-retinal fellow Dr. James J. Augsburger in 1980. Both have contributed extensively to the ophthalmic literature on ocular neoplasms and simulating conditions and are nationally and internationally known. Dr. Augsburger joined the Retina Service in 1990 as Consultant. In 1999 he left Wills to become Chairman of the Department of Ophthalmology of the University of Cincinnati.

Increasing experience with fluorescein angiography and argon laser photocoagulation resulted in marked improvement in the diagnosis and management of conditions such as diabetic retinopathy, retinal vein occlusions, and choroidal neovascular membranes. Reflecting these advances, the Retinovascular Unit was formed in 1975. The initial Director was Dr. Richard E. Goldberg. One year later, Dr. Larry E. Magargal finished his retinal fellowship and become co-Director. Dr. Gary C. Brown was named Director in 1990. This unit has made many significant contributions to the retinovascular literature. Dr. Goldberg retired in 2000 and Dr. Magargal in 2001.

The 1980s

The increasing importance of immunology in ophthalmology and the complexity of the multiple causes of ocular inflammation led to the establishment of the Uveitis Unit in 1981 under the direction of Dr. David H. Fischer, an ex-retinal fellow who also studied at the famous Proctor Institute in San Francisco and at the Moorfields Eye Hospital in London. In 1982, Dr. Jonathan B. Belmont, an ex-resident who also studied at the Proctor Foundation and at the Scripps Clinic in La Jolla, California, was named co-Director.

We celebrated the Wills Eye Retina Service's 25th Anniversary in 1985 with a scientific program and convocation at which we were fortunate to honor some of the giants of our profession. Thomas Jefferson University awarded degrees to the late Professor Gerd Meyer-Schwickerath from Essen, Germany, who, as discussed above, invented the xenon arc photocoagulator; the late Dr. Edward W. D. Norton from the Bascom Palmer Eye Institute in Miami, Florida, who contributed mightily to the surgical management of retinal detachment and who trained and nurtured many of today's leaders in the management of retinal diseases; Dr. Arnall Patz from the Wilmer Institute, Johns Hopkins University in Baltimore, who was a pioneer in the understanding of retinopathy of prematurity and various retinovascular diseases; and Dr. Schepens, mentioned above, one of the all-time greats in the management of retinal detachment.

The 1980's also saw the addition of some more excellent teachers and clinicians: Dr. Peter V. Palena (1980) who was the Director of the Retina Service of the Department of Ophthalmology of Thomas Jefferson University until its merger with Wills; Dr. J. Arch McNamara (1985), who has been invited to talk about retinopathy of prematurity at the United Nations; Dr. Joseph I. Maguire (1989), who has written important papers on boxing injuries and indocyanine green angiography; and Dr. Robert C. Kleiner (1989), who wrote one of the initial papers on choroidal polypoidal dystrophy.

The 1990s

In 1992, Dr. Benson, an ex-retinal fellow at the Bascom Palmer Eye Institute, who came to Wills in 1977 after serving as Director of the Retina Service of the Scheie Eye Institute for two years, was named Director of the Retina Service. Drs. Federman and Sarin were named co-Directors. The 1990s also saw the addition of still more excellent teachers and clinicians: Dr. James F. Vander (RS, 1990), who wrote one of the first papers on TPA-assisted removal of submacular hemorrhages; Dr. Arunan Sivalingam (1991), one of our leading surgeons; Dr. Tamara R. Vrabec (1994) who has written several important papers on AIDS-related retinopathies; and Dr. Carl D. Regillo (1998), and Dr. Allen C. Ho (1999) who have re-energized our research efforts, have published many scientific articles and have co-authored valuable textbooks.

The 21st Century

In March 2000, we celebrated our 40th Anniversary with a scientific symposium, entitled "Current Concepts in the Management of Macular Degeneration," program. At a concurrent convocation, we were again fortunate to honor more of the giants of our profession. Degrees were awarded to Professor J. Donald M. Gass of Bascom Palmer, who is the unquestioned "King" of macular diseases and medical ophthalmology; Dr. Charles D. Kelman of New York Medical College, a Wills alumnus who invented not only cryoextraction but also phacoemulsification of cataract; and Dr. Robert Machemer, Professor and Chairman emeritus of Duke University, who invented pars plana vitrectomy. In 2001, the service expanded to its current strength of 20 active members by adding more young blood: Drs. Brian P. Connelly (ex-Wills resident and fellow), Richard S. Kaiser, and Adam Martidis. All three have already made a strong impact on our academic program. Finally, in August 2002, Dr. Mitchell Fineman (ex-Wills resident and fellow) joined the service.

Diagnostic & Imaging Services

Retinal photography began on the Retina Service in the late 1960s as a legacy of the pioneering work of Dr. Arthur J. Bedell. Fluorescein angiography, which was popularized by Dr. Gass in the early 1960s, soon became an important part of our diagnostic armamentarium under Mr. Johnny Justice in 1966 and Mr. Terry Tomer in 1968. In 1970 Drs. Federman and Shields established weekly fluorescein conferences, which have helped to make diagnostic photography a major resident and fellow teaching resource. Mr. Bob Curtin has been the Director of the Photography Service since 1998.

Another unit vital to the Retina Service is Visual Physiology. Dr. Sarin introduced ultrasonography to the Retina Service in 1964. In 1973, Dr. Lucier began electrophysiology testing with the help of Dr. David Pao, work that led to the establishment of a full ERG/EOG testing facility on the Service in 1980 under the direction of Dr. Joseph I. Markoff. More recently, ultrasonic biomicroscopy and optical coherence tomography have been added. Ms. Libba Affel joined the Service in 1985 and has been technical director since then.

Other Members of the Retina Service

We would like to acknowledge the contributions of four ex-fellows who began their careers on the Retina Service and have continued them elsewhere: Dr. Richard Lanning (1978–1980), Dr. Hermann Schubert (1987–1990), Dr. Eric Shakin (1985–1989), and Dr. Tien Wong (1993–1997). All are excellent teachers and clinicians. We are grateful for the time they spent with us.

Contributions of the Retina Service

Members of the Retina Service have played strong leadership roles at Wills Eye Hospital. Drs. McDonald, Annesley, Tasman, Belmont, and Brown have been Presidents of the Wills Alumni Society. Drs. Annesley, Tasman, Sarin, Federman, Benson and Lucier have been Presidents of the Wills Medical Staff. Dr. Tasman has been the Ophthalmologist-in-Chief since 1985.

The Retina Service is very proud of the national recognition awarded to its past and current members. Drs. Tasman and Benson have served as Chairman of the American Board of Ophthalmology. Dr. Tasman has also served as President of the American Academy of Ophthalmology. Six members have met the requirements of the American Ophthalmological Society (Annesley, Tasman, Federman, Benson, Augsburger, and Brown) and Dr. Tasman is a past President and past Editor of the *Transactions*, as well as a recipient of the Howe Medal. Fifteen members have been elected to the Retina Society (Drs. Annesley, Tasman, Sarin, Goldberg, Federman, Benson, Augsburger, Fischer, Brown, McNamara, Lucier, Kleiner, Regillo, Ho, and Vander). Dr. Tasman is an ex-President. Ten members have been elected to the Macula Society (Drs. Tasman, Goldberg, Federman, Benson, Augsburger, McNamara, Brown, Kleiner, Regillo, and Ho). Thirteen members belong to the Vitreous Society (Drs. Augsburger, Belmont, McNamara, Brown, Kleiner, Fischer, Vander, Regillo, Ho, Maguire, Sivalingam, Vrabec, and Wong). Drs. Fischer, Belmont, and Vrabec are members of the Uveitis Society.

Research at the Retina Service

In 1984 Dr. Larry Donoso, an internationally esteemed investigator who has contributed hundreds of articles to the literature, was named Director of Retina Research. Dr. Donoso subsequently became the Director of the Research Department of Wills, and served in that capacity until 2002. To financially support research, the Philadelphia Retina Endowment was established in 1984, the Bower Laboratory in 1988, and the Vitreoretinal Foundation in 1990.

The Retina Service has made many contributions to ophthalmic research. Several members have been Principal Investigators for national collaborative trials. Dr. Tasman was Principal Investigator (PI) of the Diabetic Retinopathy Study (DRS) and with Drs. Brown and McNamara the PI of the CRYO-ROP study of which Dr. Tasman helped to write the protocol. Dr. Benson was PI of the Early Treatment Diabetic Retinopathy Study (ETDRS). Dr. Federman was PI of the Diabetic Retinopathy Vitrectomy Study (DRVS) and of national studies on intravitreal silicone oil, gases, and perfluorocarbon liquids. Dr. Brown was PI of the Endophthalmitis Vitrectomy Study (EVS). Dr. Vander was PI of the posterior ROP early treatment trial.

Under the guidance of the current Director of the Retina Clinical Research Unit, Dr. Regillo, the Service is involved in numerous clinical trials. The following clinical trials and their Principal Investigators are ongoing:

- A phase IIB/III, multicenter, randomized, double-masked, controlled study to evaluate the safety and efficacy of an intravitreal fluocinolone acetonide insert in patients with uveitis. (Drs. Belmont and Ho)
- A phase II randomized, open-label, multicenter controlled trial to assess the safety and efficacy of dexamethasone posterior segment drug delivery system. (Dr. Federman)
- An evaluation for safety and efficacy of anecortave acetate sterile suspension versus placebo following a single sub-Tenon's injection for the inhibition of choroidal neovascularization in patients with exudative age-related-macular degeneration. (Dr. Ho)
- A phase IB open-label multi-center trial to establish the safety and pharmacokinetic profile of an intravitreal injection of an anti-VEGF aptamer in eyes with age-related macular degeneration. (Dr. Ho)
- A phase II/III randomized, double-masked, controlled, dose-ranging, multicenter comparative trial, in parallel groups, to establish the safety and efficacy of intravitreal injections. (Dr. Ho)
- A phase III multicenter, randomized, masked, controlled study to evaluate the safety and efficacy of Retisert™, an intravitreal fluocinolone acetonide implant in the treatment of patients with diabetic macular edema undergoing vitrectomy. (Dr. Ho)
- A pilot, randomized, masked, controlled study to evaluate an intravitreal fluocinolone acetonide implant for the treatment of predominantly occult subfoveal choroidal neovascularization in patients with age-related macular degeneration. (Dr. Ho)
- Laser to Drusen Trial sponsored by the Commonwealth of Pennsylvania. (Dr. Ho)
- A pilot randomized masked controlled study to evaluate an intravitreal fluocinolone acetonide implant for the treatment of predominantly classic subfoveal choroidal neovascularization in patients with age-related macular degeneration. (Dr. Kaiser)
- Intravitreal corticosteroid for the treatment of macular edema. (Dr. Martidis)
- Transpupillary thermotherapy of occult subfoveal choroidal neovascular membranes in patients with age-related-macular-degeneration (The TTT study). (Dr. Regillo)
- Purlytin photodynamic therapy for choroidal neovascularization, a multicenter trial. (Dr. Regillo)
- Intravitreal Vitrase (hyaluronidase) injection for clearance of severe vitreous hemorrhage, a multicenter trial. (Dr. Regillo)
- A study to assess the effects of transpupillary thermotherapy on normal human retinas of eyes scheduled for enucleation. (Dr. Regillo)
- A phase II/III multicenter, randomized, masked, controlled study to evaluate Retisert™, an intravitreal fluocinolone acetonide implant, in the treatment of patients with diabetic macular edema. (Dr. Regillo)
- Feeder vessel photocoagulation for predominantly occult subfoveal choroidal neovascularization due to age-related macular degeneration. (Dr. Sivalingam)
- A phase III clinical trial for protein kinase C beta inhibitor for diabetic retinopathy. (Dr. Vander)
- A 3-month randomized, placebo-controlled, double-masked, multicenter, phase II study of the effects of adjunctive diclofenac therapy after Visudyne PDT in patients with predominantly classic subfoveal CNV secondary to age-related macular degeneration. (Dr. Vander)

We have had countless papers accepted by peer-reviewed national and international journals and have been authors or editors of many textbooks including:

- *Retinal Detachment. Diagnosis and Management* (1st and 2nd editions) (Dr. Benson)
- *Diabetes Mellitus and Its Ocular Complications* (Drs. Benson, Brown & Tasman)
- *Retina and Vitreous,* Section 4 of the Basic & Clinical Science Course, American Academy of Ophthalmology (Dr. Benson, editor)
- *Annual of Ophthalmic Laser Surgery* (Dr. Benson, co-editor with Drs. Marshall and Spaeth)
- *Current Techniques in Ophthalmic Laser Surgery* (Dr. Benson, co-editor with Drs. Coscas and Katz)
- *Congenital Anomalies of the Optic Disc* (Drs. Brown & Tasman)
- *Laser Therapy of the Anterior Segment* (Dr. Brown, with Drs. Spaeth and Schwartz)
- *Recognizing Patterns of Childhood Diseases* (Dr. Brown, with Drs. Nelson and Arentsen)
- *Retina and Vitreous, Section 4 of the Basic & Clinical Science Course*, American Academy of Ophthalmology (Dr. Brown, editor)
- *Value-Based Health Care* (in press) (Dr. Brown, with Dr. M. Brown and S. Sharma)
- *Retina: Color Atlas and Synopsis* (Drs. Ho, Brown, McNamara, Regillo, Vander & Franco Recchia)
- *Retina & Vitreous* (Drs. Federman and Vrabec, co-editors with Drs. Gouras, Schubert, & Slusher) (Part of a multivolume text: *Textbook of Ophthalmology*, Podos & Yanoff, editors)
- *Retinal Detachment. Diagnosis and Management* (3rd Edition) (Drs. Regillo and Benson)
- *Ocular Posterior Segment Imaging* (Dr. Regillo, with Drs. T. A. Ciulla and A. Harris)
- *Vitreoretinal Disease: The Essentials* (Dr. Regillo with Dr. Brown and Dr. H.W. Flynn, editors)
- *Retinal Diseases in Children* (Dr. Tasman, editor)
- *Diseases of the Peripheral Fundus* (Dr. Tasman, editor with Dr. Shields)
- *Duane's Clinical Ophthalmology* (Dr. Tasman, editor)
- *Retinopathy of Prematurity* (Dr. Tasman, co-editor with Dr. J. Flynn)
- *Clinical Decisions in Medical Retinal Disease* (Dr. Tasman, editor)
- *Wills Eye Hospital Color Atlas of Ophthalmology* (Dr. Tasman, editor)
- *Secrets of Ophthalmology*, 1st and 2nd edition (Dr. Vander, co-editor with Dr. J. Gault)

The Training Program

The Retina Service over the last 25 years has been committed to resident training. Today's residents quickly become proficient in indirect ophthalmoscopy and see a wealth of fundus disease. They learn laser therapy of proliferative and macular retinopathies and are trained in the repair of primary retinal detachments.

Between 1962 and 1975 the Retina Service trained residents from the Philadelphia Naval Hospital. Each resident would spend about six months on the Retina Service. The first to rotate through our service was Dr. James Rosborough, followed shortly thereafter by Drs. Bernard Blais, Donald Roy, Carol Reinert, and Ray Townsend. The tradition of contributing to the ophthalmologic care of our nation's servicemen and servicewomen by teaching military physicians has been continued recently by training Drs. Raul Moreno, Gordon Byrnes, Thaddeus Krolicki, Carl Regillo, Jeffrey Blice, Mark Nelson, Kent Blade, and Gary Lane.

As indicated earlier, fellowship training began in 1960 with Dr. Sarin. With developments in laser therapy and the treatment of tumors, vascular disease, and uveitis, it became obvious that a one-year training period was too short. So, in 1980, it was changed to two years and remains that today. As of July 2002, 129 ex-fellows are practicing in 32 states, the District of Columbia, and Puerto Rico and in five other countries (Canada, Great Britain, Saudi Arabia, the Philippines, and Brazil). Dr. Regillo has been the Retina Fellowship Program Director since 1999.

The first 42 years of the Retina Service were years of growth, development, teaching, and productivity. With the excellent staff we now have (Fig. 15-8), we are confident that the next 42 years will see even more exciting developments.

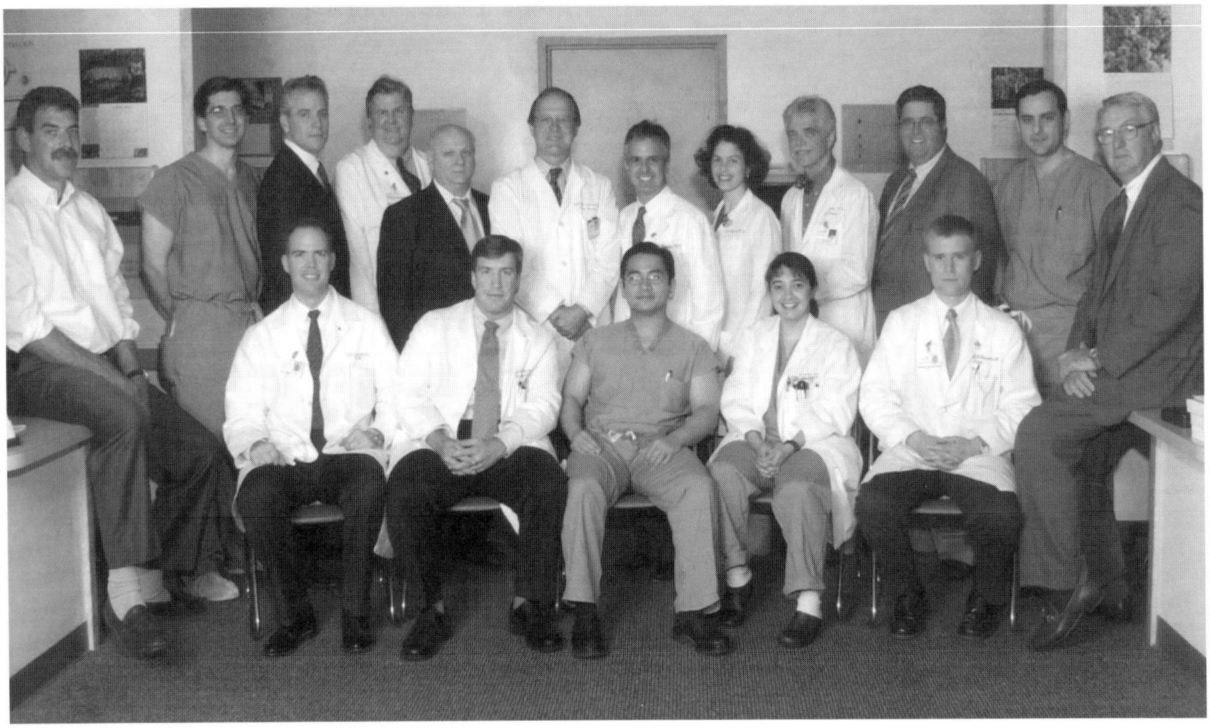

FIGURE 15-8

The Retina Service in 2002. Front Row (all fellows): Blade, Nelson, Borrillo, Schuler, Tennant. Rear Row: Belmont, Kaiser, Maguire, Fischer, Donoso, Benson, Regillo, Vrabec, Federman, McNamara, Martidis, Lucier. Absent: Brown, Connolly, Fineman, Ho, Kleiner, Sivalingam, Tasman, Vander.

Chapter 16

The Glaucoma Service

A History of the Glaucoma Service

George L. Spaeth, M.D., Director

The William and Anna Goldberg Glaucoma Service and Research Laboratories has evolved from a single room in which tonography was performed in 1960 by the single employee of the Glaucoma Service, to a department which is larger, more complex, and more productive than many entire departments of ophthalmology. For approximately the first 40 years the service grew in a manner fairly characteristic of Wills Eye Hospital. Specifically, its major driving force was its clinical strength, both in patient care and teaching. As the medical staff increased from one to double digits, the geographic area served by the Glaucoma Service and the facilities offered also increased, so that by the start of the 21st Century, Glaucoma Service physicians were caring for patients from south of Wilmington, Delaware, north to the center of Pennsylvania, west to the center of Pennsylvania, and throughout the southern half of New Jersey.

The Wills Eye Hospital itself, however, continued to be the vital center of this activity, with the Glaucoma Research Laboratory,

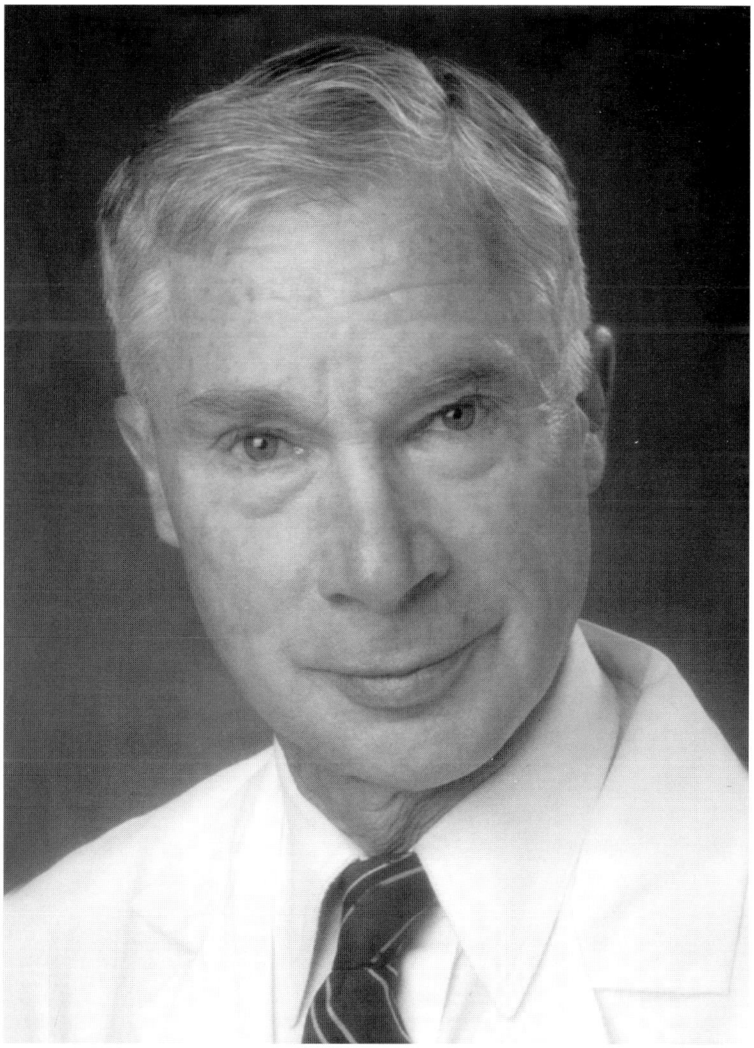

FIGURE 16-1
George L. Spaeth, M.D..

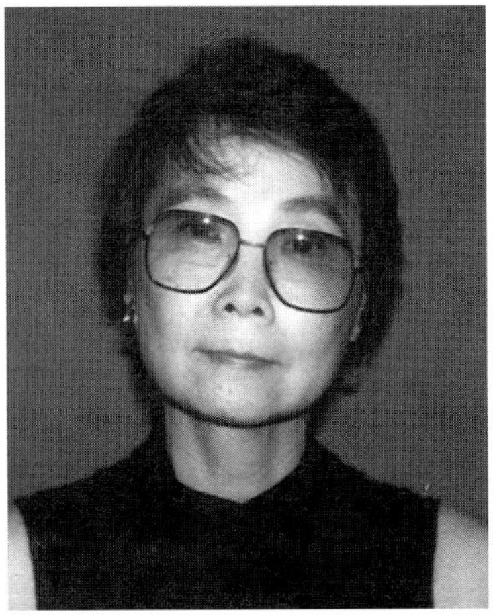

Anne K. Chan, M.D.

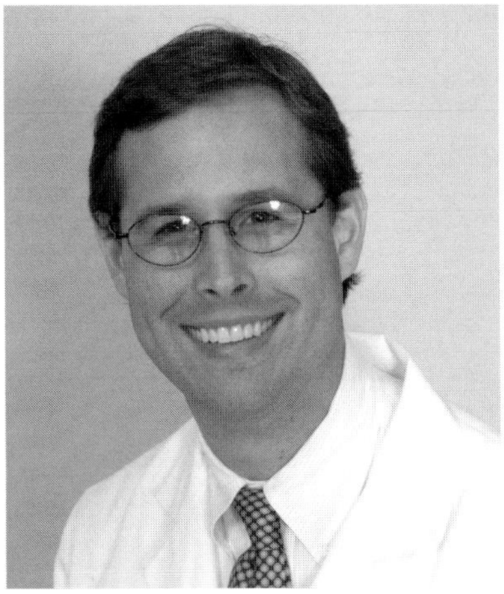

Jeffrey D. Henderer, M.D.

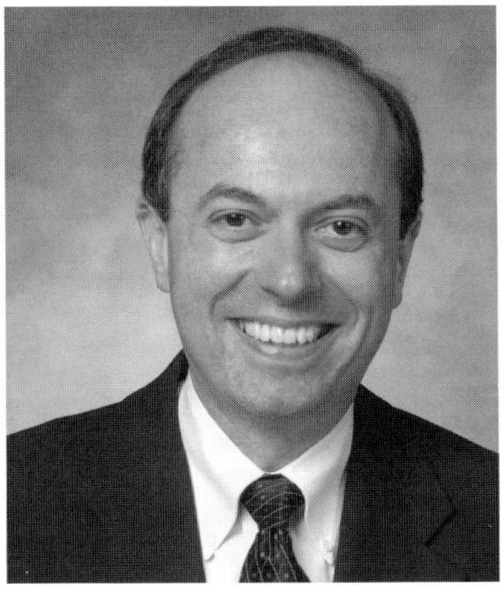

L. Jay Katz, M.D.

extensive facilities to study blood flow and perform clinical research, and a body of clinical and research fellows actively involved in training superb ophthalmologists from around the world in how to diagnose and manage patients with glaucoma. Additionally, patients from around the world came in increasing numbers to the hub at Wills Eye Hospital to obtain care with its unique Wills Eye Hospital character: superb, personalized care based on the recognition that each person is unique and that "standardized care" is never the best care. Because of their close working relationship with each other and their vast experience, the physicians on the Glaucoma Service of Wills Eye Hospital/Jefferson Medical College bring to every patient a level of competence that may be matched, but probably is not exceeded by any institution in the world.

The teaching on the Glaucoma Service reflects the same passion and competence; it is no wonder, then, that physicians from around the world come to train there. Finally, while research has been an important part of the Service from the start, initially under the innovative and productive direction of Irving Leopold, one of the great ophthalmic researchers, the breadth and depth of research gradually increased, recognizing the special strengths of Wills Eye Hospital in the field of clinical research, culminating in the appointment of Dr. William Steinmann as Research Director in 2000 and the development of the full-service Glaucoma Service Research Center with a dedicated and highly trained staff.

The creation of the Research Center would not have been possible without the remarkably generous support of William and Anna Goldberg, whose gift of $500,000 early in the history of the Service, established a research unit, and subsequent bequests and contributions such as the gift of $2 million of Walter Morgan in honor of Richard and Karen Wilson. What follows is a brief iteration of some of the events that have led up to the Service as it stands today, in which there continues to be a passion for trying to provide skilled, knowledgeable, compassionate patient care, teaching based on profoundly meaningful mentoring relationships, research which is innovative, practical, evidence-based, highly scientific, and humane, and, finally, public service in many areas. The physicians and staff of the Glaucoma Service are aware that their unit is one of a great number of excellent centers, many of which are under the direction of graduates of the Wills Eye Hospital Glaucoma Service.

Furthermore, the Wills Eye Hospital has a long history of providing excellent care for patients with glaucoma. Important contributions to the literature about glaucoma were made by Wills physicians over 150 years ago. Laboratory research was not an important part of the early history of Wills Eye Hospital. However, primary research, closely related to pharmacology, was initiated in the 1960s. Leopold worked in a small research building located on the north side of Brandywine at the rear of the main hospital, where Harry Green performed seminal research regarding the mechanism of action of

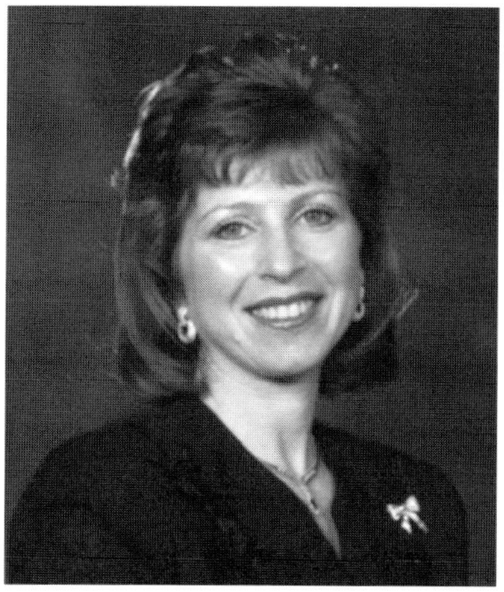

Marlene R. Moster, M.D.

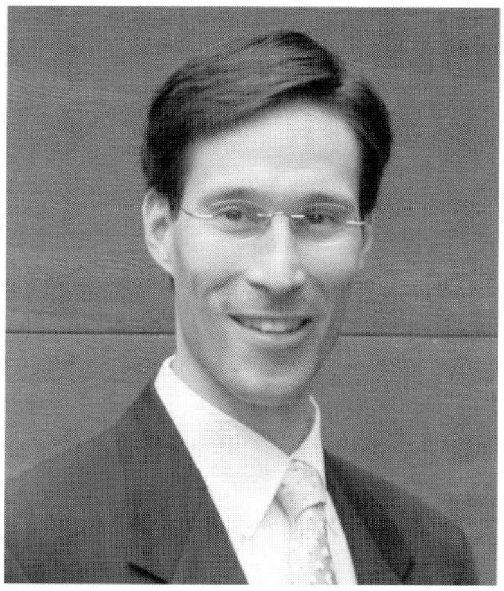

Jonathan S. Myers, M.D.

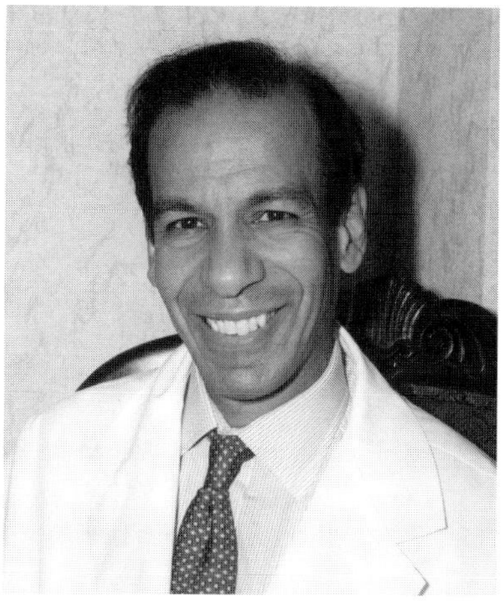

Joseph M. Ortiz, M.D.

the carbonic anhydrase inhibitors as well as other topics. Leopold himself had earlier been the discoverer of the intraocular-pressure-lowering effects of echothiophate iodide, a useful drug in the treatment of the noninflammatory glaucomas, especially in people who have had their cataracts removed.

Leopold, a pioneer in medical education in the U.S., was one of the first ophthalmic leaders to understand the importance of developing a unified approach to a particular entity, such as retinal disease or glaucoma. In 1961, he established the first fellowship for providing specialized training in the field of glaucoma at the Wills Eye Hospital. Such fellowships, now routine, were rare in the field of ophthalmology at the time. Leopold started these training positions at Wills Eye Hospital.

Dr. Clay Evatt was the first postdoctoral fellow appointed at Wills Eye Hospital for the study of glaucoma, and about the same time Dr. Anne Chan was hired by Dr. Leopold as a full-time glaucoma specialist. Dr. Chan had as her office a space about four feet wide and ten feet long beside the elevator shaft on the second floor of the Hospital, and it was here that the major test of that period of time was performed, specifically, tonography. A tonography technician was hired by the Hospital, although she also had a variety of other responsibilities.

Gonioscopy was performed by Dr. George Dublin in another small room elsewhere on the mezzanine. Slit-lamp gonioscopy was just starting to become popular, and those who employed it were few and self-taught. The direct method of gonioscopy with a Koeppe lens was used in the operating room by a handful of individuals, notably Dr. Dublin, who had a special interest in glaucoma. A separate room was also used for studying visual fields through the use of an arc perimeter and a tangent screen. Patients with any type of condition thought to need a visual field examination were seen here. The typical plot of the visual field seemed to be concentric circles of varying sizes, usually with a carefully drawn oval blind spot on the appropriate side. But the tonography room was of special significance because the patients referred there were patients with one specific diagnostic entity—glaucoma. Patients were routinely seen in the general clinics, with no segregation based on diagnostic entity.

It is vitally important to remember, when considering the care of patients at Wills Eye Hospital (and other institutions), that until the late 1960s the diagnosis and management of glaucoma was straightforward. Specifically, glaucoma was a disease that was present when the intraocular pressure was above 21 mm Hg, and the treatment was designed to lower the intraocular pressure below 21 mm Hg. Diagnosis and management were almost completely on the basis of intraocular pressure or a corollary of intraocular pressure, the determination of the coefficient of aqueous outflow, ie, how easily the fluid in the front of the eye ran out of the eye through drainage canals as measured by tonography. At an

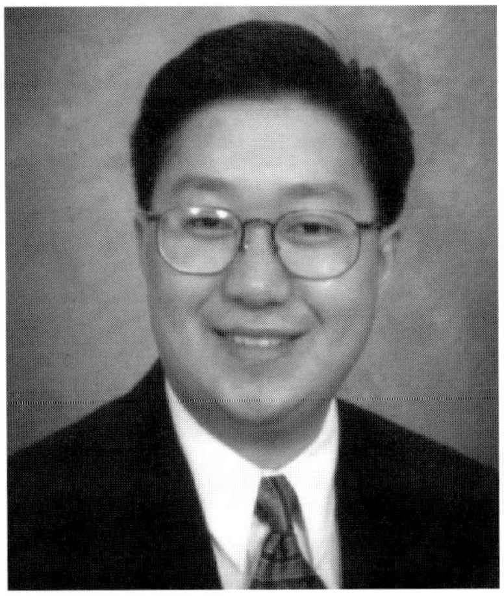

Douglas J. Rhee, M.D.

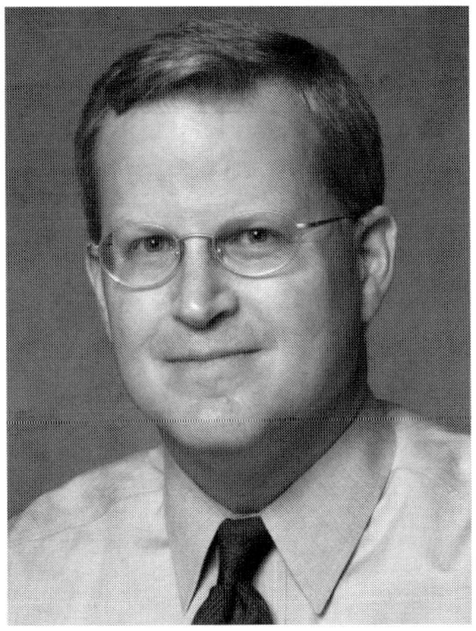

Courtland M. Schmidt, M.D.

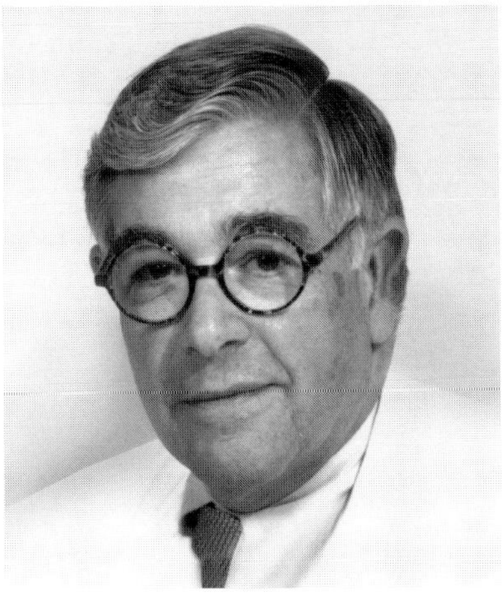

Louis W. Schwartz, M.D.

early conference held at the Wills Eye Hospital, the tonography machine was mentioned as the most important instrument in the diagnosis and management of glaucoma. While the development of optic nerve damage had long been recognized as an essential part of what happened to patients with glaucoma, the concept of using changes in the appearance of the optic disc as a way to manage patients with glaucoma was still in the future.

The patients at Wills Eye Hospital who were seen on an outpatient basis were evaluated in three separate large rooms, called the clinics I, II, and III. A resident and one or more members of the attending staff would see about 80 patients, largely during the afternoon; this consisted of a history and an examination with a penlight.

The standard entry into the clinic patient's chart would include determination of visual acuity, intraocular pressure (as measured with a Schiotz tonometer) in the large outpatient clinic, and a recommendation as to what treatment was appropriate. Comments regarding the optic disc were rare. Usually, the total entry on a patient occupied one line in the chart. If further special testing was thought necessary, an appointment was made for that; for example, if dilation was thought necessary the patient was dilated and was checked later in a "dark room" adjacent to the large clinic. A slit-lamp was also available for examination in that room. Dr. Leopold, then ophthalmologist-in-chief of the Hospital, recognized the advantages to patients and to the training process to segregate patients with glaucoma. This was followed up by the second ophthalmologist-in-chief, Arthur H. Keeney. Consequently, one of the three clinics, specifically Clinic III, was transformed into "the glaucoma clinic."

Dr. Keeney invited Dr. George Spaeth to work full-time at Wills Eye Hospital with the glaucoma patients. That year, Spaeth, who had been practicing with his brother Philip and his father, Edmund, assumed responsibility for the care of patients with glaucoma and the development of the Glaucoma Service. Clinic III was a large room, around 40 by 80 feet, filled with chairs for the patients and long tables beside which the physicians sat to examine the patients. Gloria Stephens, the clinic clerk, knew all the patients and kept the physicians organized. A social worker, Anne Sommer, also provided invaluable assistance. Patients were examined with a penlight, and intraocular pressures were measured with the head held back, using a Schiotz tonometer. The usual entry in the chart consisted of one line listing visual acuity, intraocular pressure, and the drugs employed in treatment.

While Dr. Spaeth provided teaching and patient care, the responsibility for supervision lay with the staff of each of the weekday Services. Patients requiring admission for any reason were admitted under the care of the daily Service chief. There was one resident surgeon in each clinic and usually two staff members. Around eighty patients were seen each afternoon. Those requiring slit-lamp examina-

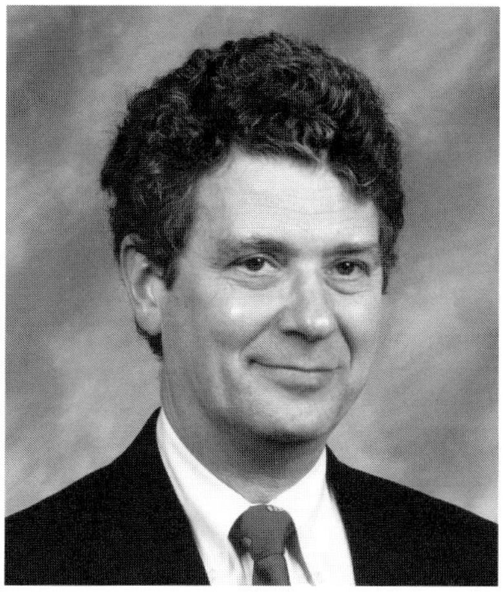

Elliot Werner, M.D.

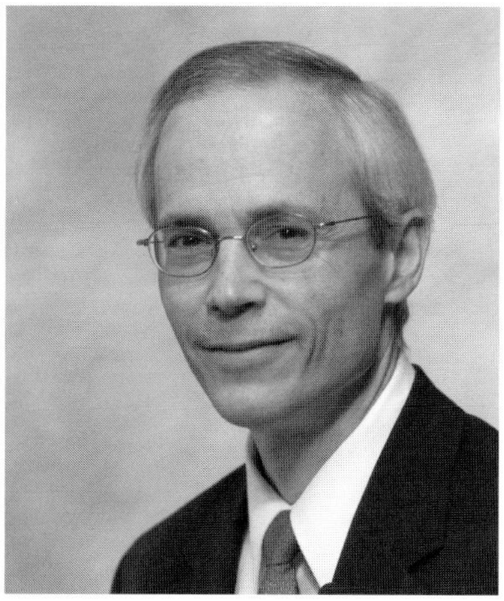

Richard P. Wilson, M.D.

tions or fundoscopy were examined later in the afternoon in the dark room adjacent to the clinic. Those needing gonioscopy, tonography, or a visual field examination were referred to the appropriate unit.

Around 1970 Curtis Pritchard was given $60,000 by William and Ann Goldberg to buy new equipment and build individual examination rooms for Clinic III. These plasterboard cubicles were simple and stark, but they provided privacy and permitted the use of slit lamps. This change was accompanied by one that was even more important in the history of the Glaucoma Service—the decision of Dr. Harold Barnshaw, one of the Chiefs of the Charity Care Services at Wills Eye Hospital to have his Service glaucoma patients cared for entirely by the staff of the Glaucoma Service. Thus, not only the outpatient care of these "charity" patients, but their inpatient and surgical care as well, became the responsibility of the Glaucoma Service staff, which at that point consisted of Dr. Spaeth and Dr. Anne Chan. A short while later, Dr. Patrick Kennedy, another one of the five Chiefs, made the same decision. The result was a real Glaucoma Service, with a space of its own, equipment of its own, staff of its own, and patients of its own. A short while later, Dr. Philip Spaeth became one of the weekday Chiefs and also turned his Service patients over to the Glaucoma Service. Finally, there was a *bona fide* service with opportunities for meaningful training and clinical research.

Since that time, the Service has grown in all aspects. Basic research has included investigations of aqueous humor to characterize the factor that appears to inhibit cell growth and the pharmacokinetics of 5-fluorouracil incorporated into liposomes, as well as molecular histological study of the mechanisms that affect the basic control of intraocular pressure. Early in the history of the Service, clinical research was varied but has been directed primarily to three areas: (1) methods of examination of the optic nerve, characterization of the changes observed during examination of the optic nerve, and correlation with the type, state, and stage of disease; (2) development and interpretation of static perimetry with the Octopus Computerized Perimeter, and (3) development and evaluation of surgical technique for the management of glaucoma.

The Wills Eye Hospital Glaucoma Service was largely responsible for the popularization in the United States of computerized perimetry. The first instrument in the United States was used at Baylor University in Dallas. Very shortly thereafter, the first Octopus Computerized Perimeter #201 was purchased for the Wills Eye Hospital Glaucoma Service. The obvious advantages that this provided for both patient care and research led to the purchase of a second 201. The following year a third was purchased for the Glaucoma Diagnostic Laboratory. Wills now has by far the greatest experience in the use of the Octopus Computerized Perimeter, and the first book published on the subject was co-authored by Drs. Whalen (a former fellow on the Glaucoma Service) and George Spaeth.

The Glaucoma Service obtained the first commercially available neodymium:YAG laser and led in investigating and then popularizing peripheral iridectomy with this instrument. This laser was also used by Dr. Gary Brown of the Retina Service and Dr. Stephen Lichtenstein of the General Ophthalmology Service in pioneering work in the vitreous and posterior capsule. It was the prototype instrument used in developing new techniques of glaucoma surgery, including a filtration procedure that avoids cutting the conjunctiva (laser trabeculostomy), developed by Dr. Jay Katz and Dr. Louis Schwartz, and transscleral cyclodiathermy, developed by Drs. Schwartz and Marlene Moster. This latter technique holds great promise for patients with aphakic secondary glaucomas, and Wills clinicians were uniquely experienced in the use of this technique.

The Glaucoma Service has continued its work in the development of laser surgery, most specifically with a holmium laser, and more recently with a neodymium yttrium lithium fluoride laser. The holmium laser found a place for a short while in treating specific kinds of glaucoma such as the glaucoma that occurs in patients who have had intraocular lens implants. The neodymium yttrium lithium fluoride laser can be used to create openings in the sclera as part of glaucoma surgery. This was used with some success by one of the previous fellows on the Glaucoma Service of the Wills Eye Hospital, specifically, Dr. Ronald Gross, who is now Professor of Ophthalmology and Director of the Glaucoma Service at Baylor.

Another advance for the Wills Eye Hospital Glaucoma Service was the purchase in 1985 of the PAR Image Analyzer, permitting quantitative study of the appearance of the optic disc. This highly sophisticated instrument is capable of representing changes that occur in the optic disc in a way that was not possible before. The ability to study images quantitatively can be applied to other fields as well, such as intraocular tumors, the configuration of the anterior chamber angle, and the size of the heart. This department of image analysis has grown with the acquisition of other instruments such as the Heidelberg Retina Tomograph (HRT), the Heidelberg Retinal Flow-Meter, the Nidek Scheimpflug anterior segment camera in the Glaucoma Service, and Siemens ultrasound imaging equipment for measuring blood flow to the optic nerve by the Neuro-Ophthalmology Department. Image analysis of the optic nerve, is still an evolving art and science that has become an accepted part of the clinical research of patients with glaucoma. Some ophthalmologists now use the HRT in clinical care, believing that the instrumentation is sufficiently reliable and the information it provides sufficiently reproducible that it can be used with confidence to detect changes in the appearance of the optic nerve, permitting more accurate determination of whether the optic nerve is getting worse or getting better. Since change in the nature of the optic nerve is one of the most important measurements to be made in a patient with glaucoma or suspected of having glaucoma, this is an important step ahead. Indeed, the Director of the Glaucoma Service at Wills Eye Hospital has proposed that management be based on improvement in appearance of the optic disc. This is a radical new concept, which may prove to be an important contribution. However, unless it is possible to document validly small improvements, such a methodology remains only theoretical.

Members of the Glaucoma Service at Wills Eye Hospital have contributed articles in American, European, and Asian journals, as well as such textbooks as *Diagnosis and Management of Early Primary Angle Glaucoma*, with chapters by the members of the Glaucoma Service staff; *Laser Therapy of the Anterior Segment*, by Brown, Schwartz, and George Spaeth; *Atlas of Itraocular Surgery*, by Spaeth and Koch; *Complications of Glaucoma Treatment*, by Sherwood and Spaeth; and *Ophthalmic Surgery: Principles and Practices*, edited by Spaeth.

In addition, the Glaucoma Service has provided educational materials for the American Academy of Ophthalmology in the form of modules, manuals, and television tapes. Recognition has come in the form of invitations to speak at American and European teaching institutions and such awards as the Sir Stewart Duke-Elder Award of the International Congress of Ophthalmology, the Senior Lifetime Achievement Award of the American Academy of Ophthalmology, and the Greek Glaucoma Society Agnostakis and Trantas Medal of Merit and Honor. The first President of the American Glaucoma Society was the Director of the Wills Eye Hospital Glaucoma Service and the current President is Dr. Richard Wilson.

Training ophthalmologists in the field of glaucoma has been one of the major purposes of the Wills

Eye Hospital Glaucoma Service. Its former fellows have headed glaucoma departments in the U.S. at Yale Medical School, Albany Medical School, North Carolina Medical School, Fort Knox Medical Center, Montefiore-Albert Einstein University, the University of Indiana, the University of Florida at Gainesville, the University of Florida at Jacksonville, the Naval Medical Center, San Diego; Baylor University, Houston; and other institutions. Glaucoma-Service-trained Fellows are Heads of the Department of Ophthalmology at the University of Florida, Gainesville; the State University of New York Health Science Center at Brooklyn, and the Naval Medical Center at San Diego. The Glaucoma Service has had an especially close relationship with Moorfields Eye Hospital's glaucoma specialists in London, Windsor, and Birmingham, all of whom got their glaucoma training at Wills. Mr. Roger Hitchings, a leader in the study of the early surgery for glaucoma and long head of the Moorfields Glaucoma Unit, is now head of the research unit at Moorfields.

The staff of the Glaucoma Service itself at Wills Eye Hospital has expanded consistently. It has become internationally renowned, and its members are frequently invited to speak at international conferences. The Director of the Service is on the European Board of Opthalmology. Other members are continuing active participants in conferences in South America, Africa, the Middle East, and Asia. At least four of the members of the staff have been repeatedly listed in "The Best Doctors of America." The members of the staff now include George Spaeth, Anne K. Chan, Richard Wilson, L. Jay Katz, Marlene R. Moster, Ralph Sando, Courtland Schmidt, Louis Schwartz, Jeffrey Henderer, Jonathan Myers, Douglas Rhee, Elliott Werner, Eugene Fernandes, and Jose Ortiz.

Publications continue to be produced by members of the Glaucoma Service staff and in the appendix are listed just those publications for the two years prior to publications of this text. Dr. Wilson, as an editor of the *Yearbook of Ophthalmology*, has exerted a great influence on what ophthalmologists around the world read about glaucoma and the Director of Service, as editor of *Ophthalmic Surgery*, has through his editorials and editing policy influenced the thinking of ophthalmologists world-wide. Many of the texts, such as *Ophthalmic Surgery: Principles and Practice* have become the standard textbooks utilized by residency training programs everywhere. The members of the Glaucoma Service have become leaders in the administrative aspects of the field of glaucoma. The Director was among the founders and was the first president of the American Glaucoma Society, and many of the members of the service occupy leadership positions in the American Academy of Ophthalmology, the American College of Surgeons, the Association for Research in Vision and Ophthalmology, and other ophthalmic and medical organizations.

In the field of research, the Glaucoma Service continues to be productive. Recent association with Alon Harris, PhD, of the University of Indiana has proved especially fruitful. Grants from the National Institutes of Health (National Eye Institute) have been obtained for the Collaborative Initial Treatment of Glaucoma Study, the Advanced Glaucoma Intervention Study, and the Glaucoma Laser Trial. The Wills Eye Hospital Glaucoma Service served as the disc reading center for the Glaucoma Laser Trial. Many pharmaceutical grants have been obtained, primarily through Dr. L. Jay Katz. Dr. William Steinmann has become the Research Director of the Glaucoma Service Research Center, teaching the Fellows about the design, implementation, and analysis of clinical research. His weekly conferences have become an essential part of the training program on the Glaucoma Service.

The William and Ann Goldberg Glaucoma Service at Wills Eye Hospital/Jefferson Medical College has grown from a small back room to a large and expanding unit providing patient care, training at all levels, and fundamental and clinical research. It has been responsible for over 500 articles in refereed journals as well as numerous books and book chapters. The Service is moving into yet more exciting areas of patient care, research and training in the 21st century.

Chapter 17

The Cornea Service

Elisabeth J. Cohen, M.D., Director

The Cornea Service at Wills Eye Hospital began in the late 1950s when one of the attending surgeons, Wilfred E. Fry, M.D., demonstrated an expertise in corneal diseases. Dr. Fry was an enthusiastic ophthalmic pathologist and an initial member of the Verhoeff Society. Thirty of his 50 publications concerned ophthalmic pathology. He served as President of the American Ophthalmological Society in 1966, one of the very few Wills physicians to hold this post. He was editor of the *Transactions of the American Ophthalmic Society* from 1942 to 1949.

At first, the Cornea Service met one afternoon a week on the balcony of the second floor of Wills Eye Hospital at 16th & Spring Garden Streets. This had been the area of the hospital designated as the Gonioscopic Clinic and was supervised by Dr. George Dublin. There was one small examining room containing a Bausch & Lomb Thorpe slit lamp. This area had been designated the Slit Lamp Clinic before slit lamps were routinely used in the General Ophthalmology Service.

The attending physicians on the Cornea Service

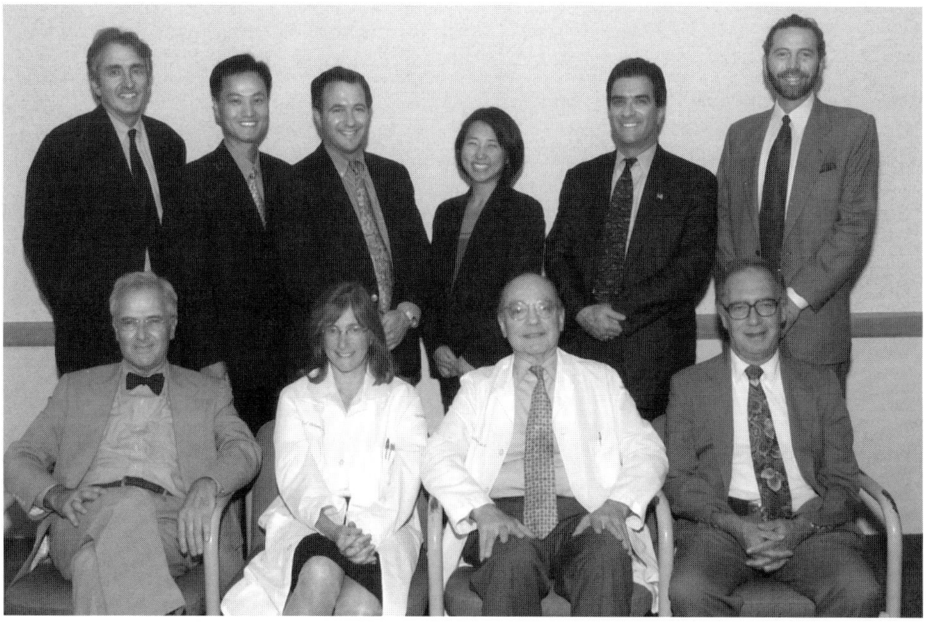

FIGURE 17-1

Members of the Cornea Service in 2002

Front Row: Michael A. Naidoff, M.D., Elisabeth J. Cohen, M.D., Peter R. Laibson, M.D., H. Thomas Dodds, M.D. Back Row: Irving M. Raber, M.D., Stephen Y. Lee, M.D., Christopher J. Rapuano, M.D., Christine W. Chung, M.D., Sadeer B. Hannush, M.D., Melvin I. Roat, M.D. Missing: Anita I. Miedziak, M.D.

would gather once a week to evaluate a few patients referred from the General Ophthalmology Service with corneal problems that needed further expertise for diagnosis and management. The members of the Cornea Service in the late 1950s and early 1960s, in addition to Dr. Fry, were Robert Mulberger, M.D., Philip Spaeth, M.D., and Oram Kline, M.D. All of these physicians eventually became attending surgeons at Wills Eye Hospital. They were joined in 1963 and 1964 by Dr. Richard Keates, who had completed a six-month corneal fellowship, which was standard for this time, studying as a Heed Ophthalmic Fellow with Drs. Ramon Castroviejo and Townley Paton in New York City and Max Fine in San Francisco. The Heed Ophthalmic Fellowship consisted of observing these surgeons in their office and in the operating room for two months each.

The Cornea Service did not have residents at first, but when Dr. Tadeu Cvintal from Sao Paulo, Brazil, was first appointed as a fellow on the Cornea Service in 1963 by Dr. Wilfred Fry, a senior resident was assigned to the Cornea Service to work with Dr. Cvintal. Dr. Cvintal completed his fellowship after two years and returned to Sao Paulo, Brazil, where he is now in clinical practice and is head of a residency program. Dr. Cvintal would prepare the cases for presentation to Dr. Fry each week and Dr. Fry and the other members of the Service would evaluate them together. It was usually the final word of Dr. Fry whose dictation was taken by Dr. Cvintal and placed in the clinic chart that determined the diagnosis and treatment for these patients.

The first full-time Cornea Service physician was Peter R. Laibson, M.D., who joined the Cornea Service in October 1965, after completing a residency at Wills Eye Hospital and a fellowship at Massachusetts Eye & Ear Infirmary with Claes H. Dohlman, M.D. This was the first one-year corneal fellowship in the United States. Dr. Laibson was the first salaried corneal physician at Wills Eye Hospital and he joined the Cornea Service at the request of Arthur Keeney, M.D., who had replaced Irving H. Leopold, M.D. as Ophthalmologist-in-Chief.

At that time, the Cornea Service consisted of Dr. Laibson and one secretary. He established a regular clinic which met each afternoon at 1:30 and supervised a resident who rotated through the Cornea Service on each of these afternoons. He saw private patients in the morning in the same setting as the Cornea Service.

The second corneal fellow, Dr. Guillermo Ortolan, from Heberon, Brazil, began his training with Dr. Laibson and the other cornea attendings in 1967. Dr. Ortolan remained for a year as a cornea fellow, having served the previous year as a fellow on the Retina Service.

Dr. Fry remained the head of the Cornea Service until 1968, when he was replaced as Director by Robert Mulberger, M.D., one of the five attending surgeons who supervised the Thursday Clinic. Dr. Laibson became the third Director of the Cornea Service in 1973.

The cornea fellows continued to be appointed at the rate of one per year until the early 1970s. At that time the Service expanded with more examining rooms and facilities. Two, then three fellows were appointed for one-year clinical fellowships. In recent years there are also usually three international research fellows. The great majority of the fellows spend one year on the Cornea Service, although several have spent up to two years in clinical and basic sciences. There have been 12 Heed scholars who have served as fellows on the Cornea Service, as well as six recipients of the McLaughlin Fellowship and four recipients of the E.A. Baker Foundation Fellowships, the latter two from Canada, and one Fulbright Scholar from Turkey.

Dr. Juan Arentsen became the second full-time member of the Cornea Service, joining Dr. Laibson in 1976. Dr. Arentsen served his first residency with his father, Dr. Juan Arentsen Sr., in Santiago, Chile, did a second residency with Dr. Edward Maumenee at Johns Hopkins University, then a one-year Pathology Fellowship with Dr. William Richard Green at Hopkins and then a further year as a corneal fellow with Dr. Laibson before joining the geographic full-time faculty at Wills Eye Hospital. He also was the half-time director of the residency program, replacing Dr. Guy Chan who had left to become Professor and Chairman of Ophthalmology at Temple University School of Medicine.

Elisabeth J. Cohen, M.D. became the third full-time member of the Cornea Service in 1981. She graduated from Harvard Medical School in 1975 and then did a medical internship at the Hospital of the University of Pennsylvania (1975–1976). She completed a residency at Wills Eye Hospital in 1979, and then a two-year fellowship at the Massachusetts Eye & Ear Infirmary in Boston specializing in immunology and contact lens fittings for keratoconus and post keratoplasty. Dr. Cohen became Co-Director of the Cornea Service in 1993 and Director of the Cornea Service in 1999.

After spending 14 years on the geographic full-time faculty at Wills Eye Hospital in the Cornea Service, Dr. Arentsen left to return to Chile in 1989. He was replaced by Kent Leavitt, M.D., who had done his residency at Wills Eye Hospital and a cornea fellowship on the Cornea Service at Wills Eye Hospital. Dr. Leavitt returned to the west coast in 1991.

Christopher J. Rapuano, M.D. joined the Cornea Service as the fifth full-time member of the staff in 1991. An ex-resident of Wills Eye Hospital, he completed a cornea fellowship with Jay Krachmer, M.D. at the University of Iowa. He was a 1990 graduate of Brown University and Columbia College of Physicians and Surgeons. Dr. Krachmer had been a fellow of Dr. Laibson's on the Cornea Service at Wills Eye Hospital in 1973. Dr. Cohen trained under Dr. Laibson's mentor, Claes Dohlman M.D., and Dr. Rapuano trained under Dr. Laibson's student!

The current full-time faculty of the Cornea Service includes Elisabeth J. Cohen, M.D., Director, Peter R. Laibson, M.D., Co-Director, and Christopher J. Rapuano, M.D., Co-Director of the Refractive Surgery Department. The part-time faculty consists of Christine W. Chung, M.D., H. Thomas Dodds, M.D., Sadeer B. Hannush, M.D., Stephen Y. Lee, M.D., Anita I. Miedziak, M.D., Michael A. Naidoff, M.D., Irving M. Raber, M.D. and Melvin I. Roat, M.D. The part-time faculty on the Cornea Service at Wills Eye Hospital consists of doctors who staff the Cornea Clinic each afternoon of the week and who have private practices outside of Wills Eye Hospital. The main requirements for a cornea staff position is satisfactory completion of a one-year cornea fellowship and a willingness to teach the residents in the Cornea Clinic and the operating room, and to cover the Wills Eye Hospital Emergency Room.

The members of the Cornea Service have served on numerous editorial boards of the major ophthalmic journals published in the U.S. Elisabeth J. Cohen, M.D. was the editor of the *Contact Lens Association of Ophthalmology Journal* and the *Yearbook of Ophthalmology*. She serves on the editorial board of the *Archives of Ophthalmology* and the journal, *Evidence-Based Eye Care*. She was on the editorial board of the journals *Cornea* and *Ophthalmic Surgery*. Dr. Laibson was editor of the *Yearbook of Ophthalmology* and *Key Ophthalmology*. He was on the editorial boards of *Archives of Ophthalmology* and the journal *Cornea*, and the *Video Journal of Ophthalmology*, as well as the new *Journal of the Ocular Surface*. Christopher J. Rapuano, M.D. is the current editor of the *Yearbook of Ophthalmology*, and is on the editorial board of *Evidence-Based Eye Care*, *Current Opinion in Ophthalmology* and the journal *Cornea*. He was the first editor of the best-selling Wills Manual and the author of the Anterior Segment volume in the Requisites of Ophthalmology series. Drs. Cohen, Laibson and Rapuano are each authors of over 150 papers published in peer reviewed ophthalmology journals.

Drs. Cohen, Laibson and Rapuano are leaders locally and nationally in cornea and ophthalmology professional organizations. Dr. Cohen was president of the Wills Eye Physicians Organization. Dr. Rapuano is Chairman of the Facilities Committee, organizing the transition into the new Wills. He was chairman of the Wills Eye Hospital Annual Conference. Drs. Cohen and Laibson are Co-Medical Directors of the Lions Eye Bank of Delaware Valley. Drs. Rapuano and Hannush serve on the Medical Advisory Board of the Eye Bank. Drs. Cohen, Laibson and Rapuano are full Professors of Ophthalmology at Jefferson Medical College of Thomas Jefferson University. Dr. Laibson served as president of the Castroviejo Cornea Society, the international cornea society. Dr. Cohen was a member of the Board of the Castroviejo Cornea Society and Dr. Rapuano is currently on the Board. Dr. Rapuano has also been Co-Director of the Refractive Surgery Department at Wills Eye Hospital since 1996.

Drs. Laibson and Cohen are recipients of the Silver Tray award of the Wills Eye Ex-residents' Society, recognizing their contribution to Wills Eye Hospital and in the residency training program. Dr. Rapuano is a recipient of the Golden Apple Award in recognition of his contributions to teaching the residents. Doctors Raber and Hannush have also been recognized by the residents for their contributions to resident teaching.

The physicians on the Cornea Service have participated in several N.I.H. funded multicenter prospective randomized research projects, including the prospective evaluation of radial keratotomy (PERK), the Herpetic Eye Diseases Study (HEDS) and the Cornea Donor Study (CDS). Dr. Laibson was the recipient of an ROI Basic Science grant on Recurrent Herpetic Keratitis in 1966–69. They have served on various committees for the American Academy of Ophthalmology. Dr. Laibson was a member of the Board of Councillors of the American Academy of Ophthalmology for six years. Currently, Dr. Rapuano is chairman of the Refractive Surgery Ophthalmic Technology Assessment Committee (OTAC) at the Academy. Drs. Laibson, Cohen and Hannush have served on Advisory Panels for the FDA.

There have been 13 Biennial Cornea Conferences organized by the Cornea Service of Wills Eye Hospital. At the last six conferences there have been Wilfred E. Fry, M.D. Memorial Lectures, given by George Waring, M.D., Jay Krachmer, M.D., Mark Speaker, M.D., Harminder Dua, M.D., Eric Donnenfeld, M.D. and Peter R. Laibson, M.D.

Our fellows have come from many states and numerous foreign countries. A number of ex-fellows are currently heads of eye departments. Jay Krachmer, M.D. is Professor & Chairman, Department of Ophthalmology, University of Minnesota, in Minneapolis. Dr. Harminder Dua is Professor and Chairman at the University of Nottingham in Nottingham, England. Helia Angotti, M.D., PhD, is Head Professor and Chairperson Faculdade de Medicina do Triangulo Mineiro, Brazil. Yaacov Rozenman, M.D. is Chairman at Shaare Zedek Hospital in Jerusalem. Patricia Laughrea is Professor de Clinique and Program Director of Ophthalmology at Laval University in Quebec. Many more have academic affiliations and are very involved in the training of cornea fellows and ophthalmology residents across the United States (see appendix).

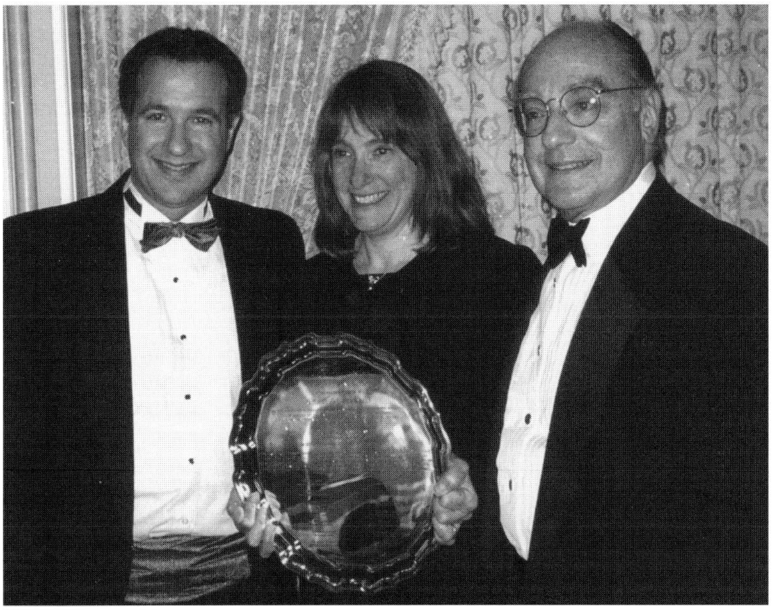

FIGURE17-2

Elisabeth J. Cohen, M.D., recipient of the Silver Tray at the Wills Eye Hospital Annual Conference 2002, with Christopher J. Rapuano, M.D. and Peter R. Laibson, M.D. (photo courtesy of John Siliquini, M.D.)

Chapter 18

The Pediatric Ophthalmology Department

Joseph H. Calhoun, M.D., Director

The history of pediatric ophthalmology at Wills Eye Hospital as a separate specialty begins with the arrival of Dr. Robison D. Harley. In 1966, he retired after 20 years of private practice in Atlantic City to begin another career in Philadelphia. During those 20 years, he had come one day a week to St. Christopher's Hospital for Children, teaching and providing ophthalmic care to children. At the urging of Dr. Waldo Nelson, then the chairman of the hospital, Dr. Harley began a pediatric ophthalmology section there. In 1967, Dr. Arthur Keeney, the ophthalmologist-in-chief, enticed Dr. Harley to begin a pediatric ophthalmology department at Wills. For many years thereafter, Dr. Harley divided his time between the two institutions. Until the mid 1970s, the residents and fellows trained at both facilities. It was the wealth of clinical material in unusual and rare diseases and the association with other pediatric subspecialists that led to the first *Pediatric Ophthalmology* textbook.

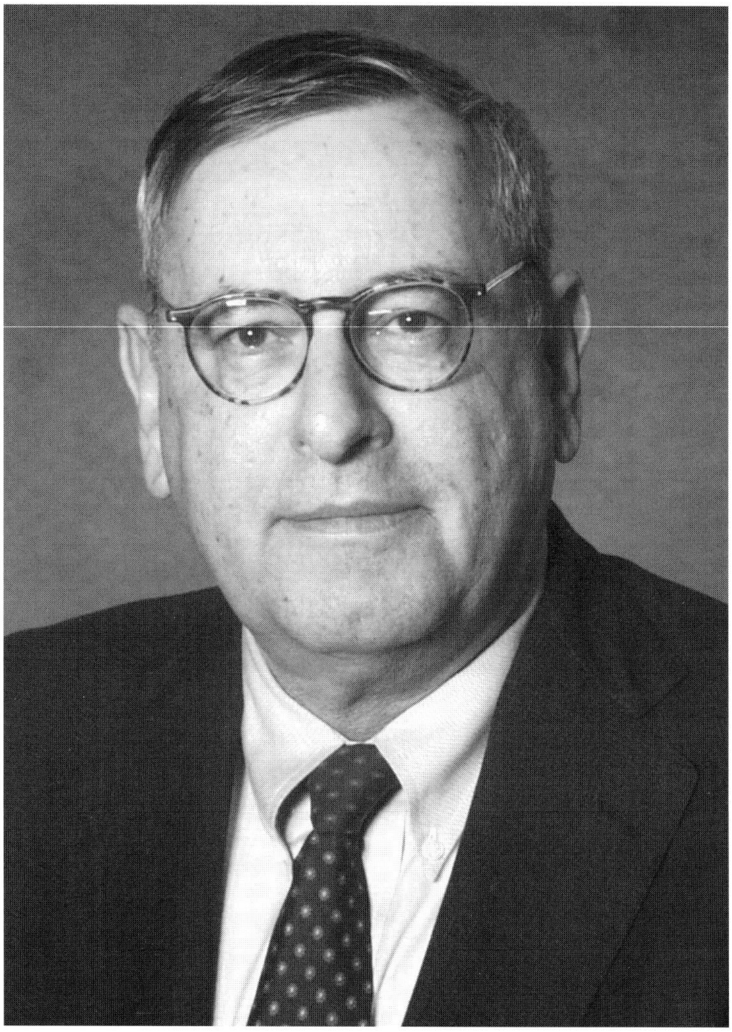

FIGURE 18-1
Joseph H. Calhoun, M.D., first fellow and current Director of the Pediatric Ophthalmology Department.

Prior to the formation of the Pediatric Ophthalmology Department, most of the evaluation of strabismus was performed in the Orthoptics Department headed by Miss Moffit and Miss Haddon. Dr. William Krewson was the physician in charge of that department. Dr. Harley introduced the concept—rather radical for that time—of having ophthalmologists themselves examine infants and children with strabismus. Initially the Pediatric Ophthalmology Department shared with the nascent Retina and Cornea Services offices on the west side of the second floor of the old Wills Eye Hospital at 16th and Spring Garden Streets.

As more and more residents were trained to examine children, the need for an Orthoptic Department gradually decreased. In the early 1970s, the Orthoptic Department was closed and its space was occupied by the Cornea Service.

In the first several years of the Pediatric Ophthalmology Department, patients were seen only on referral from one of the five horizontal services, one for each day of the week. Patients would be assigned to a horizontal service based entirely on what day they first came to Wills Eye Hospital. These services would refer the infants and children for evaluation, surgery, or both.

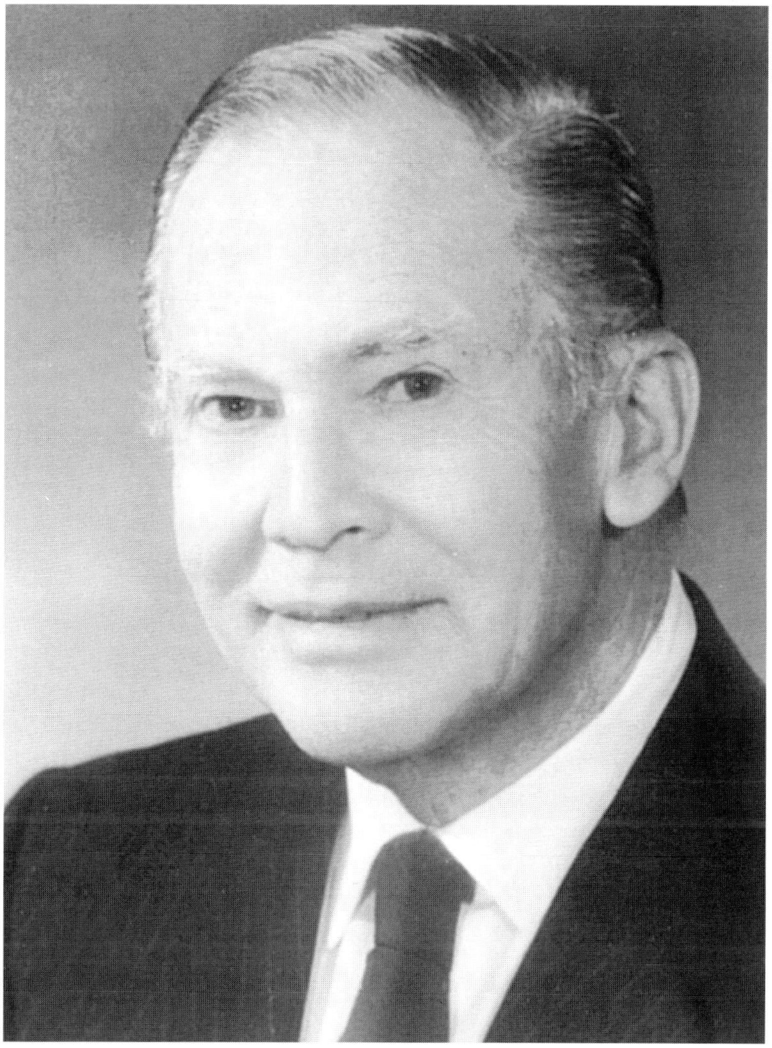

FIGURE 18-2
Robison D. Harley, M.D., founder and first Director of the Pediatric Ophthalmology Department.

The Monday service, under the direction of Dr, Patrick Kennedy, was the first of the horizontal services to direct that all children from that service be managed by the Pediatric Ophthalmology Department. Over the next several years, each of the other horizontal services followed its example. It is probably safe now to reveal that during these transitional years the covering charts of many children were altered to indicate a different horizontal service origin so that the children could be followed in the Pediatric Ophthalmology Department.

About 1967, Fight For Sight, Inc., of New York, a philanthropic organization dedicated to the improvement of children's eyesight, began its long association with Wills Eye Hospital. This organization provided the funding for examining rooms, equipment, and the creation of an area appropriate for children. In recognition of the organization's support, the pediatric ophthalmology area has been informally named Fight for Sight by many ophthalmologists.

As the need for more space for the vertical services increased, the Pediatric Ophthalmology

Department expanded first into the Retina Service area when the latter department moved to larger quarters and eventually into a small room that had been used for the Ear, Nose and Throat Clinic in Wills Eye Hospital.

Dr. Donelson Manley joined the staff of the Pediatric Ophthalmology Department in 1967 after finishing a one-year fellowship with Dr. Marshall Parks in Washington, D.C. He combined a part-time practice at Wills Eye Hospital with active involvement in teaching. Subsequently Dr. Leonard Nelson also joined the Pediatric Ophthamology staff. He has made major contributions as a teacher and surgeon.

In 1968, Dr. Harley initiated what would now be called programs of continuing medical education. The first was a two-day symposium on pediatric ophthalmology held at the Philadelphia County Medical Society Building, several blocks down Spring Garden Street from the old Wills Eye Hospital. Now such programs by the various services are a regular feature at this institution.

In 1968, the Pediatric Ophthalmology Department purchased the first operating microscope for use for surgery in Wills Eye Hospital, a floor-mounted Zeiss microscope. Its acquisition was prompted by the need for good magnification and co-axial illumination in the removal of cataracts in children. At that time, the surgical technique was the discission-aspiration method. Gradually more and more surgeons not in the Pediatric Ophthalmology Department were using it for surgical procedures. The oculars were kept in a drawer by the head nurse of the operating room and were given only to surgeons who had approval to use this instrument.

The first vitrectomy machine used at Wills was purchased by the Pediatric Ophthalmology Service in 1973. Dr. Nicholas Douvas of Port Huron, Michigan, created the Roto-extractor, the second such instrument commercially available. Each purchaser had to go to Port Huron to take a course, not only in the surgical techniques, but in the care and maintenance of the instrument, since it was new to operating nurses also. With funds provided by the Pediatric Ophthalmology Department, Dr. Calhoun took the course and bought the machine for use for cataracts in infants and children. That instrument, and others that quickly followed, radically changed the surgical technique for infantile cataracts. Prior to these types of instruments, in the discission-aspiration technique the posterior capsule was always left intact. In time it became opacified, so at least one discission or cutting of the secondary membrane was required. With these new instruments the cataract, the posterior capsule, and some of the anterior vitreous were removed at the first and only surgery.

From these humble but auspicious beginnings, the Pediatric Ophthalmology Department has grown to its present size. Its staff of eight pediatric ophthalmologists is actively involved in patient care, teaching, and research at Wills Eye Hospital. In the current facilities the support of Fight For Sight is still evident in the attractive playroom for children that greets visitors to the area. New facilities, new faces, and new techniques have not lessened the dedication to the care of children's eye diseases started three decades ago by Dr. Harley.

Chapter 19

The Oculoplastic Department

Edward H. Bedrossian, Jr., M.D., Joseph C. Flanagan, M.D., Director, and Marie B. Moore

Early History

The early plastic work done at Wills Eye Hospital was limited to the correction of eyelid deformities resulting from infection, burns, or trauma. Early surgeons used the crudest of techniques and equipment. Nevertheless, by the Civil War, Wills Eye Hospital had become known for its excellence in cataract extractions and plastic surgery.

An early Wills Eye physician, Dr. George C. Harlan, had great skill both as a surgeon and as an author. Many of his papers were read at meetings of the ophthalmology section at the Philadelphia College of Physicians and at annual meetings of the American Ophthalmological Society, of which he was president in 1893. About that time he wrote a chapter entitled "Surgery of the Eyelids," published in Norris and Oliver System. As a result of his extensive Army experience in general surgery, Harlan devised several flap operations, including one for the treatment of ectropion using pedicle flaps.

Nasolacrimal duct obstruction and problems with epiphora were as prevalent at the turn of the century as they are today. Meller in his 1908

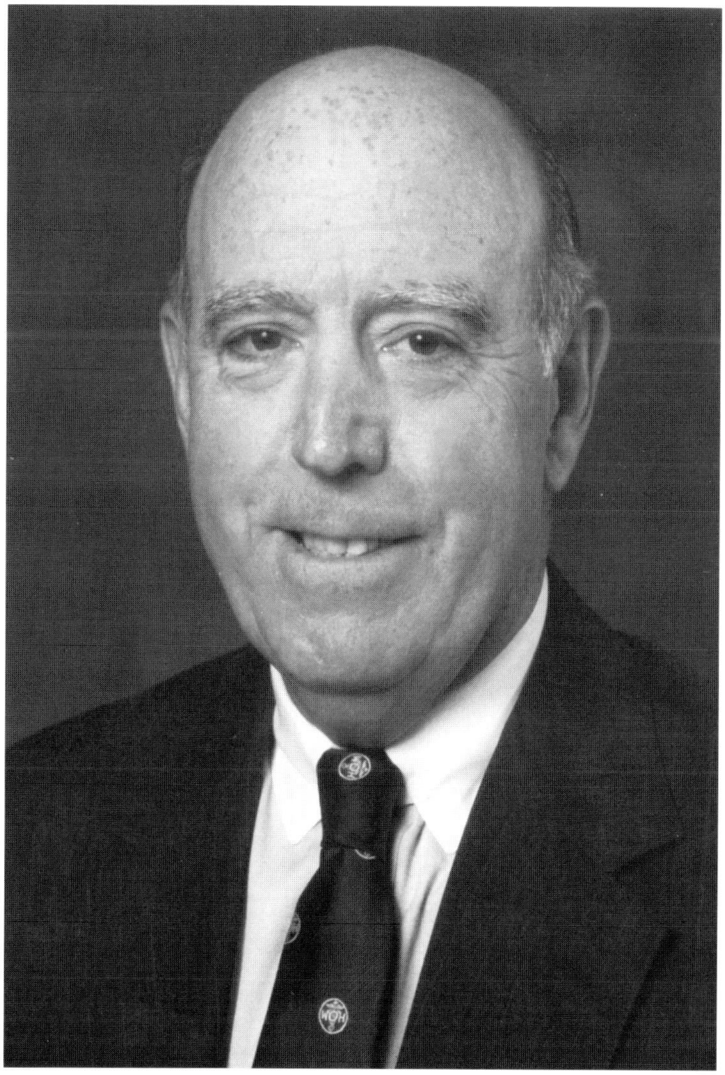

FIGURE 19-1
Dr. Joseph C. Flanagan, director of the Oculoplastic Department.

Ophthalmic Surgery described a procedure for removal of nasolacrimal sac (dacryocystectomy). This procedure was extensively utilized by surgeons at Wills Eye Hospital, even though it was not widely favored elsewhere at the time.

World War I greatly increased the number of cases requiring skin grafting. Socket reconstruction, using dermal grafts as described by Weeks and epidermal grafts as described by Wheeler, was performed by Wills surgeons during this period.

Form the 1930s to the 1960s, Wills Eye Hospital, now in a newly constructed building at 16th and Spring Garden Streets, was organized around several general eye services, each headed by a chief. One of its chiefs, Dr. Edmund B. Spaeth, was noted for his ophthalmic surgery, particularly in the fields of plastics and motility.

Oculoplastic Consultant

Edmund Benjamin Spaeth attended the Army Medical School in Washington, D.C. In 1917 he went with the Sixth Division of the Army to France, where he served as a medical officer in the trenches. On his return to the United States in 1918, he was assigned to Walter Reed Army Medical Center.

Dr. Spaeth spent the next seven years treating traumatic injuries and devising various operations and prostheses. He became the first Chief of Ophthalmology at Walter Reed Hospital. In 1924, he obtained a six-month leave of absence to return to Europe for further study in ophthalmology with Drs. Linder, Fuchs, Worth, and Axenfeld. Returning to Washington, he published in 1925 his first book, *Newer Methods of Ophthalmic Plastic Surgery*. For this textbook, a classic of its day, he received the Lucien-Howe Award of the University of Buffalo.

In 1927 he resigned his commission and moved to Philadelphia, bringing with him enormous energy, confidence, creativity, and willingness to approach any problem.

In 1939 Dr. Spaeth (Fig. 19-2) became an attending surgeon at Wills Eye Hospital and published his scond book, *Ophthalmic Surgery*, while also at the Graduate School of Medicine of the University of Pennsylvania.

Although his interests and activities encompassed all of ophthalmology, his particular domain was ophthalmic plastic surgery. He gave structure to the discipline by helping to found the American Society of Ophthalmic Plastic and Reconstructive Surgery (ASOPRS) in 1970.

The Oculoplastic Surgery Department

In 1969, the Oculoplastic Service was officially established, and Dr. Gerard Shannon was appointed its first director.

Gerard Michael Shannon (Fig. 19-3) received his M.D. in 1949 from Jefferson Medical College in Philadelphia. Following an internship at Nazareth Hospital, Philadelphia, he served as a captain in the

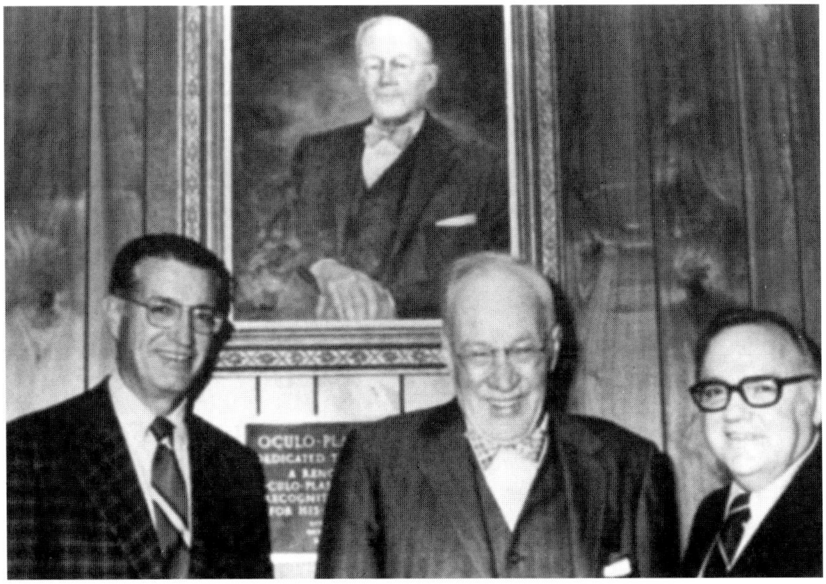

FIGURE 19-2
Left to right: the late Dr. Thomas D. Duane (then ophthalmologist-in-chief), the late Dr. Edmund B. Spaeth, and the late Dr. Gerard M. Shannon at dedication of Oculoplastic Department, February 14, 1974.

U.S. Army Medical Corps until 1952. His interest in ophthalmology became even more fervent during his residency at Wills Eye Hospital from 1953 to 1956. In 1957, encouraged by Dr. Spaeth, Dr. Shannon pursued an interest in ophthalmic plastic surgery as a Heed Ophthalmic Fellow under the supervision of Dr. Byron Smith of New York. He returned to Philadelphia to receive his Master of Science degree in ophthalmology from the Graduate School of Medicine of the University of Pennsylvania in 1958.

Dr. Shannon's talents and willingness to accept challenges extended to local, state, and national meetings. He was president of the Eye Section of the Philadelphia County Medical Society; chaired the Plastic Surgery Committee of the Pennsylvania Academy of Ophthalmology and Otolaryngology; and was a director of the National Examining Board of Ocularists. His academic appointments included Clinical Professor of Ophthalmology, Jefferson Medical College and Assistant Clinical Professor of Ophthalmology, Temple University, both in Philadelphia. He was a Fellow of the American Academy of Ophthalmology, American College of Surgeons, and American Society of Ophthalmic Plastic and Reconstructive Surgery. In addition to lecturing in the United States and abroad, he authored more than forty articles and co-authored *Practical Ophthalmic Plastic and Reconstructive Surgery*, published in 1976.

It was at Dr. Shannon's invitation that Drs. Cyril M. Luce and John J. Siliquini organized the first formal oculoplastic service at Wills Eye Hospital. Dr. Luce, who served his residency under the direction of Dr. Spaeth, was a member of the staff until his death in 1975. On February 14, 1974, two years after Wills Eye Hospital affiliated with Thomas Jefferson University, the Oculoplastic Department was formally dedicated to Dr. Edmund B. Spaeth (Fig. 19-2). Once the hospital moved to its 1980 location, the Oculoplastic Department, under Dr. Shannon's leadership, was able to expand its examination and minor surgery rooms on the hospital's third floor.

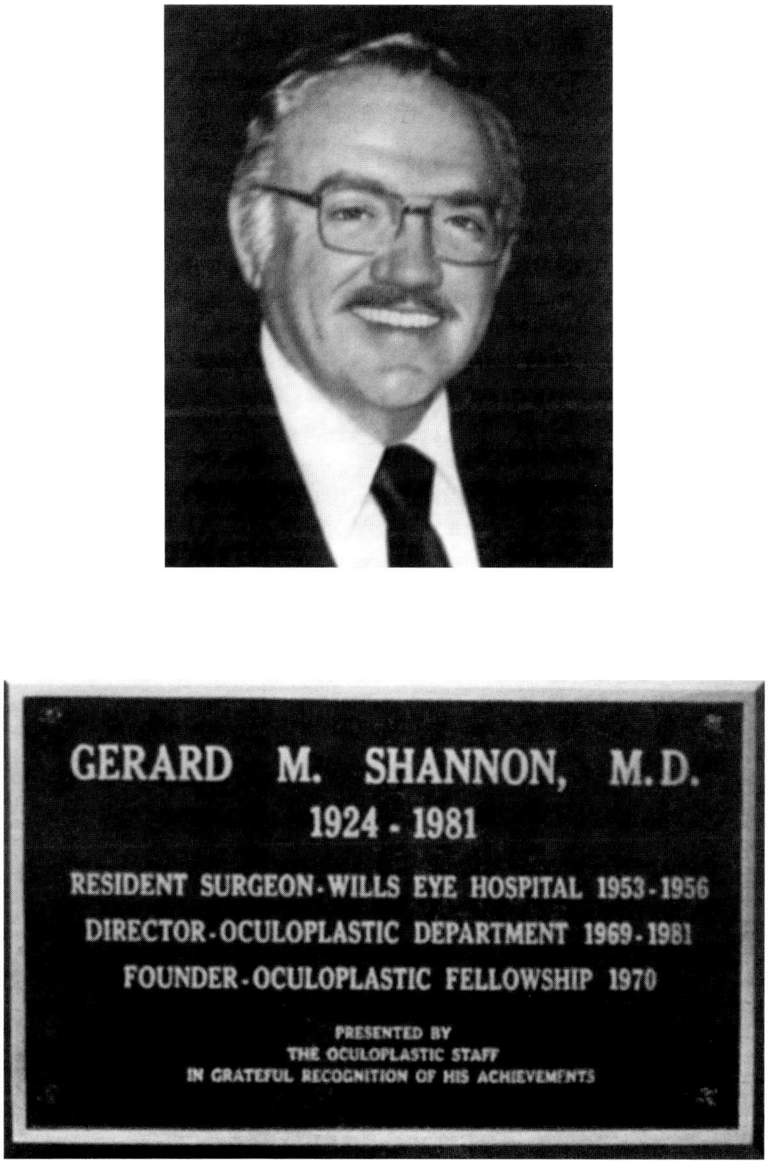

FIGURE 19-3
The late Dr. Gerard M. Shannon.

On July 29, 1981, at the age of 57, Gerard M. Shannon, M.D., F.A.C.S., died suddenly while fishing in Iceland with a group of ophthalmologists. He is remembered and respected for his knowledge, his ethics, and his skill as an oculoplastic surgeon.

The Oculoplastic Department Today

After the untimely death of Dr. Gerard Shannon Wills Eye Hospital looked internally. In 1981 Doctor Joseph C. Flanagan, F.A.C.S., assistant director of the Oculoplastic Department, was appointed Director.

Dr. Flanagan's outstanding contributions to the field of oculoplastic surgery have been recognized by the various organizations to which he belongs and he has been the recipient of numerous distinguished awards. A Heed Fellow, he has also received the Alumni Achievement Award from Jefferson Medical College, the highest honor that the University bestows on one of its graduates, and he was honored by The State Department in 1984 with a Certificate of Accommodation for performing reconstructive plastic surgery on the victims of the U.S. Embassy bombing in Beirut. Probably his most treasured award was induction into the LaSalle College Hall of Fame.

The medical staff of the Oculoplastic Department, under the direction of Dr. Flanagan, includes Drs. John J. Siliquini, Ignatius S. Hneleski, Jr., Christine L. Zolli, Susan M. Hughes, Edward H. Bedrossian, Jr., Mary A. Stefanyszyn, Thaddeus Nowinski, Robert B. Penne, Marc S. Cohen, Marlon Maus, Jurij R. Bilyk and Ignatius S. Hneleski, III. (Dr. Christine Zolli has the distinction of being the first woman physician to be granted a fellowship in oculoplastic surgery at Wills Eye Hospital.)

Edward H. Bedrossian Jr., M.D., F.A.C.A. joined the Oculoplastic Surgery Service at Wills Eye Hospital in July of 1983 and he is currently an Attending Surgeon. From 1987–2002, Dr. Bedrossian, Jr. served as the founding director of the Wills Eye Hospital Fascia Lata Bank. This facility brought national recognition to the Oculoplastic Surgery Department by providing banked irradiated homologous fascia lata to oculoplastic surgeons nationwide and abroad.

Dr. Stefanyszyn, a graduate of Harvard Medical School, joined the Wills Eye Hospital Department in 1985. She has published numerous articles and lectures nationally and internationally on various oculoplastic and orbital topics. Her special areas of expertise are the treatment of patients with Graves' orbitopathy and cosmetic eyelid and brow surgery. She is a member of the Orbital Society, the International Society for Orbital Disorders, Society of Heed Fellows, and a Fellow of the American College of Surgeons.

Dr. Penne joined the Oculoplastic Service on July 1, 1990 after completing his residency at Wills Eye Hospital, a Neuro-orbital fellowship at Wills Eye Hospital and a fellowship in Oculoplastic and Orbital Surgery at Wills Eye Hospital. He was a co-founder of the ocular pemphigoid clinic in the 1990s and has been an Associate Editor of the *Yearbook of Ophthalmology* since 1998. Dr. Penne has also been Chairman of the Wills Eye Hospital Conference since 2000.

Dr. Cohen completed his residency at Wills Eye Hospital in 1988 at which time he was Co-Chief Resident. He then completed a Neuro-ophthalmology fellowship at Wills Eye Hospital and was awarded a Fight For Sight Fellowship grant. This was followed by an Oculoplastic Surgery fellowship with Norman Schorr at UCLA. In 2001 Dr. Cohen presented a lecture on the cosmetic use of Botox at the national meeting of the American Academy of Cosmetic Surgery and was awarded the prestigious "Presidents Award" for the best scientific presentation at the meeting.

Marlon Maus, M.D. graduated from Jefferson Medical College in 1985. He did his residency in Ophthalmology at Wills Eye Hospital from 1986 to 1989 and from 1989 to 1990 he had a combined fellowship in Oculoplastic Surgery, Neuro-Ophthalmology and Ocular Pathology at Wills Eye Hospital. Dr. Maus was a staff member of the Oculoplastic Department from 1990 to 2001 and also served as co-Director of Resident Education. He worked very closely with the residents especially on surgical emergencies and trauma cases and introduced many innovative ideas to the program. His service was invaluable. Dr. Maus left Wills Eye Hospital in 2000 to pursue a career in Public Health where he currently is seeking advanced degrees at the University of California San Francisco.

Dr. Bilyk joined the Oculoplastic Service in July 1994 and in addition to general oculoplastics concentrates on orbital disease, including Graves' orbitopathy and trauma. He also works closely with the Otolaryngology and Neurosurgery Departments at Jefferson University Hospital in the management of skull base processes. At Wills, Dr. Bilyk has been awarded the Wills Resident Award for Excellence in Surgical Teaching twice and most recently he won the 2002 Golden Apple award.

Dr. Hneleski, III, is interested in thyroid eye disease as well and also reconstructive eyelid surgery. He enjoys instructing residents in complex eyelid surgery and lecturing on eyelid and lacrimal disorders.

With a department also including John Siliquini and Susan Hughes, the Oculoplastics Service is well equipped to provide comprehensive care for all aspects of eyelid, lacrimal and orbital diseases. Surgical treatment is offered for congenital anomalies, degenerative diseases, inflammatory diseases, trauma, tumors and endocrine disorders. Cosmetic and reconstructive surgery of eyelids, lacrimal system and orbit are available and, in many cases, on an out-patient basis and a Cosmetic Surgery Unit has been fully operational since July 1994.

The Oculoplastic Department has also pioneered in the use of specialized treatments such as cryotherapy for trichiasis, argon laser therapy for vascular skin lesions, Botulinum toxin injections for essential blepharospasm, and microsurgical blepharopigmentation.

The Wills Eye Hospital Fascia Lata Bank, as mentioned earlier, was established within the Department of Oculoplastic Surgery at Wills Eye Hospital in November 1987 under the directorship of Edward H. Bedrossian Jr., M.D., F.A.C.S. to meet a growing demand for homologous fascia lata protected against the transmission of communicable disease. Regrettably the Fascia Lata Bank closed its doors in 2000 because of the decreased availability of donor tissue and increase in commercial production.

Dr. Robert Penne was instrumental in establishing an Ocular Cicatricial Pemphigoid Clinic which is now in its fifth year. This joint venture of the Cornea, Oculoplastic and Dermatology Departments meets on the second Friday of each month. A variety of different conjunctival scarring diseases are seen for evaluation including Pemphigoid, Stevens-Johnson Syndrome, ocular burns, and atopic diseases among others. The Clinic has become extremely busy and has proved to be a valuable resource for the management of these difficult patients, as well as for the training and teaching of residents and fellows. Wills Eye Hospital residents, Thomas Jefferson dermatology residents, and cornea and oculoplastic fellows all spend time rotating through the service.

With the establishment of the Neurosurgery Unit at Wills Eye Hospital it became possible for the Oculoplastic Department to participate in combined procedures. It was a natural collaboration since the orbit and brain are separated by the thinnest of bones. Several disease processes involve areas that straddle neurosurgery and oculoplastics. Some examples include tumors of the orbit that invade the brain, such as neurofibromas, squamous cell carcinoma, and other neural tumors.

The two departments have pioneered several approaches that make use of highly advanced technology that is available at Wills Eye Hospital. Drs. Warren Goldman, who is now at Hahnemann, and Marlon Maus described a transorbital approach to brain tumors, minimizing trauma to the brain and allowing for minimal scarring and deformity. A transorbital approach is also being utilized to cannulate the superior ophthalmic vein to close vascular abnormalities in the cavernous sinus that are not otherwise accessible. Neurovascular surgeon, Dr. Robert Rossenwasser, together with Dr. Joseph C. Flanagan and Dr. Marlon Maus, of the Oculoplastic Department at Wills, are responsible for introducing this approach at Wills Eye Hospital.

The education of Wills Eye Hospital residents is a priority in the department. A comprehensive lecture series is presented yearly. During their oculoplastic rotation, Wills residents are exposed to patient evaluation, as well as to all other areas of patient management. They are taught meticulous oculoplastic surgical techniques as well as post-operative care. In addition, under the auspices of Dr. Edward H. Bedrossian, Jr., in conjunction with the Department of Anatomy of Jefferson Medical School, there is a yearly orbital dissection course utilizing cadaver specimens. Recently, this has expanded to include anatomy of the forehead, face and neck. With the increasing demand for cosmetic surgery, members of the oculoplastic department have expanded aesthetic surgical procedures to including blepharoplasty, brow lift, mid-facelift liposuction, Botox injections, fat-transfers, laser skin resurfacing, chemical peels and mini-incision facial enhancement procedures.

A two year ASOPRS-approved fellowship under Dr. Flanagan's supervision is offered. The department provides continuing medical education for the staff of Wills Eye Hospital and for the ophthalmic community at large through updates, courses, and symposia featuring prominent guest speakers held throughout the year.

The staff contributes scientific presentations to the Wills Eye Hospital Annual Clinical Conference and the annual meeting of the American Academy of Ophthalmology. Individual staff members also present papers and speak at local, regional, national and international meetings. The Oculoplastic Service further contributes to medical knowledge through its achievements in clinical and basic research.

The Oculoplastic service is truly grateful to their support staff in the department, namely Laura Webb and Rosemary Bernard, as well as to all of the support staff from the many private offices that assist the physicians on their respective days. Thanks too to Marie B. Moore, who had been with the department from its inception in 1968. She retired in 2000 after 32 years of dedicated service, but currently assists Dr. Flanagan part-time and continues to provide support to the department as well.

Chapter 20

The Oncology Service

Jerry A. Shields, M.D., Director

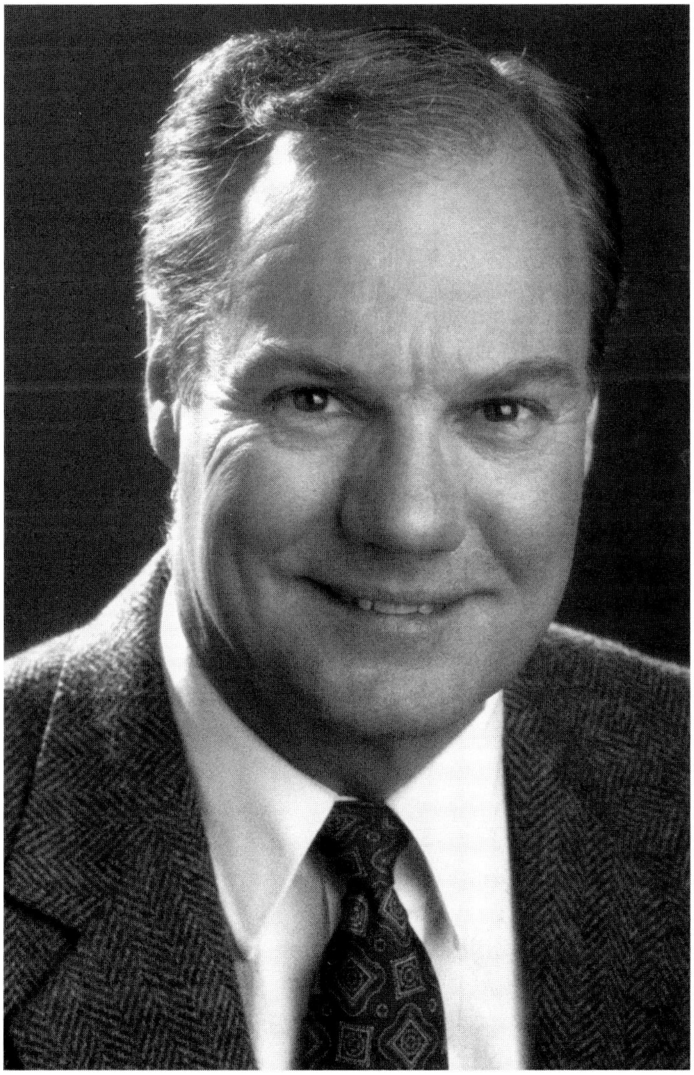

FIGURE 20-1
Jerry A. Shields, M.D., director of the Oncology Service.

The Ocular Oncology Service at Wills Eye Hospital is perhaps the leading facility in the world for the diagnosis and management of patients with ocular tumors. This chapter reviews briefly the history of the Oncology Service and describes its role in patient care, research, academic ophthalmology, and education.

History of the Oncology Service

Several years ago, most patients with ophthalmic tumors were managed by general ophthalmologists. Since no individual or service had a specific expertise in ocular tumors, only a few such patients were referred to Wills Eye Hospital for diagnosis and treatment. During the early 1970s Dr. Jerry A. Shields (Fig. 20-1), an ex-resident and retina fellow at Wills Eye Hospital, completed an additional fellowship in ophthalmic pathology and returned to the hospital with a strong interest in ocular oncology. With the support of members of the Retina Service, Dr. Shields began to develop a unit on that service devoted specifically to ocular oncology. It was soon apparent that the number of patients with eye tumors and pseudotumors referred to Wills Eye Hospital had increased dramatically. Hence, in 1978, the Ocular Oncology Service, devoted exclusively to the diagnosis and management of patients with

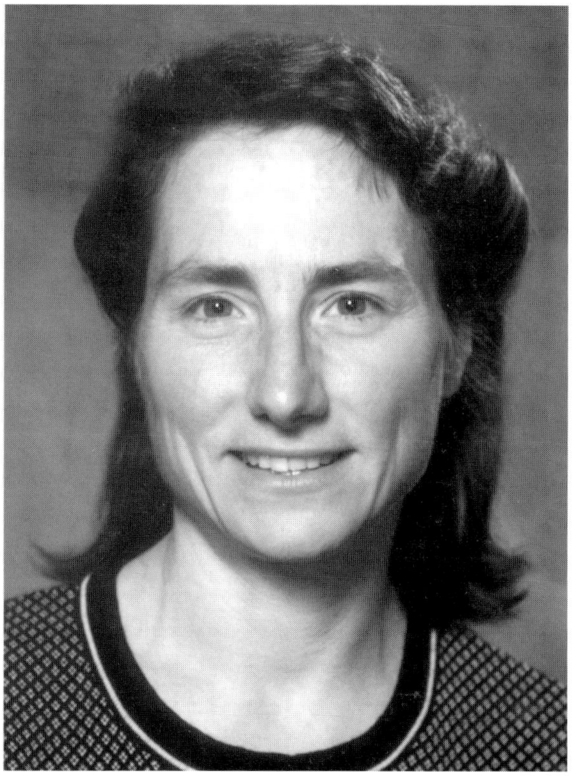

FIGURE 20-2
Dr. Carol Shields

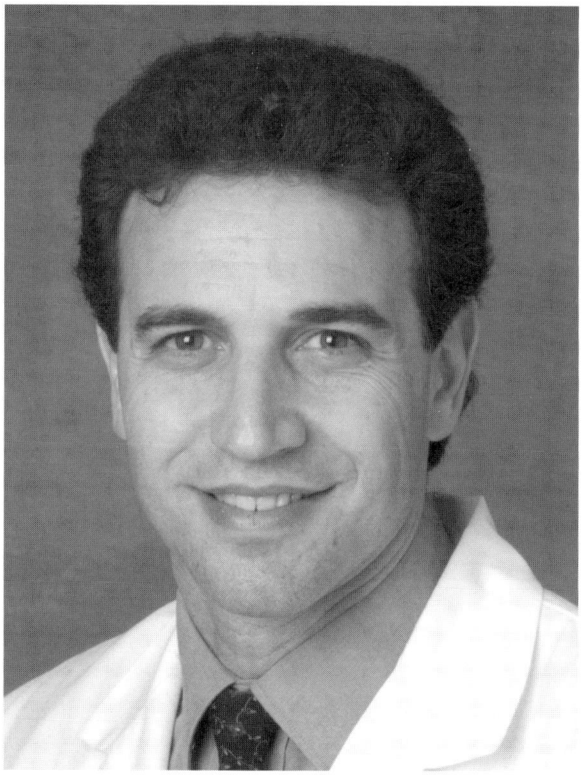

FIGURE 20-3
Dr. Miguel Materin

ocular tumors, was officially established at the hospital.

During the early days of the Oncology Service, most patient care was rendered by Dr. Shields with the residents, retina fellows and other physicians who rotated through and worked for a period of time on the service. As an increasing number of patients were referred to the Oncology Service, it became apparent that more staff physicians were needed. In 1980 Dr. James Augsburger, an ex-Retina Service fellow, joined the staff under the direction of Dr. Jerry Shields. He subsequently returned to the Retina Service until he became director of the Department of Ophthalmology at the University of Cincinnati.

In 1988, Dr. Carol Shields (Fig. 20-2), an ex-resident at Wills Eye Hospital and the wife of Dr. Jerry Shields, joined the full-time Oncology Service. She was well prepared for treating patients with ocular tumors because of post residency fellowship training in ophthalmic pathology and orbital and eyelid disease, as well as a fellowship on the Oncology Service. Dr. Carol Shields has subsequently developed great expertise in the diagnosis and management of ocular tumors and currently directs the retinoblastoma branch of the oncology service. She has been highly active in patient care and has spearheaded an extraordinary number of clinical research projects in all branches of ocular oncology, mostly related to diagnosis and management of uveal melanoma and retinoblastoma.

The Oncology Service continued to grow and attract more patients with ocular tumors. In 1992, Dr. Patrick De Potter, a native of Belgium, completed ocular oncology fellowships in Switzerland and on the Oncology Service and joined the full-time staff. He brought to the service a unique interest in magnetic resonance imaging of ocular tumors. After four years, he was offered a chair of ophthalmology that prompted his return to his home country of Belgium. Dr. Arun Singh, an ex-fellow on the Oncology, then joined the staff. He had a special interest in genetics of ophthalmic tumors and spearheaded clinical research in that field. In 2000 Dr. Singh was given a position in ocular oncology in England and currently continues to practice ocular oncology there.

The newest members of the service include ex-fellows added to the staff in 2001, Dr. Miguel Materin (Fig. 20-3), and Dr. Brian Marr (Fig. 20-4). The number of patients managed on the Ocular Oncology Service continues to increase and more physicians will probably be added to the staff in the future.

Patient Care

The main emphasis of the Oncology Service is on the diagnosis and treatment of patients with tumors and related conditions of the intraocular structures, eyelids, conjunctiva, and orbit. The most common conditions treated include uveal melanoma and retinoblastoma. About 500 new patients with uveal melanoma and 120 new patients with retinoblastoma are currently evaluated and managed each year. In addition, many patients with benign and malignant lesions of the conjunctiva, orbit, and eyelid are managed weekly on the service. The physicians on the Oncology Service have a strong tradition of performing a thorough ocular history and examination on every patient and they have developed particular expertise in counseling patients with ocular tumors.

Clinical Research

In conjunction with colleagues in other medical specialties, the members of the Oncology Service have played a major role in improving methods of diagnosis and treatment of ocular tumors. With regard to diagnosis, they have been continually involved in treatment of methods and interpretation of untrasonography, fine needle aspiration biopsy, indocyanine green angiography, computed tomography and magnetic resonance imaging.

Concerning uveal melanoma, the most notable therapeutic contributions by the Oncology Service include the avoidance of enucleation by the use of radioactive plaques, local resection, and laser and thermotherapy. Concerning retinoblastoma, improved methods of treatment with laser techniques, cryotherapy, plaque radiotherapy, chemoreduction and chemothermotherapy are being applied. Improved methods of surgical treatment of conjunctival malignancies have been employed.

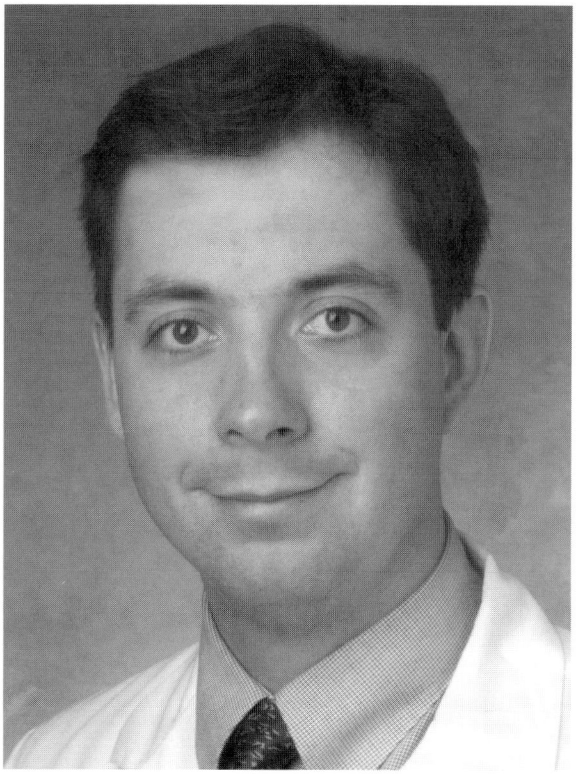

FIGURE 20-4
Dr. Brian Marr

Academic Endeavors

The members of the Oncology Service are highly active in national and international meetings that relate to ocular oncology. Major papers, courses and workshops related to clinical research have been presented at several international symposia on intraocular and orbital tumors, at the American Academy of Ophthalmology, and numerous retinal, pediatric ophthalmology, and oculoplastic meetings. In 1999, the Oncology Service hosted in Philadelphia the biennial meeting of the International Society of Ocular Oncology. The three-day meeting was a great success, with papers and posters presented by contributors from 40 countries. In the subsequent meeting in Amsterdam in 2001, Dr. Jerry Shields was elected as the first president of the International Society of Ocular Oncology.

More than 1100 articles and textbook chapters have been written by current members of the Oncology Services. In addition to many textbook chapters, important textbooks that have been authored or co-authored by members of the service are as follows:

1. Tasman WS, Shields JA: *Diseases of the Peripheral Fundus*. Hagerstown, Harper & Row, 1979.
2. Shields JA: *Diagnosis and Management of Intraocular Tumors*. St. Louis, CV Mosby, 1983.
3. Shields JA: *Diagnosis and Management of Orbital Tumors*. Philadelphia, Saunders, 1989.
4. Shields JA, Shields CL: *Intraocular Tumors. A Text and Atlas Philadelphia*, Saunders, 1992.
5. Sanborn G, Gonder J, Shields JA. *Atlas of Intraocular Tumors*. Philadelphia, Saunders, 1993.
6. Shields JA (Ed): *Management of Malignant Ocular Tumors*. International Ophthalmology Clinics. Boston, Little, Brown Co. 1993.
7. DePotter P, Shields JA., Shields CL: *MRI of the Eye and Orbit*. Philadelphia: JB Lippincott, 1994.
8. Guyer DR, Yannuzzi L, Chang S, Shields JA, Green WR (Eds): *Retina-Vitreous-Macula. A Color Text*. Philadelphia, WB Saunders 1997.
9. Shields JA, Shields CL. *Atlas of Eyelid and Conjunctival Tumors*. Philadelphia, Lippincott Williams and Wilkins, 1999.
10. Shields JA, Shields CL. *Atlas of Intraocular Tumors*. Philadelphia, Lippincott Williams and Wilkins. 1999.
11. Shields JA, Shields CL. *Atlas of Orbital Tumors*. Philadelphia, Lippincott Williams and Wilkins. 1999.

Training and Education

Since its inception in 1974, all Wills residents and retinal fellows have had teaching rotations through the Oncology Service and a number of physicians have done specific training in ocular oncology on the service. Physicians who were fellows on the Oncology Service are now practicing part-time or full-time ocular oncology in Argentina, Australia, Belgium, Brazil, Canada, Colombia, England, Egypt, Germany, India, Iran, Ireland, Mexico, Philippines, Taiwan, Turkey, Venezuela, and in various parts of the United States. Short-term visitors have come to the Oncology Service from many parts of the world. An endowed chair for research in ocular oncology has recently been established through donations from Dr. Luther Brady and others, and it is expected to be filled in the near future. Much of the support for research has been provided through the Eye Tumor Research Foundation, organized by Dr. Carol Shields.

The Oncology Service at Wills Eye Hospital of Thomas Jefferson University is now widely considered to be one of the leading facilities in the world for treatment of ophthalmic tumors. Continued improvements in patient care, research and education are anticipated.

Chapter 21

The Neuro-Ophthalmology Service

Peter J. Savino, M.D., Director, Robert C. Sergott, M.D., Co-Director

Neuro-ophthalmology existed at the Wills Eye Hospital long before it was recognized as a specialty. Dr. William Campbell Posy, an ophthalmologist at the Wills Eye Hospital, co-authored with Dr. William G. Spiller, professor of neuro-pathology and at that time associate professor of neurology at the University of Pennsylvania, the classic 1906 work entitled *The Eye and Nervous System*. This is recognized as one of the original works in neuro-ophthalmology, but since the term did not exist at that time, the authors describe their effort as being "to present Ophthalmo-Neurology in such a form that general practitioners may without difficulty become conversant with its symptomatology."

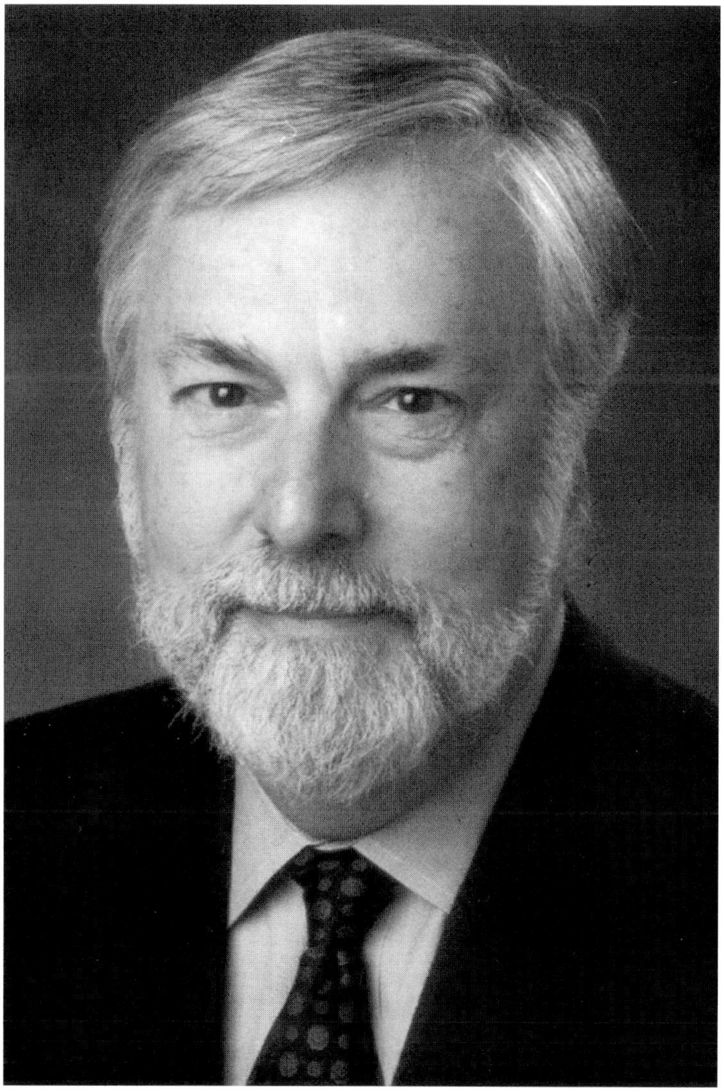

FIGURE 21-1
Dr. Peter J. Savino, director of the Neuro-Ophthalmology Service.

Early History

The official beginning of Neuro-ophthalmology at Wills Eye Hospital occurred in 1927 when the Neurology Department was formally established. The first director of that department was Dr. Theodore Weisenburg, who was a clinical neurologist at the University of Pennsylvania and at the Poly Clinic and Medico-Chirurgical Hospital (known today as Graduate Hospital).

The department's consultative

service was headed by Dr. William Duane, a neurosurgeon from Thomas Jefferson University. In 1938, Dr. Nathan Schlezinger, a neurologist, joined the Department and became responsible for its day-to-day functioning. Four years later, Dr. Bernard Alpers was appointed chief of neurology at Wills Eye Hospital, although Dr. Schlezinger was still responsible for delivering neurologic care to ophthalmologic patients.

The Neuro-Ophthalmology Service

In 1976, a major revision occurred when the Neurology Service became the Neuro-ophthalmology Service and an official subspecialty of the Wills Eye Hospital. Dr. Norman J. Schatz was named the first director of neuro-ophthalmology and served in the capacity until 1983, when Dr. Peter J. Savino (Fig. 21-1) was appointed director. In 1998, Dr. Robert C. Sergott was appointed Co-Director of the Neuro-Ophthalmology Service.

The Neuro-Ophthalmology Service instituted fellowship training in 1976. The first fellows trained were Dr. Robert Osher, who was a preresidency fellow and Dr. Tulay Kansu, a neurologist from Ankara, Turkey. Since that time, there have been a total of 49 fellows who have been trained on the Neuro-Ophthalmology Service. Many of these fellows hold academic positions in universities in the United States, but several are involved in academic medicine in other countries, such as Turkey, Australia, New Zealand, Saudi Arabia, Canada and Japan. Presently, the Neuro-Ophthalmology Service at Wills Eye Hospital is recognized as the single largest center for the subspecialty both nationally and internationally.

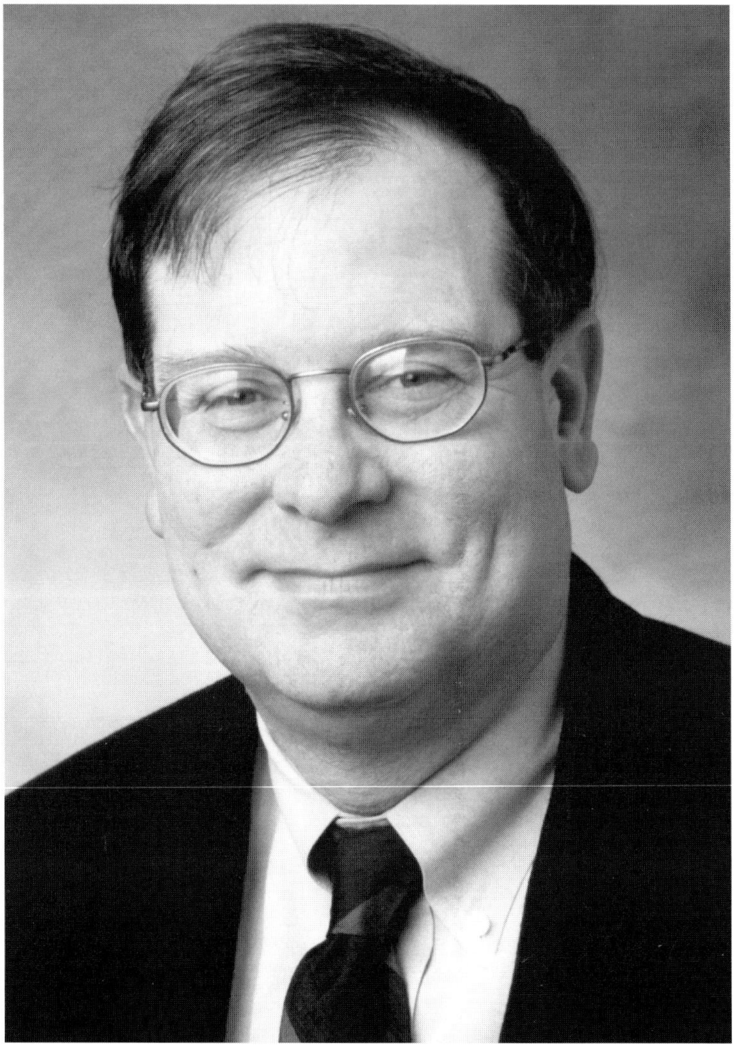

FIGURE 21-1
Dr. Robert C. Sergott, co-director of the Neuro-Ophthalmology Service.

Research

The Neuro-Ophthalmology Service has conducted research on a variety of neuro-ophthalmologic topics that have been published in major journals. The Service has also been part of multi-centered trials, including the Optic Neuritis Treatment Trial (ONTT), the Longitudinal Optic Nerve Study (LONS), and the Leber's Hereditary Optic Neuropathy Study. In addition, a study on Giant Cell Arteritis in cooperation with Johns Hopkins University is in progress.

Vascular Studies Laboratory

In 1988 the Vascular Studies Laboratory was founded. In February of 1990 Color Doppler capability was employed to measure blood flow to the optic nerves. The Vascular Studies Laboratory has been a major innovator in this technology. Many scientists have come here and have taken the technology back to their own institutions. In a large part because of original studies performed at the Wills Eye Hospital Vascular Studies Laboratory in conjunction with the Glaucoma Service, ocular blood flow has become an important investigative tool in glaucoma.

The Vascular Studies Laboratory continues to concentrate its investigation on optic neuropathies, such as giant cell arteritis, carotid artery disease and strokes. In conjunction with the Neurological Surgery Service at Wills Eye Hospital, transcranial Doppler studies have been added to the spectrum of studies performed.

Under the leadership of Dr. Robert C. Sergott, the Vascular Studies Laboratory continues to venture into new areas of investigation of the blood flow to the eye and brain.

The Future

The move to a fourth structure will provide challenges and opportunities to the Neuro-Ophthalmology Service. We believe that it will provide us with the substrate to advance our patient care, teaching and research activity.

Chapter 22

The Ophthalmic Pathology Laboratory

Ralph C. Eagle, Jr., M.D., Director

Born of scientific curiosity, the pathology laboratory at the Wills Eye Hospital evolved into a clinical necessity. As early as 1893, the staff entered a plea for a laboratory, insisting that "a pathological laboratory is sadly needed, that the scientific side of the hospital may keep pace with the humanitarian." Dr. W. F. Norris was appointed curator and pathologist in 1900, but his title was largely a sinecure. The small room that had been set aside for laboratory purposes was first utilized in 1903 when Dr. H. G. Von Goldberg became pathologist. According to Dr. Von Goldberg, his work "consisted largely in the preparation of specimens for gross and microscopic study, the bacteriological examination of smears and occasional cultures. This later work was conducted principally for the study of infection, rather than for the prevention of disease, so that it was of no special clinical importance except as a matter of interest and scientific investigation."

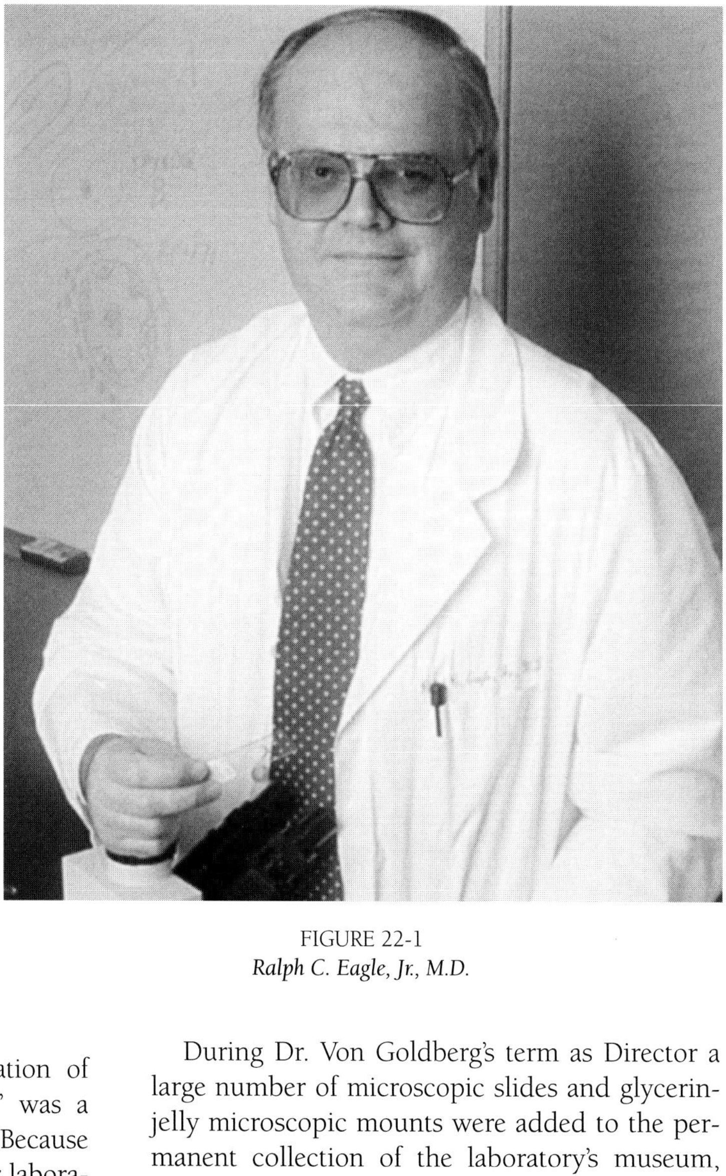

FIGURE 22-1
Ralph C. Eagle, Jr., M.D.

A laboratory budget was established in 1907 and funds were appropriated for the purchase of "proper apparatus" for the laboratory. "Examination of secretions in preparation for operation" was a major role of the laboratory at that time. Because no provision had been made for a regular laboratory technician, Dr. Nelson Brinkeroff donated his services.

During Dr. Von Goldberg's term as Director a large number of microscopic slides and glycerin-jelly microscopic mounts were added to the permanent collection of the laboratory's museum, and a library of microphotographic plates was established. Many embryological and zoological specimens were collected, as well as normal eyes from executed criminals. A freezing microtome also was purchased.

Dr. Brinkeroff succeeded Dr. Von Goldberg in December 1913 and was given a salary. Dr. Brinkeroff introduced the use of autogenous vaccines and the Wassermann test for syphilis. The volume of histopathological specimens and microbiological cultures and smears increased. Dr. Blinkeroff resigned in March 1932 and was succeeded by Dr. Perce DeLong.

The number of tests performed continued to increase dramatically during Dr. DeLong's tenure. Dr. DeLong was a great educator who headed the pathology laboratory for 30 years. Under his leadership ophthalmic pathology began to play an important role in medical education. The laboratory participated in the instruction of ophthalmology residents at Wills and physicians enrolled in the University of Pennsylvania's Graduate School of Medicine. When the Wills Eye Hospital moved from Logan Square to a new building on Spring Garden Street in 1932, Dr. Delong supervised the expansion of the laboratory.

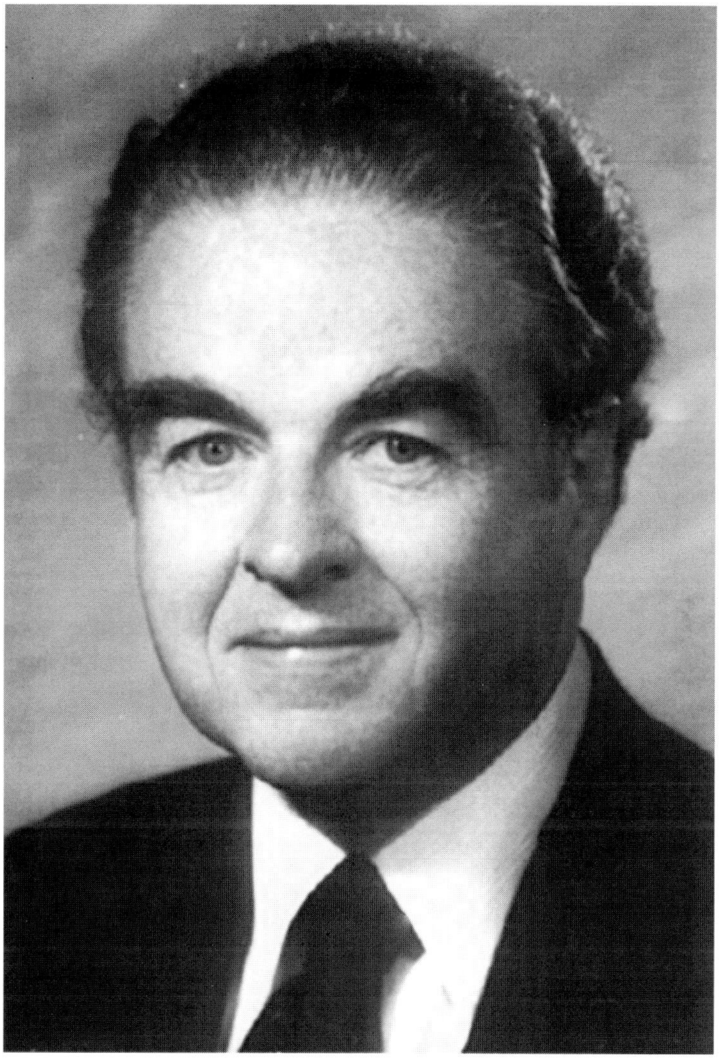

FIGURE 22-2
Charles Steinmetz, M.D.

Dr. John McGavic began to work with Dr. DeLong at Wills in 1950, and assumed leadership of the Pathology Department in 1954. Dr. McGavic was an early member of the Verhoeff and Eastern Ophthalmic Pathology Societies. He initially described Bowen's disease of the cornea and the development of orbital sarcoma after radiation therapy for retinoblastoma. Dr. McGavic left Wills in 1957, but continued to serve as a consultant to the Pathology Laboratory.

Dr. DeLong continued to coordinate the laboratory until a new Director could be found. Dr Charles Steinmetz (Fig. 22-2), who had been examining specimens on a part-time basis for several years, became Director in 1960. Dr. Steinmetz trained with pioneer ocular oncologist Algernon Reese and noted ophthalmic pathologists Georgiana Dvorak-Theobald and Michael Hogan. Dr. Steinmetz initiated a number of laboratory modernization projects during his ten-year term as Director. The laboratory abandoned the old celloidin technique in 1965 and began embedding eyes in paraffin. This allowed the introduction of modern automated tissue processing equipment. A modern freezing microtome for frozen section diagnosis also was secured.

While Dr. Steinmetz was Director, former Wills resident Dr. W. Richard "Dick" Green spent two

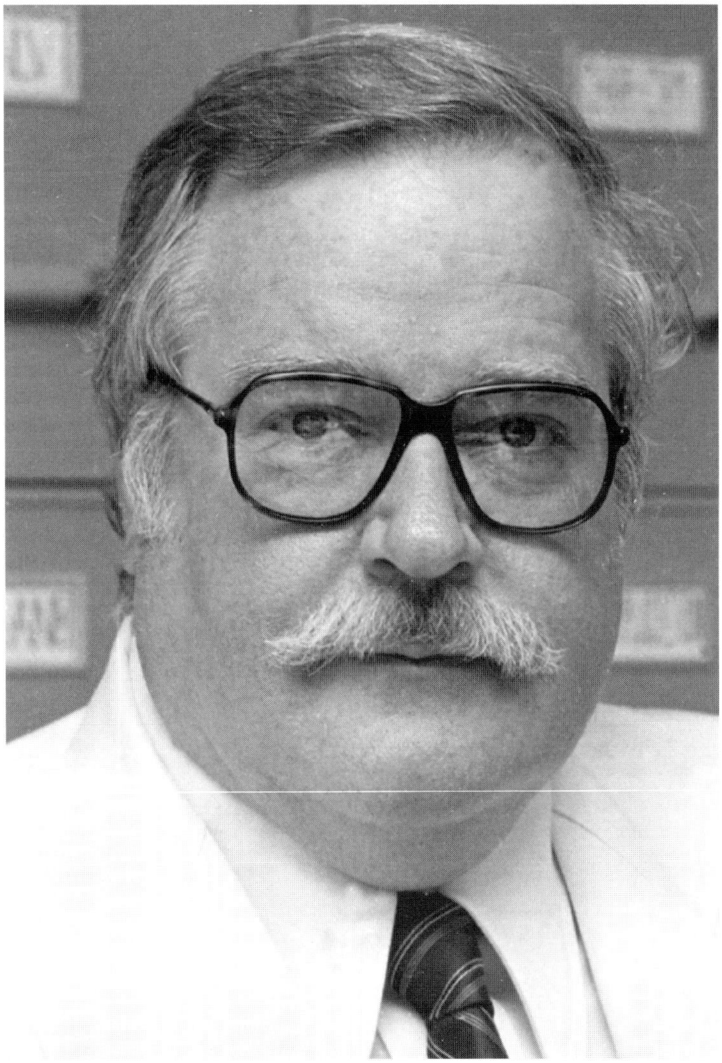

FIGURE 22-3
W. Richard Green, M.D.

and a half productive years in the Wills Pathology Laboratory after completing a second residency in Pathology. Dr. Green had intended to stay at Wills, but became the unfortunate victim of hospital politics. He moved on to Baltimore where he became the ocular pathologist at the Wilmer Institute, a great loss for Wills. Dr. Green became Professor of Ophthalmology and Pathology at Johns Hopkins and was universally considered to be the world authority on retinal pathology. (Fig. 22-3)

Dr. Merlyn Rodrigues succeeded Dr. Steinmetz in 1972 and was instrumental in establishing an active electron microscopy laboratory in 1973. A prolific researcher, she published numerous scientific papers, many dealing with the ultrastructure of corneal disease. She left Wills to become the head of the Ophthalmic Pathology Laboratory at the NIH's National Eye Institute and subsequently worked at the University of Maryland and the FDA.

Dr. Vitaliano B. ("Jun") Bernardino, Jr. (Fig. 22-4) became the laboratory's Director in 1974. Dr. Bernardino trained in both ophthalmic pathology and retina with Dr. Taylor Smith at the Massachusetts Eye and Ear Infirmary in Boston. Dr. Bernardino was in charge of ophthalmic pathology at the Jefferson Medical College before coming to Wills. When Wills became Jefferson's Department of Ophthalmology, Dr. Bernardino became the Director of Pathology. When Wills moved to Ninth and Walnut Streets in 1980, the laboratory facilities were again expanded.

In 1982, former Wills resident Dr. Robert Folberg, who also was board-certified in general pathology, was appointed full-time Co-Director of the Pathology Department (Fig. 22-5). Dr. Folberg was a pioneer in the use of information technology in ophthalmic pathology including computerized instruction and the webcasting of lectures. Dr. Folberg left Wills to become Director of the Ophthalmic Pathology Laboratory at the University of Iowa in 1984, and later was appointed Chair of the Department of Pathology of the University of Illinois in Chicago. His research interests included pigmented lesions of the conjunctiva and prognostic vascular patterns in uveal melanoma.

Dr. Folberg was responsible for increasing the quality of the anatomic pathology service at Wills. Under his leadership, the laboratory was initially accredited by the College of American Pathologists. He also recruited Mrs. Violeta Arbizo to serve as

Supervisor of the combined Anatomic Pathology and Electron Microscopy laboratories (Fig. 22-5). Mrs. Arbizo was a skilled ocular histology and electron microscopy technician who had worked in Dick Green's laboratory in Baltimore. Violeta personally trained a staff of new histology technicians who consistently produced histological sections of uniformly outstanding technical quality. She retired in 1998. Neena Panackal, who was one of Violeta's skilled pupils, was appointed chief supervisory technician at that time. Neena was noted for her literary ability as well as her histotechnical skills. While at Wills, she published a volume of short stories in Malayalam, the language of her native state of Kerala in India.

After Dr. Folberg's departure, Dr. Bernardino reassumed full Directorship and supervised a staff of several part-time staff ophthalmic pathologists. They included world renowned ocular oncologist Jerry Shields who was a former Wills resident, retina fellow and AFIP alumnus; Nognart Romayananda Chan who had trained with Dick Green at the Wilmer Institute; former AFIP fellow George Kurz; and Linda Mottow-Lippa who was a fellow in Dr. Frederick A. Jacobiec's laboratory in New York. During this period consultants in general surgical pathology from Jefferson including Drs. Arthur Patchefsky and Harry Cooper provided frozen section diagnostic services.

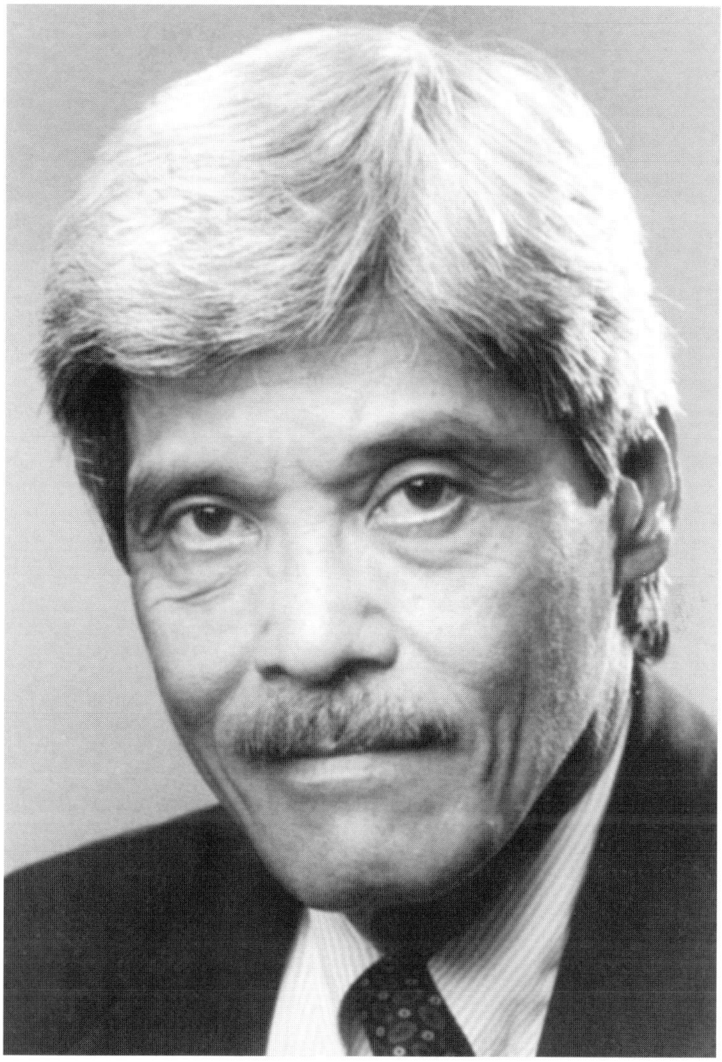

FIGURE 22-4
V. B. ("Jun") Bernardino, Jr., M.D.

Dr. Ralph C. Eagle, Jr. (Fig. 22-1) came from the Scheie Eye Institute, where he had trained, to become full-time Director of the Department of Pathology in May 1986. Dr. Bernardino continued to serve the Department as staff ophthalmic pathologist. Dr. Eagle was an Ophthalmologist who had almost three years of fellowship training in ophthalmic pathology including a pre-residency fellowship with Dr. Myron Yanoff and two years at the Armed Forces Institute of Pathology in Washington, D.C. Dr. Eagle had a prior Wills connection; in 1976 he was a retinal research fellow at the Wills Eye Hospital on Spring Garden Street for seven months before his fellowship at the AFIP.

Dr. Eagle pioneered the use of scanning electron microscopy in ophthalmic pathology as an educational aid and as an adjunct to standard pathology techniques. His original description of the iridocorneal endothelial or ICE syndrome in 1979 and an important paper on fundus flavimaculatus coauthored with Dr. "Jun" Bernardino included scanning electron micrographs as illustrations.

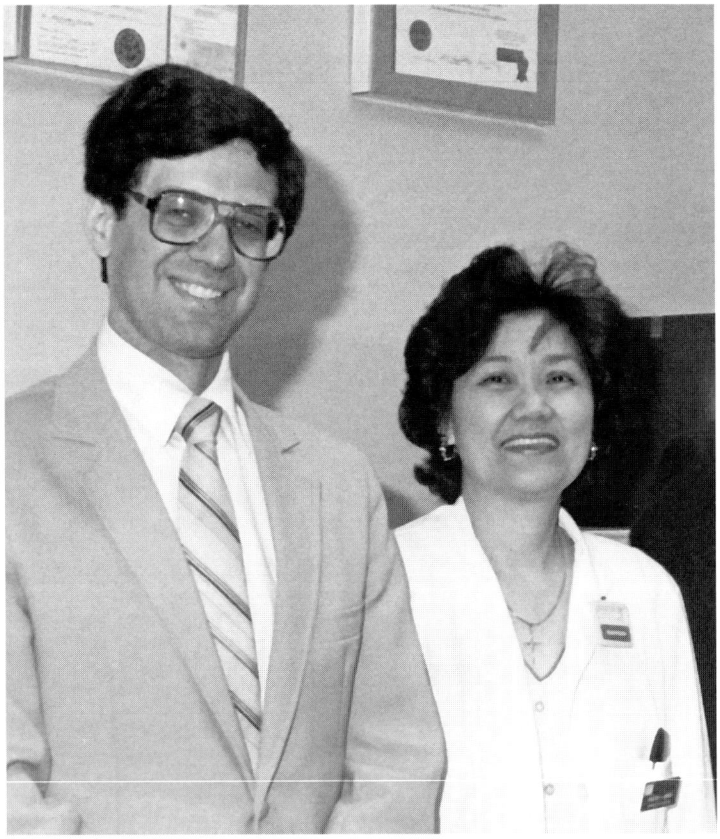

FIGURE 22-5
Robert Folberg, M.D. and Violeta Arbizo

in 1995 and is responsible for the Hospital's extremely popular Review Course, which is attended by more than 400 ophthalmologists yearly.

Dr. Eagle is a member of the Verhoeff-Zimmerman Society and served as the society's representative on the Board of the American Registry of Pathology. He subsequently was appointed to the ARP's Executive Board of Directors. An active member and officer of the American Association of Ophthalmic Pathologists, he organized and directed the AAOP's successful campaign to revise misguided federal laboratory legislation (CLIA '88) that would have decimated ophthalmic pathology by legally disqualifying ophthalmologists from the practice of that specialty. He served as AAOP President in 2000–2002. The Department hosted the annual meeting and histopathology slide seminar of the Eastern Ophthalmic Pathology Society (EOPS) in September 2000 in conjunction with Dr. Nasreen Syed of the Scheie Eye Institute and Myron Yanoff of MCP Hahnemann University (Fig. 22-6). Dr. Charles Steinmetz had hosted a previous EOPS meeting in 1980.

A dedicated teacher, Dr. Eagle gave weekly pathology lectures at Wills and was invited to give intensive reviews of ophthalmic pathology at ophthalmic institutions throughout the world. He was appointed coordinator of the Lancaster Course's ophthalmic pathology section in 1992, and also served on the faculty of the AFIP's ophthalmic pathology course for several decades. During this time the Department began to offer post-residency fellowship training in ophthalmic pathology to a select group of fellows. Jefferson Medical College also established a formal basic science elective in ophthalmic pathology at Wills, which was popular with medical students who were interested in ophthalmology. Dr. Eagle was appointed Director of the Department of Continuing Medical Education

Wills entered into a formal consultative agreement with the Department of Pathology at the Pennsylvania Hospital in 1988 after personnel problems curtailed Jefferson's ability to provide services. Consultant surgical pathologists from Pennsylvania Hospital provided frozen section diagnostic services at Wills and interpreted nonocular specimens. Pennsylvania Hospital also agreed to perform special studies for Wills including immunohistochemistry and flow cytometry. Consultant Surgical Pathologists from Pennsylvania Hospital who served at Wills included Drs. Michael Husson, Edgar Rice, Gary Stopyra, Daniel Kuo and Ray Schiffman.

In 1992 the anatomic pathology laboratory's

outdated electron microscope suite was closed during a major laboratory renovation. Although space limitations and fiscal concerns were major factors in this decision, the advent and widespread use of diagnostic immunohistochemistry had caused a marked decline in the use of diagnostic electron microscopy. The Department continued to have access to electron microscopy under the agreement with Pennsylvania Hospital. During the renovation, a separate laboratory office was constructed to isolate clerical personnel from the technical part of the lab.

Neurosurgery began to be performed in the operating rooms of the Wills Eye Hospital in 1994, and continued after the Hospital was rechristened the "Jefferson Hospital for Neurosciences" (JHN). The neurosurgical operating schedule included many craniotomies for brain tumors. Neurosurgery had major effects on laboratory services at Wills. Jefferson Neuropathologists Mark Curtis and Larry Kenyon began to provide consultative services in Neuropathology at Wills including onsite frozen section diagnosis. The presence of critically-ill neurosurgical patients and a neurosurgical intensive care unit had an even greater effect on the clinical laboratory. The volume, intensity and complexity of testing increased markedly. Clinical Laboratory Operations Manager Ms. Caroline Agnew oversaw the smooth transition of the Clinical Lab to a full-service laboratory with 24-hour coverage. The Clinical Laboratory was operated by the Clinical Laboratory Division of the SmithKline Beecham Corporation for more than a decade and a half. Dr. William C. Kashatus, Regional Medical Director for SKBL, served Wills as Co-Director for the Clinical Laboratory until his retirement and was succeeded

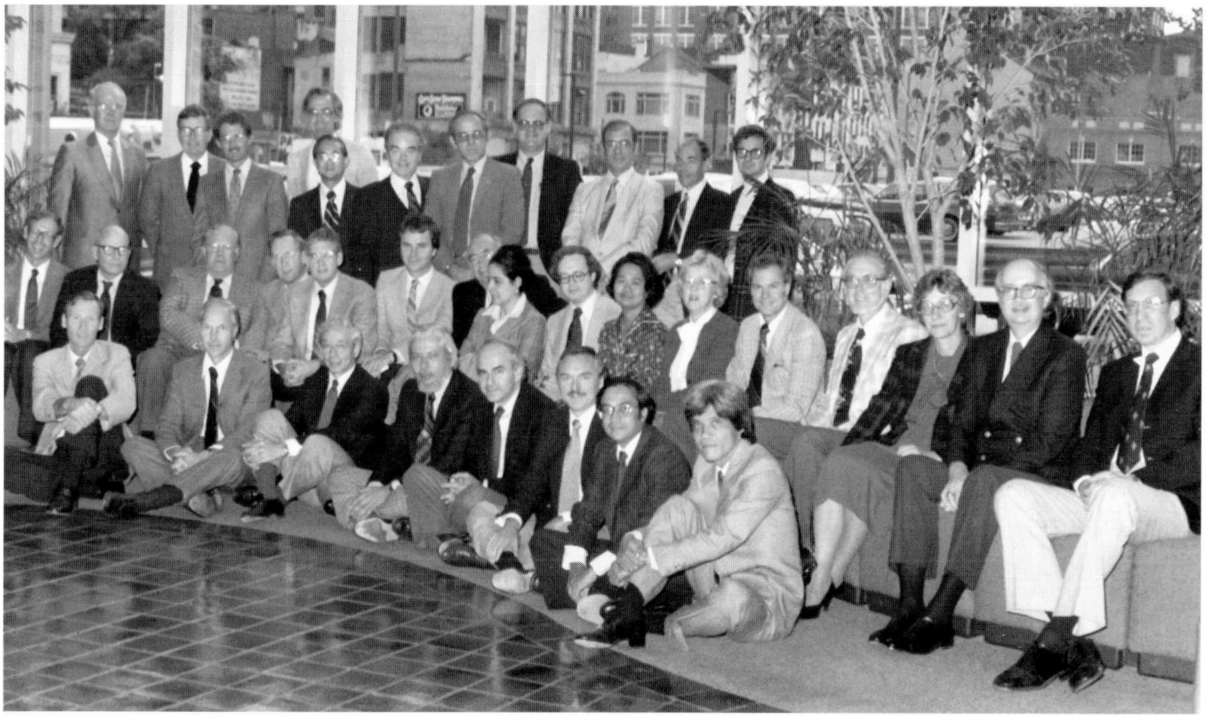

FIGURE 22-6

Eastern Ophthalmic Pathology Society. 1980 meeting at Wills Eye Hospital

Front row (from left):Victor Curtin, William Hunter, Henry Ring, Charles Lee, Alan Friedman, George Howard, Narsing Rao, V. B. ("Jun") Bernardino. Middle row (from left): Dan Albert, Taylor Smith, John McGavic, Bill Frayer, Ramon Font, Seymour Brownstein, Joseph Dixon, Merlyn Rodrigues, Norman Charles, Nongnart Romayananda Chan, Barbara Streeten, Jerry Shields, George Kurz, Elise Torczynski, Andrew Ferry, Paul Henkind. Back row (from left): Robert Collyear, N. Rod Willis, Don Nicholson, Gordon Klintworth, Mark Tso, Charles Steinmetz, Richard Smith, Ralph Eagle, Esmond Gordon, Richard Lubowitz, Ian McLean by Dr. Jack Snyder who served for several years. Jefferson's Department of Pathology assumed responsibility for the JHN Clinical Laboratory in December 2000 when Jefferson's purchase of the 900 Walnut Street building was finalized. Dr. Eagle remained the Director and licensee of the ophthalmic pathology laboratory, which moved to new, more streamlined and better designed quarters on the 14th floor of the new hospital in June 2002.

Patient care, medical education and research continue to be the three primary functions of the Ophthalmic Pathology Laboratory at the Wills Eye Hospital. The laboratory provides the hospital's patients and professional staff with high quality diagnostic services in ocular histopathology, and serves as an international referral center for the processing and diagnosis of ocular specimens, including a large number of eyes with intraocular tumors. The laboratory and its professional staff also serve as a major educational resource for medical students, ophthalmology residents and practicing ophthalmologists. Finally, the laboratory's staff makes original contributions to the medical literature, and engages in medical research projects, individually and or in conjunction with other departments and services, which are designed to advance the frontiers of medical knowledge.

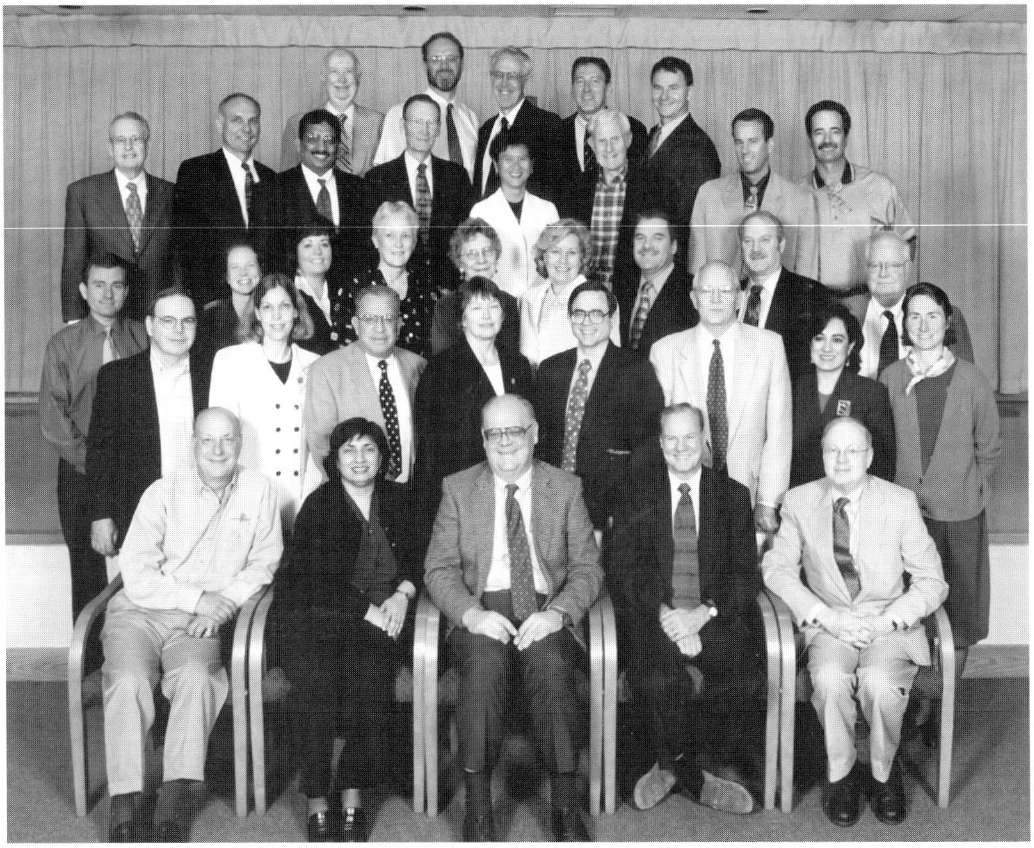

FIGURE 22-7

Eastern Ophthalmic Pathology Society. 2000 meeting at Wills Eye Hospital

Front row (from left): Myron Yanoff, Nasreen Syed, Ralph Eagle, Jerry Shields, Norman Charles. Row 2: Joseph Sassani, Pearl Rosenbaum, Ahmed Hidayat, Martha Farber, Alan Proia, Donald Morris, Patricia Chevez-Barrios, Carol Shields. Row 3: Steven McCormick, Margaret McLaughlin, Nora Laver, Ann Milam, Elise Torczynski, Ann Barker-Griffith, Victor Elner, David Bardenstein, W. Richard Green. Row 4: Ramon Font, Thaddeus Dryja, Deepak Edward, Victor Curtin, Debbie Shetlar, Lorenz Zimmerman, Guy Allaire, Henry Perry. Back Row: Andrew Ferry, Godfrey Heathcote, Gordon Klintworth, Miguel Burnier, Seymour Brownstein.

Chapter 23

Foerderer Eye Movement Center for Children

Robert D. Reinecke, M.D., Director

In 1982 Wills Eye Hospital was notified that a large bequest for children's research was included in the will of Mrs. Ethel Brown Foerderer. Various proposals concerning the use of the bequest were considered. The most suitable area for research in children, and the one least established in the United States, was that of eye movement. Dr. Robert D. Reinecke assumed directorship of the new Foerderer Center on July 1, 1985.

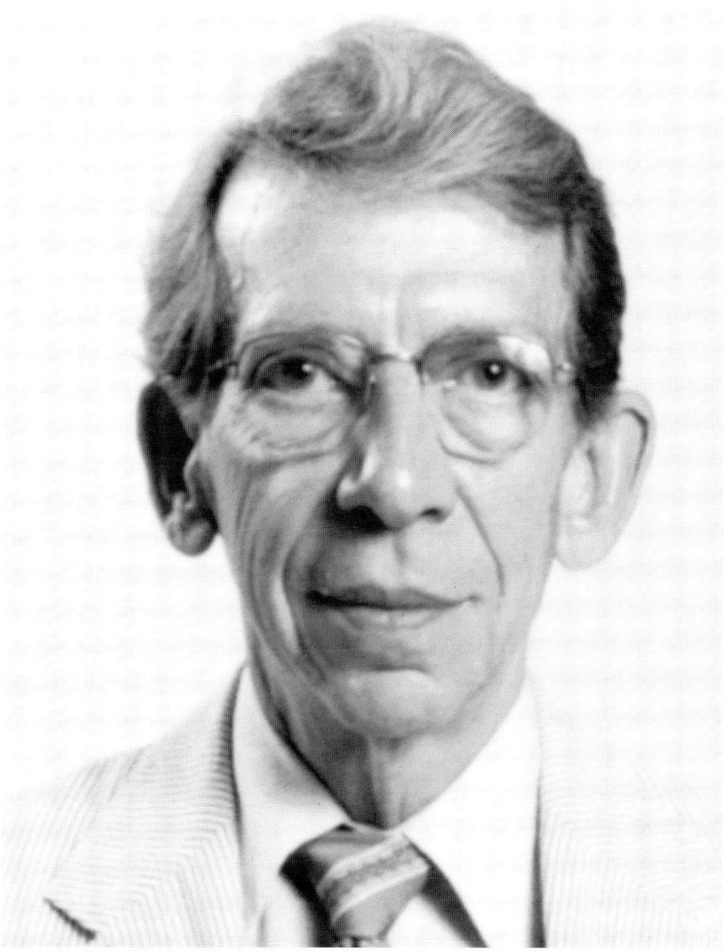

FIGURE 23-1
Dr. Robert D. Reinecke

Agreement was reached with the Board of City Trusts that the center should have a basic science component as well as a clinical side. As a result, Jefferson Medical College made space available for animal investigations related to the kinds of eye movement disorders being studied in the clinical center, and Wills Eye Hospital provided space for the clinical center and offices for the investigators. The trustees of the estate of Ethel Brown Foerderer agreed to this arrangement and further agreed that the principal should not be invaded after the laboratory was set up, but that the interest on the bequest should be used as a core operating budget.

Goals of the Center

The Center was intended to be an independent research center as well as a resource for clinicians. The independent research goals of the Center predominate in determining its operation. The specific subjects investigated depend on the investigators' talents and interests as well as on the timeliness of the particular clinical and scientific issues involved. All the investigators will be involved in clinical appraisals of the patients seen in the Center. In this way, plans for treatment and future evaluations can be made with the latest clinical and basic research findings.

Specific research areas at the Center include the following:

- Strabismus and nystagmus are the two most common eye movement disorders of children. The latter is characterized by slow drifting eye movements interrupted by fast jerk eye movements. New eye movement technology is in place and being used.
- Computer eye movement modeling is performed and evaluated, a promising approach combining the talents and experience of the scientist and the clinician.
- Coupled with the above is the need to study aspects of vision that are especially relevant to the care of children. Children with eye movement disorders commonly have amblyopia. In order to evaluate the effectiveness of eye movement treatments, the vision must be measured, a major challenge in the case of children of preverbal age (those less than age 3). Special computer driven visual evoked vertical potentials are used to access vision in the infants as well as to evaluate the degree of albinism.

Medical students, postgraduate students, residents, and fellows actively participate in research. Laboratory equipment allows clinical investigators to access state-of-the-art eye movement recording devices and employ sophisticated visual acuity measurement techniques.

The Physical Plant

Two separate laboratories carry on their work in the Foerderer Center. Because Wills Eye Hospital has no facilities for the housing of animals, it was necessary to establish one laboratory close to the animal quarters of Jefferson Medical College. The facility at Jefferson is oriented toward studying the saccadic eye movements of rhesus monkeys that have been trained to move their eyes in response to visual stimuli. Among the data recorded are neural signals that must be amplified hundreds of times. Thus, specially shielded rooms are necessary to reduce ambient electronic noise and to allow the signals to be properly interpreted. The facility was completed in June 1986, and Dr. Hershel Goldstein became its director. The machinery facilities there have allowed the fabrication of new measurement devices used in clinical assessments of patients.

The principal eye movement recording device consists of two pairs of electromagnetic coils that have their electrical fields changed about 20,000 times per second. A separate receiving coil is embedded in a contact lens that is placed on a patient's eye (or sewn on an animal's eye) for precise eye position and movement determinations. The data are sampled and stored digitally. The torsional movement of an eye can also be recorded. In addition, a newly developed "fast sweep" visual evoked potential technique that is particularly useful for assessing infant visual acuity is employed here.

The Center's laboratories have been established and developed along three lines. The first involves the establishment of resources permitting the clinical acquisition and analysis of movement recordings. The essential elements are: (1) magnetic search-coil and electro-oculographic systems that accurately record eye movements; (2) a computer system for experimental control and data processing; and (3) a galvanometer-based rear-projection system to present oculomotor stimuli. Each of these elements incorporates the most modern technologies. The Center's eye-coil system makes it one of the first centers capable of routinely measuring the torsional component of eye movements in addition to the standard horizontal and vertical components. The rear-projection system can present targets to elicit both saccadic and smooth pursuit eye movements over a 90° by 90° field. The use of a new, highly visible green laser light source permits the testing of a wider ranger of visually impaired subjects. The intensity of the target is controlled, almost instantaneously, by an acousto-optic modulator. With this equipment, visual detection thresholds (and possibly even resolution thresholds) can be determined during eye movements, thus allowing researchers to study visuo-motor interactions that have only recently been opened to scientific investigation.

The Center's second line of development involves the recording of neural activity in laboratory animals trained to make eye movements to a controlled target on demand. Approximately 770 square feet of space at the Jefferson location were renovated to accommodate this work. The area was partitioned into five rooms to house recording equipment and provide work and office areas. The recording room, as noted above, was specially designed to provide an electrically low-noise environment for recording minute neural signals.

The third line of development involves the perceptual side of the Center's research.

The Foederer Center has had a productive history and has attracted patients worldwide.

Chapter 24

Wills Eye Hospital Celebrations

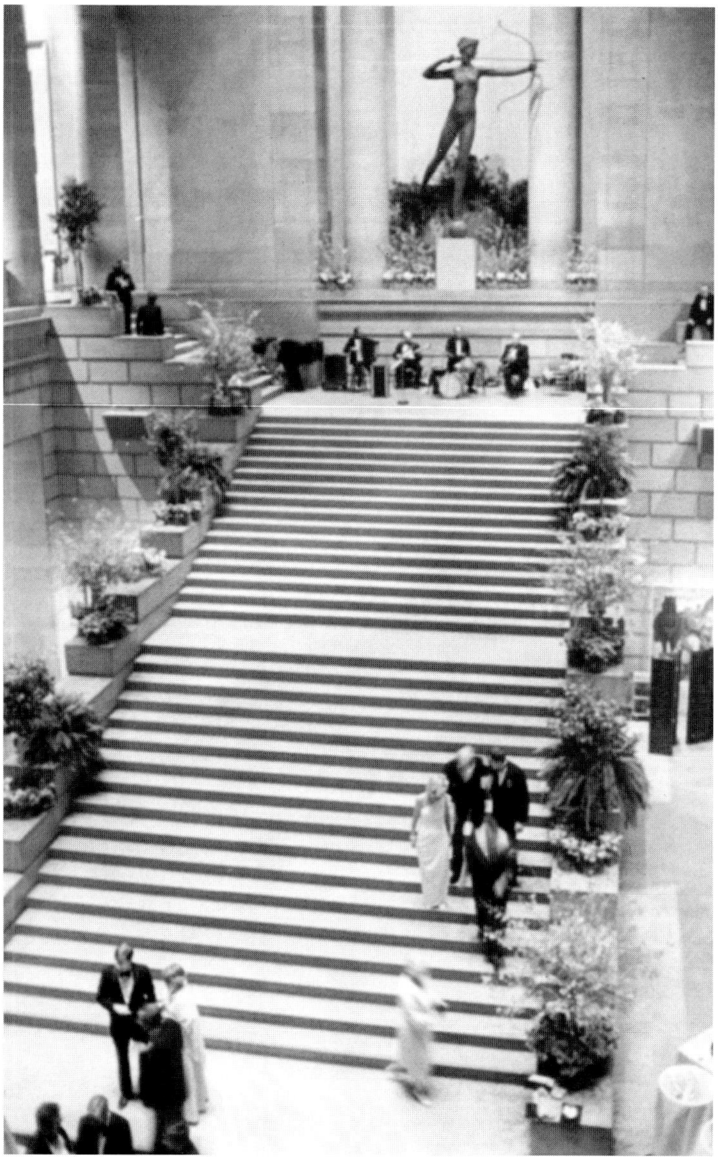

FIGURE 24-1
The grand staircase of the Philadelphia Museum of Art with the statue of Diana at the top of the picture.

25th Anniversary Retina Ball

The Wills Eye Retina Service 25th Anniversary in 1985 was highlighted by two memorable events: a scientific program topped off by a convocation, and an unforgettable gala ball at the Philadelphia Museum of Art (Figs. 24-1 and 24-2).

Several distinguished ophthalmologists attending the Retina Anniversary festivities were awarded honorary degrees by Thomas Jefferson University: the late Professor Gerd-Meyer Schwickerath from Essen, Germany; the late Dr. Edward Norton from Bascom Palmer Eye Institute in Miami, Florida; Dr. Arnall Patz from the Wilmer Instititute, Johns Hopkins University in Baltimore; and Dr. Charles Schepens from the Massuchusetts Eye and Ear Infirmary in Boston.

Wills over the years, and particularly the Retina Service, has maintained close ties with the U.S. Navy and has participated in the training of several of its residents and fellows. In a poignant moment during the scientific program, the Surgeon General of the Navy, Vice Admiral Louis Seaton, paid tribute to the Retina Service in recognition of this association.

THE WHITE HOUSE

WASHINGTON

March 13, 1985

I am pleased to send warm greetings and congratulations to all those gathered for the 25th anniversary celebration for the Wills Eye Hospital Retina Service in Philadelphia.

It is heartening and noteworthy that your directors have guided the Service's outstanding growth in the past twenty-five years to be one of the world's largest retina units. The medical and scientific excellence of this institution, along with its concern for the well-being of the individual patient, have made it justly renowned among those who care about the visual health of our Nation.

Nancy and I send our congratulations and best wishes for many more years of success in high-quality eye care.

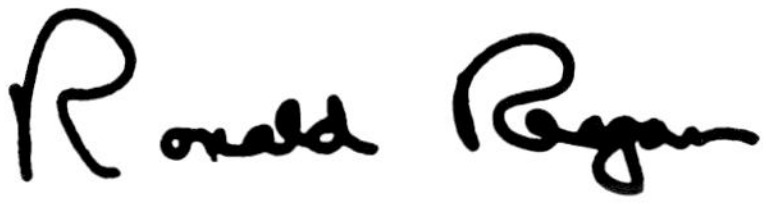

FIGURE 24-2
The 25th Retina Service Anniversary was honored by a letter from President Ronald Reagan.

A second factor that made the convocation such a success was a fascinating lecture by the late Dr. Edward Norton on some of the historical figures who influenced both medicine in general and ophthalmology in particular. He concluded with remarks on Antonio Scarpa, whose *Treatise on Principal Diseases of the Eye* was the most popular textbook of ophthalmology for the first three decades of the 19th century in Europe and America.

Dr. Norton pointed out that Scarpa was not an ophthalmologist although he had made many observations about the eye and was an excellent writer and skillful artist. He selected the paper, typeface, and bindings used in all his books, and many of his books were so expensive to produce that he had to enlist patrons to underwrite them.

Antonia Scarpa was born in 1746, and his interest in diseases of the eye was kindled by his professor at the University of Pavia, Giovanni Battista Morgagni, whose name is still associated with hypermature cataracts. Ultimately he obtained the Chair of Anatomy at the University of Pavia, which at that time was under Austrian rule. As a result of Scarpa's suggestion to Emperor Joseph II, all dead bodies from the state hospital were automatically turned over to the medical school. This was a big step forward, because in Germany one had to buy cadavers, and in England grave robbing was the order of the day. Thus, under Scarpa the University of Pavia became a center for anatomical study.

During the Napoleonic Wars the rulership of Pavia changed hands several times. By the time that the wars were over, however, Scarpa had become virtual dictator at the University. He was ruthless and eliminated from the faculty anyone disloyal to him. Even the State Police feared him.

With the wealth he obtained as a surgeon and political manipulator *extraordinaire*, he built a magnificent villa and acquired a superb collection of paintings.

Scarpa died in 1832, the same year that Wills was founded. He was almost blind at the end, a hated and forgotten man. The only witnesses at his funeral were his hired servants. When the burial was over, his body was disinterred. His cadaver was carefully dissected, except for his head, which was separated from his body. The head was preserved in a jar and remains on display at the University even today.

1995 Wills Eye Ball

Each year the Wills Women's Committee sponsors the Eye Ball to raise money for research. Every year in the spring, during the annual clinical conference, the ex-residents enjoy a black tie dinner dance. These events have become traditional galas that are eagerly anticipated each fall and spring as part of the social scene.

In September 1995 the Annual Wills Ball was again held at the Philadelphia Museum of Art. Chaired by Alice Lea Tasman and co-chairs Veronica Connor and Joan Lucier, this too was a memorable evening. Once again the star was the Philadelphia Museum of Art, this time accompanied by a new city skyline, fireworks and music by Peter Duchin.

Bob Hope was honorary chairman and special guests included then Surgeon General C. Everett Koop and famous ophthalmologist-novelist, Robin Cook, M.D. (Figs. 24-3 through 24-10).

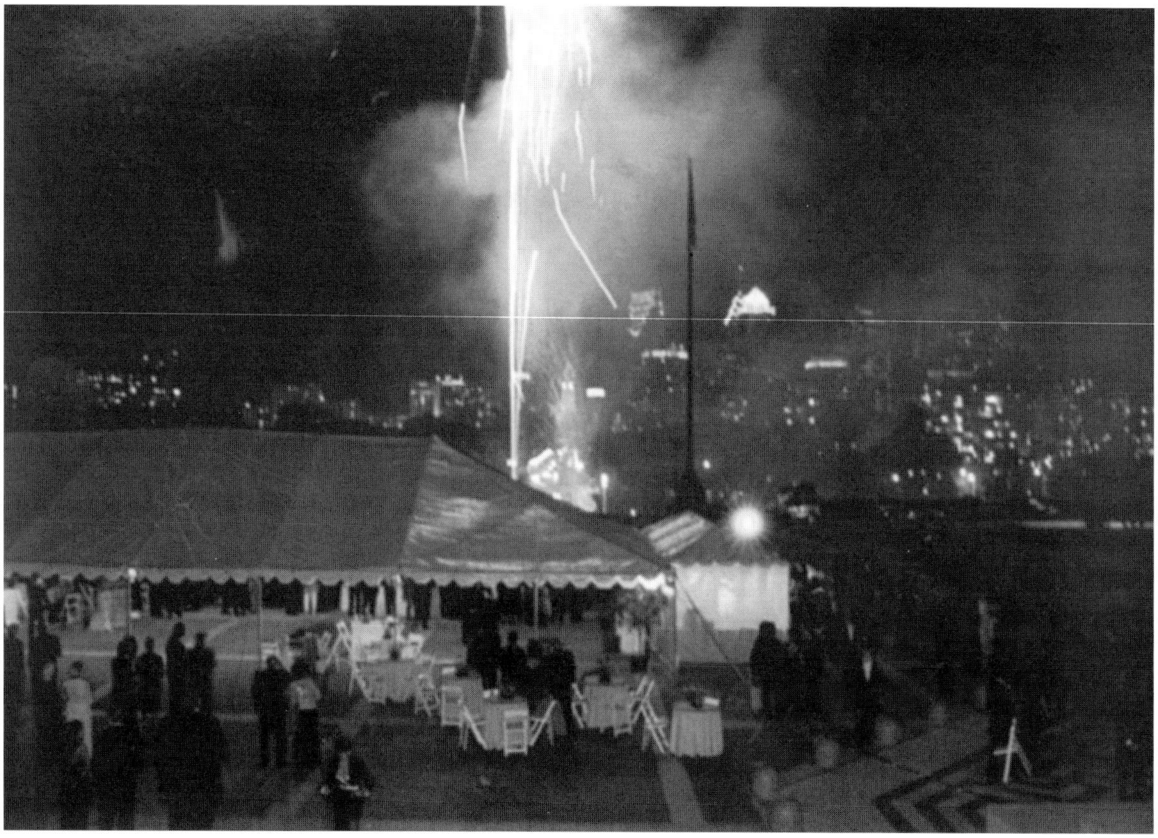

FIGURE 24-3
Fireworks from the bottom of the Art Museum stairs. 1995.

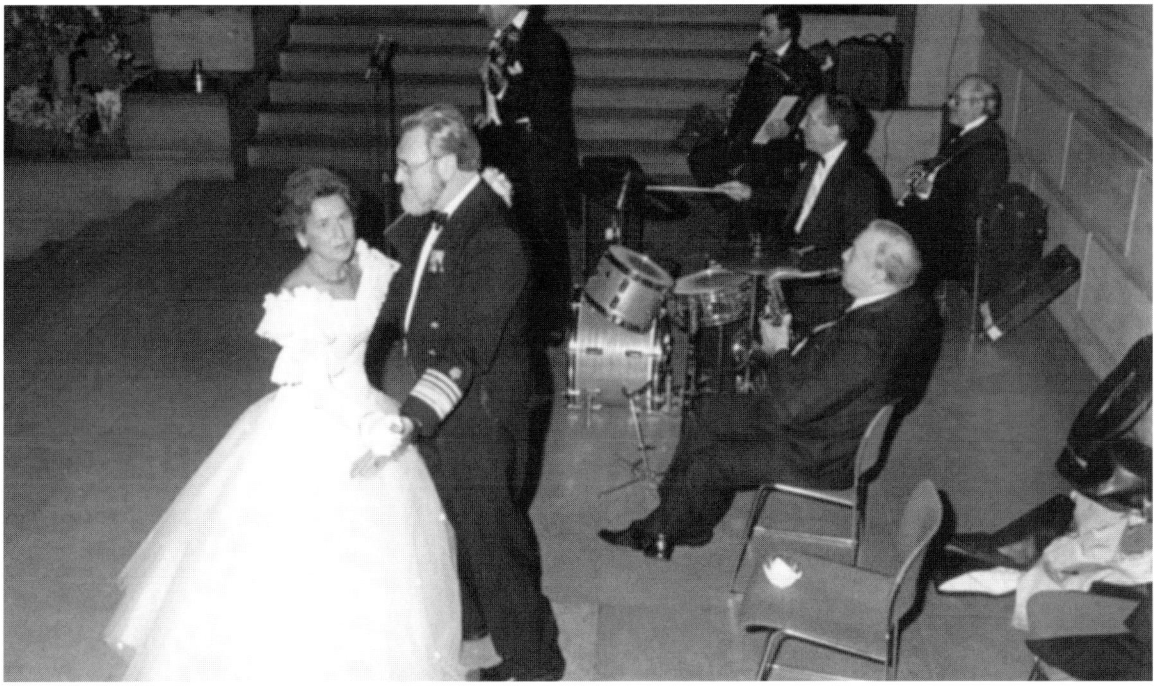

FIGURE 24-4
Alice Lea Tasman, chairman of the 1995 Ball, dances with Dr. C. Everett Koop, then Surgeon General of the United States.

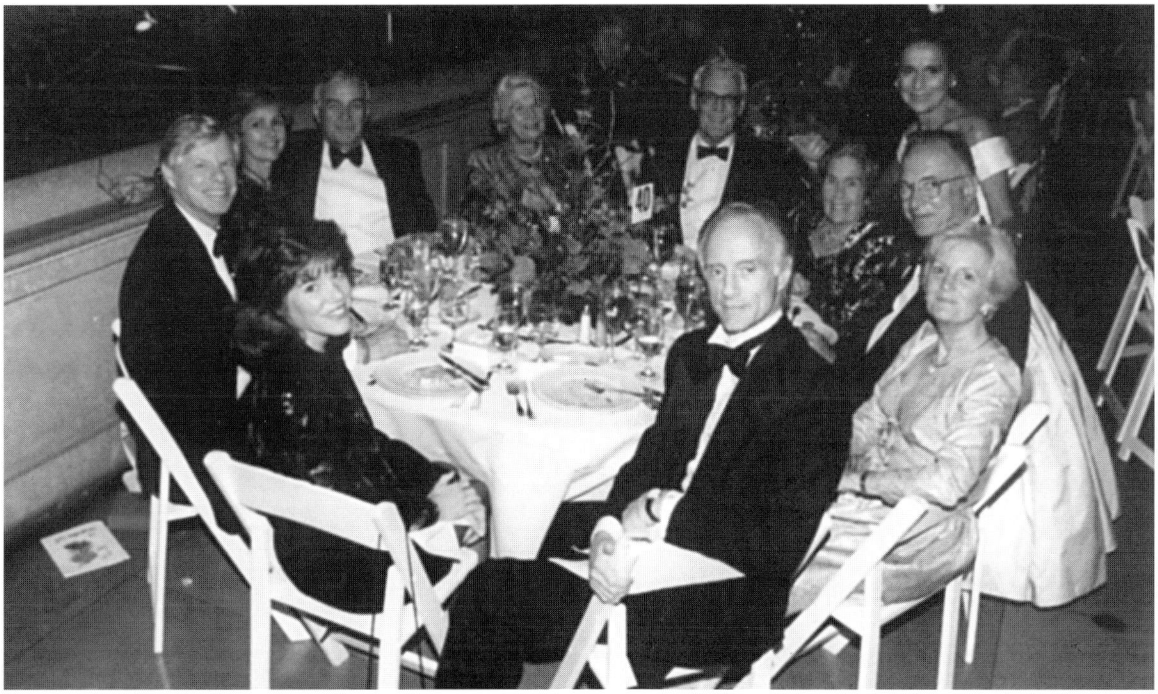

FIGURE 24-5
Clockwise: Author Robin Cook, M.D. and his wife Jean, Ambassador James Malone Rentschler and his guest Lydia, Dr. and Mrs. Thomas Langfitt, Mr. and Mrs. Thacher Longstreth, Alice Lea Tasman (standing), Dr. William Tasman, and Mrs. W. Banks (Nancy) Anderson.

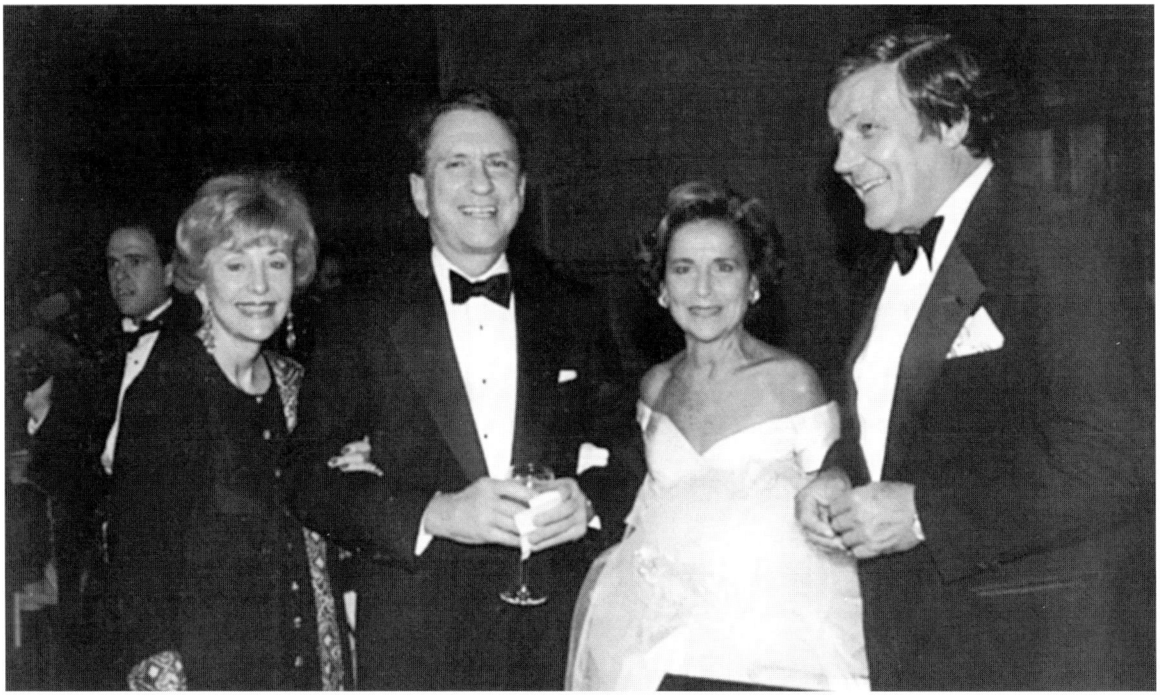

FIGURE 24-6
Senator and Mrs. Arlen Specter with Chairman Alice Lea Tasman and Peter Duchin.

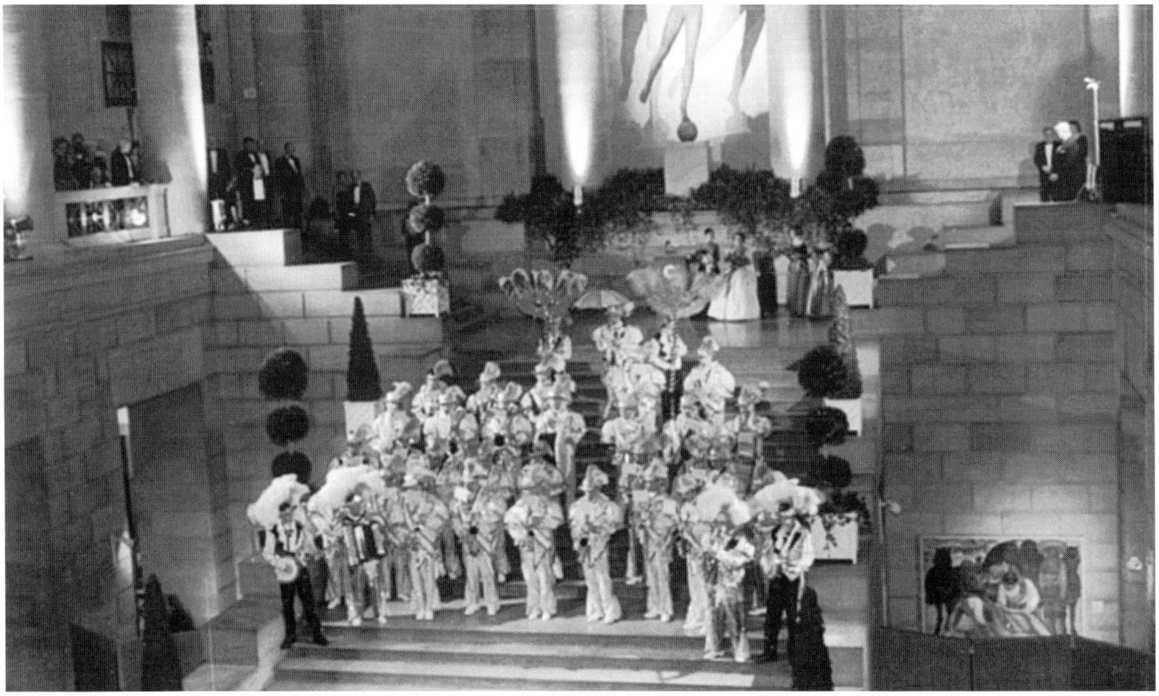

FIGURE 24-7
The Mummers, a Philadelphia institution, play on the grand staircase.

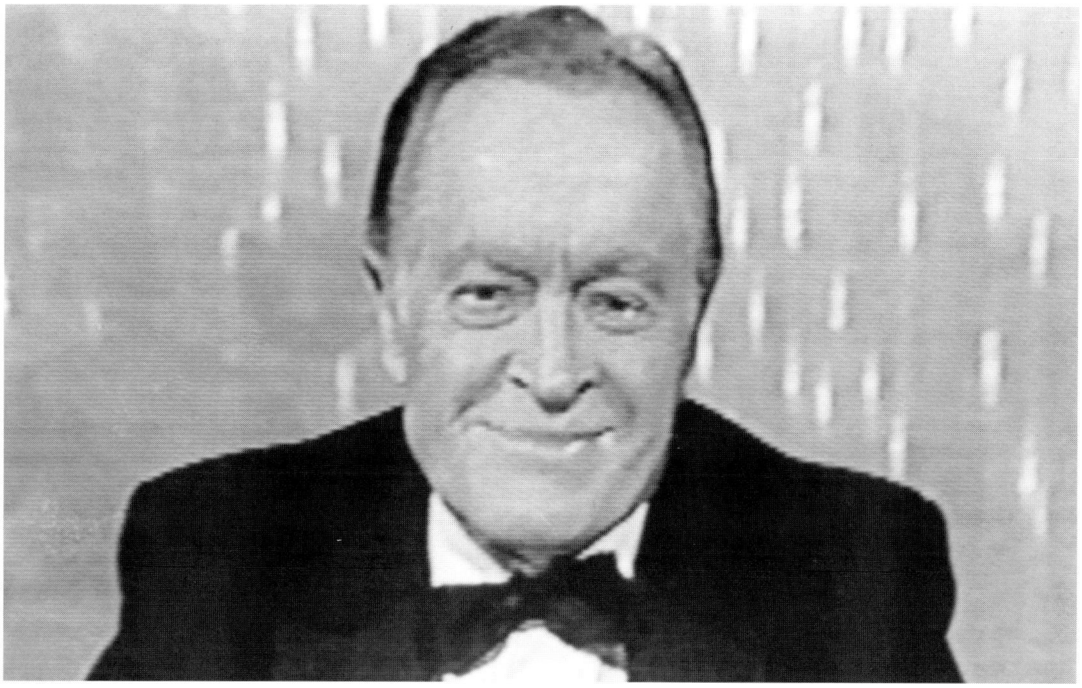

FIGURE 24-8
Bob Hope as he delivered a personal greeting via videotape in 1995.

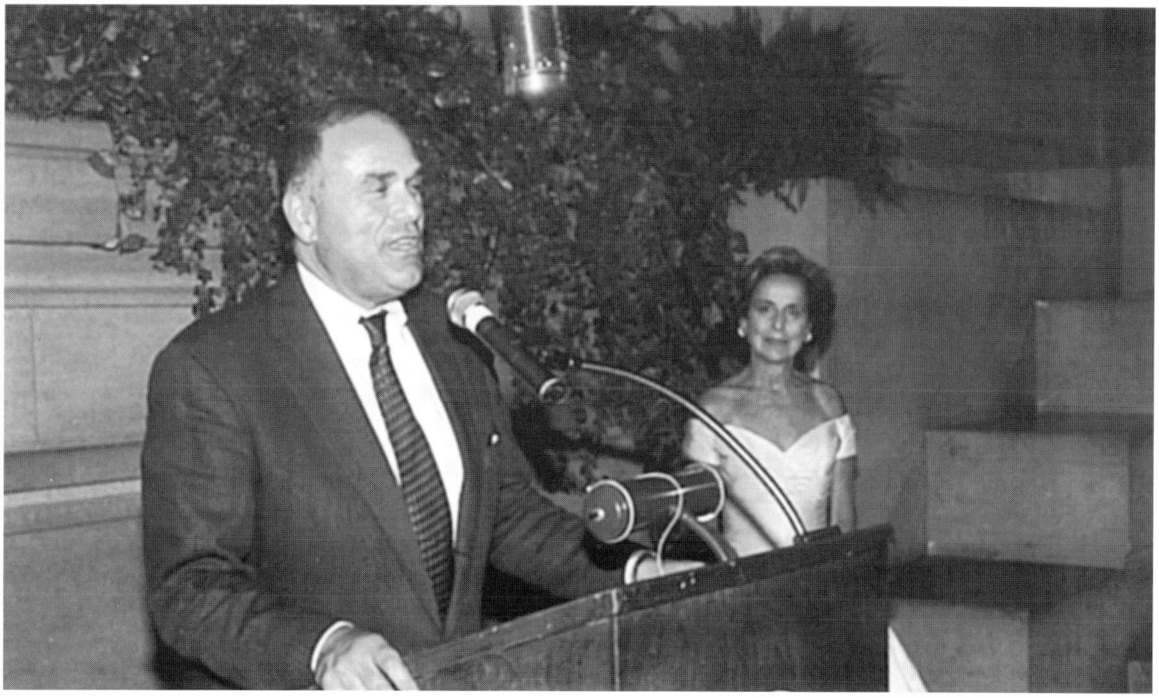

FIGURE 24-9
Ed Rendell, Mayor of Philadelphia in 1995.

Barbara Bush

September 23, 1995

Dear Friends,

I'm happy to send my best wishes to all those involved in the Wills Eye on Philadelphia Ball. Alice Lea Tasman invited me to participate in tonight's event as honorary chair, but because George and I are just returning from a three week speaking tour in Asia, I'm afraid I had to regret.

I understand Wills Eye Hospital was cited in U.S. News and World Report as one of the top three eye hospitals in the United States, but I also know that they need to keep raising funds in order to continue providing great medical care. What better way to get everyone involved than to host a black-tie dinner at the Philadelphia Museum of Art!

George joins me in sending our best wishes for a successful event.

Warmly,

Barbara Bush

Dear Alice Lea,

I shall be thinking not only of you and Bill on the evening of September 23rd but of the happy throng which will have gathered with you at the Philadelphia Museum of Art to dine and dance in a fabulous setting.

I'll be thinking, too, of the cause which all of you will be supporting - Wills Eye Hospital's crusade to eradicate blindness around the world. What a wonderful cause this is, a cause not only to sponsor but also to celebrate.

I wish all of you a memorable and joyous evening, an evening which will delight your eyes, please your palates, charm your ears, freshen your spirits, and set your feet a-dancing.

Ever,

Olivia de Havilland

Olivia de Havilland

FIGURE 24-10

Congratulatory letters from Mrs. Barbara Bush and Olivia deHavilland recognizing the 1995 Ball.

Fortieth Retina Service Anniversary and Year 2000 Ball

The year 2000 featured two landmark occasions. One was the fortieth anniversary celebration of the Retina Service in honor of Dr. William H. Annesley, Jr., former Director of the Retina Service at which time honorary degrees were presented to J. Donald M. Gass, M.D., Robert Machemer, M.D., and Charles D. Kelman, M.D., Wills illustrious alumnus. In addition to an outstanding symposium on macular degeneration organized by Dr. Jay L. Federman, there was an evening of celebration at the Pennsylvania Academy of Fine Arts to mark the occasion.

Then in October 2000 another festive Wills Eye Ball was held at the Philadelphia Museum of Art under the direction of Alice Lea Tasman, Tamara Giordano-Krugman, and Veronica Connor. Over 600 people attended. The evening, which was replete with fireworks, a laser show, and Peter Duchin's Orchestra, raised a net sum of $500,000 for Wills Research. (Figs. 24-11 through 24-17).

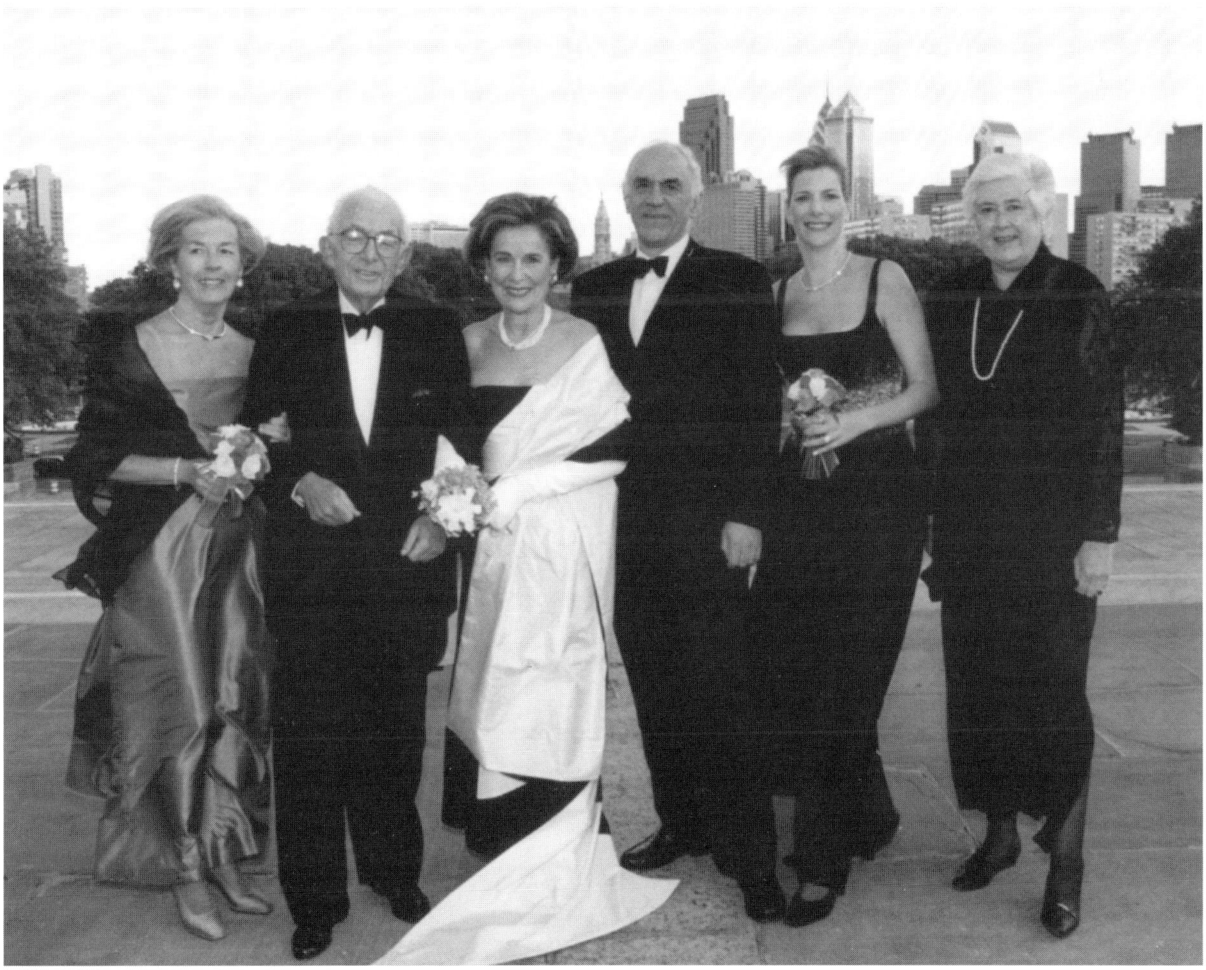

FIGURE 24-11
Left to Right: Veronica Connor, Ball 2000 Co-Chairman, Ambassador Henry Grunwald (honored guest), Alice Lea Tasman, Chair of the Ball, Professor Alan Bird of Moorfields Eye Hospital, London, England (honored guest), Tamara Krugman, Ball 2000 Co-Chairman, and Mrs. Bird.

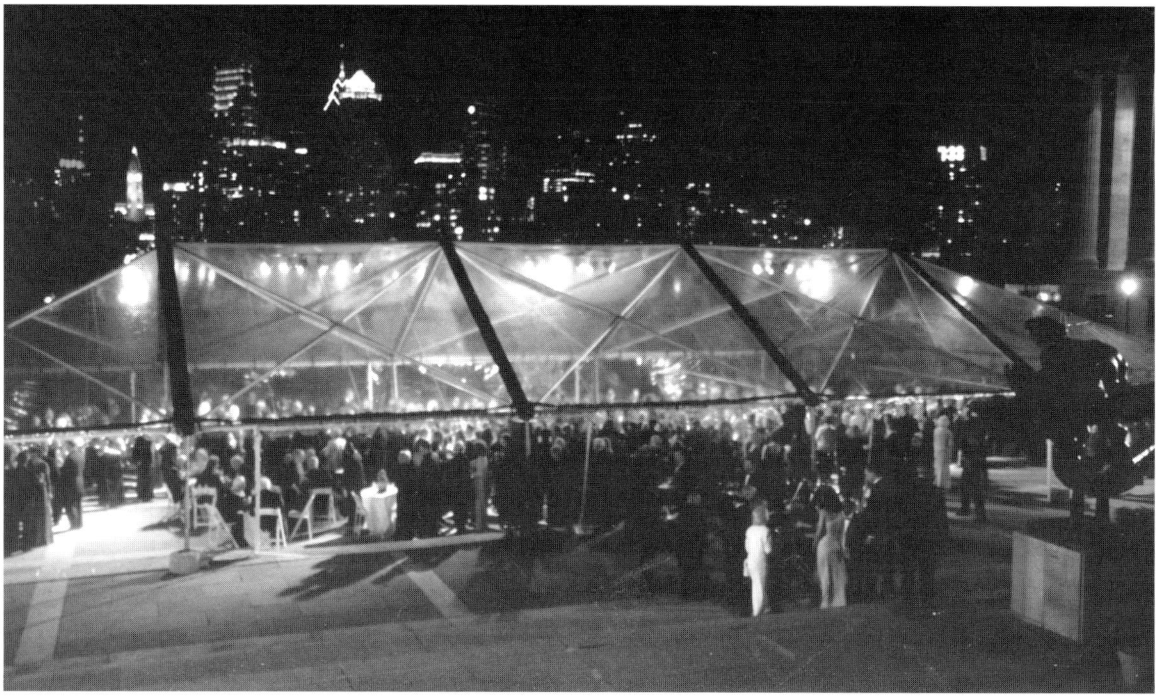

FIGURE 24-12
Cocktails on the steps of the Art Museum.

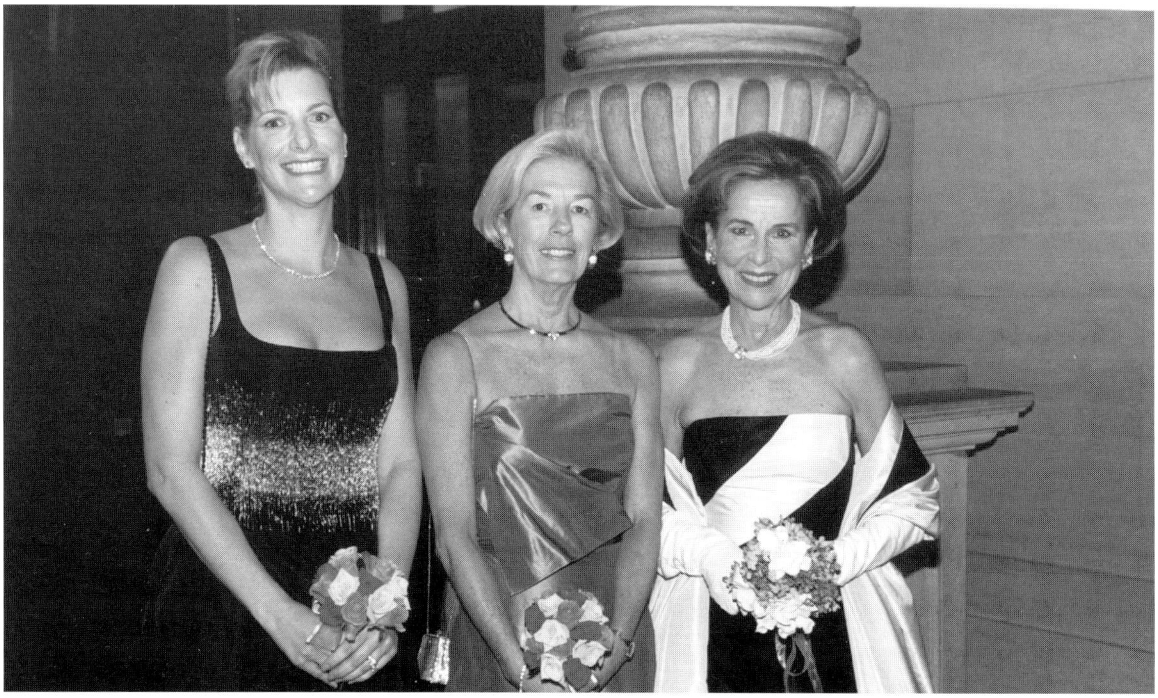

FIGURE 24-13
Tamara Krugman, Veronica Connor, and Alice Lea Tasman.

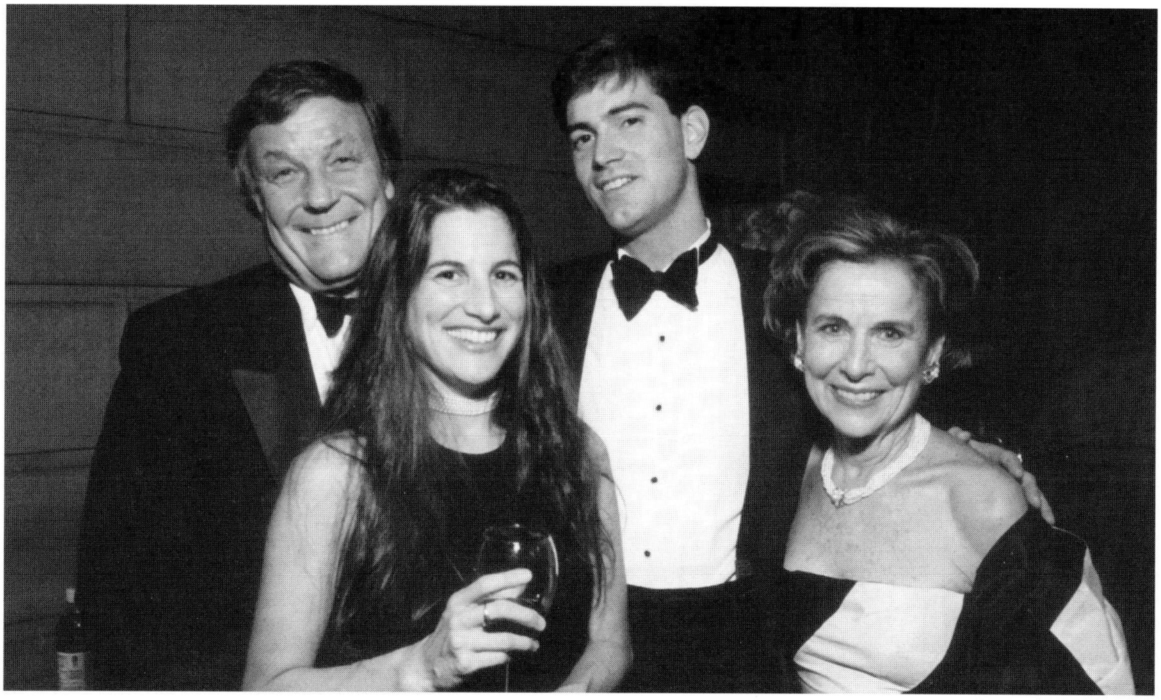

FIGURE 24-14
Bandleader Peter Duchin with Alice Tasman Morris, Richard Morris and Alice Lea Tasman.

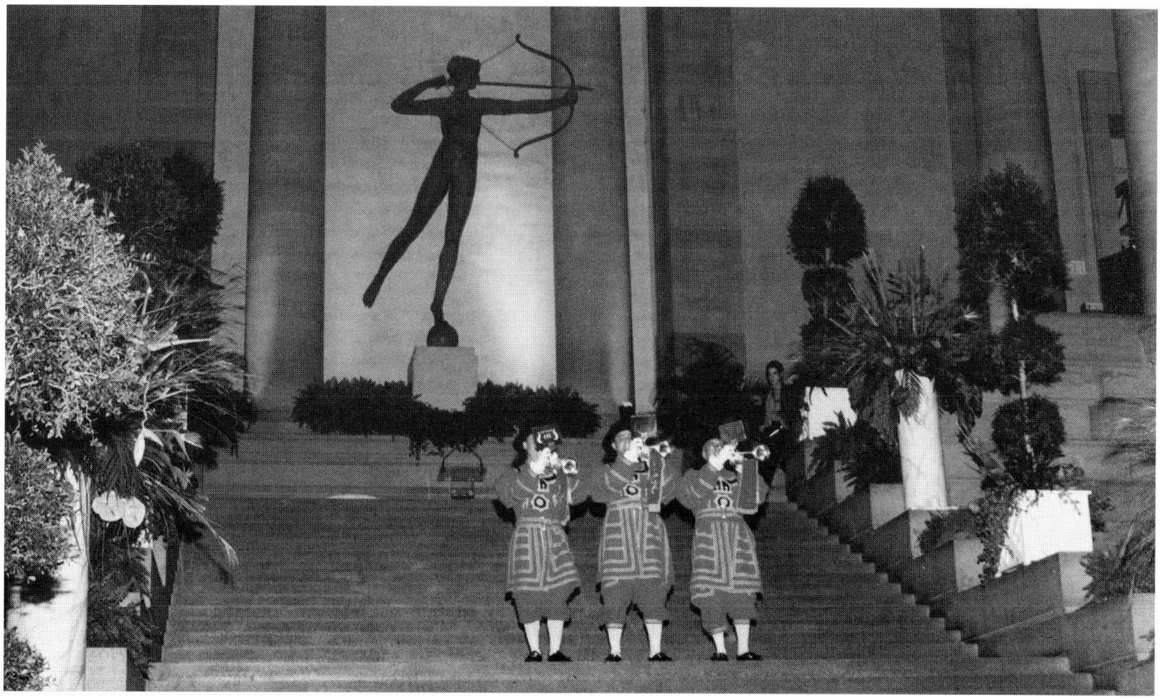

FIGURE 24-15
Trumpeters sounding the call for dinner.

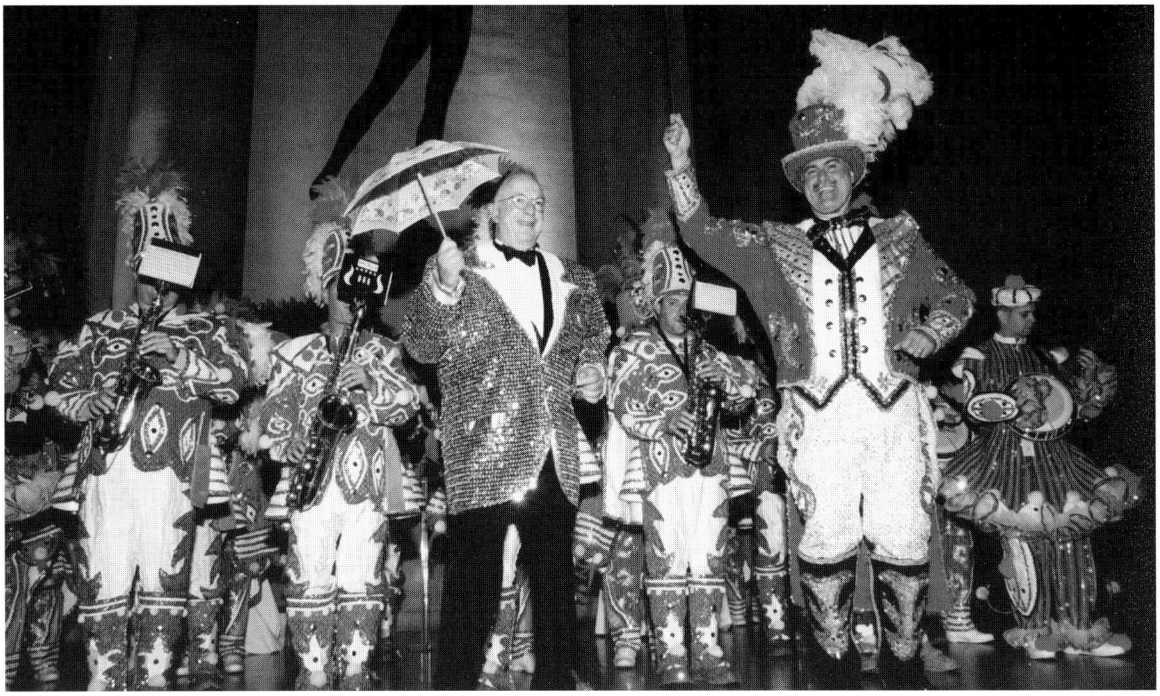

FIGURE 24-16
The Quaker City Street Band adds to the festivities.

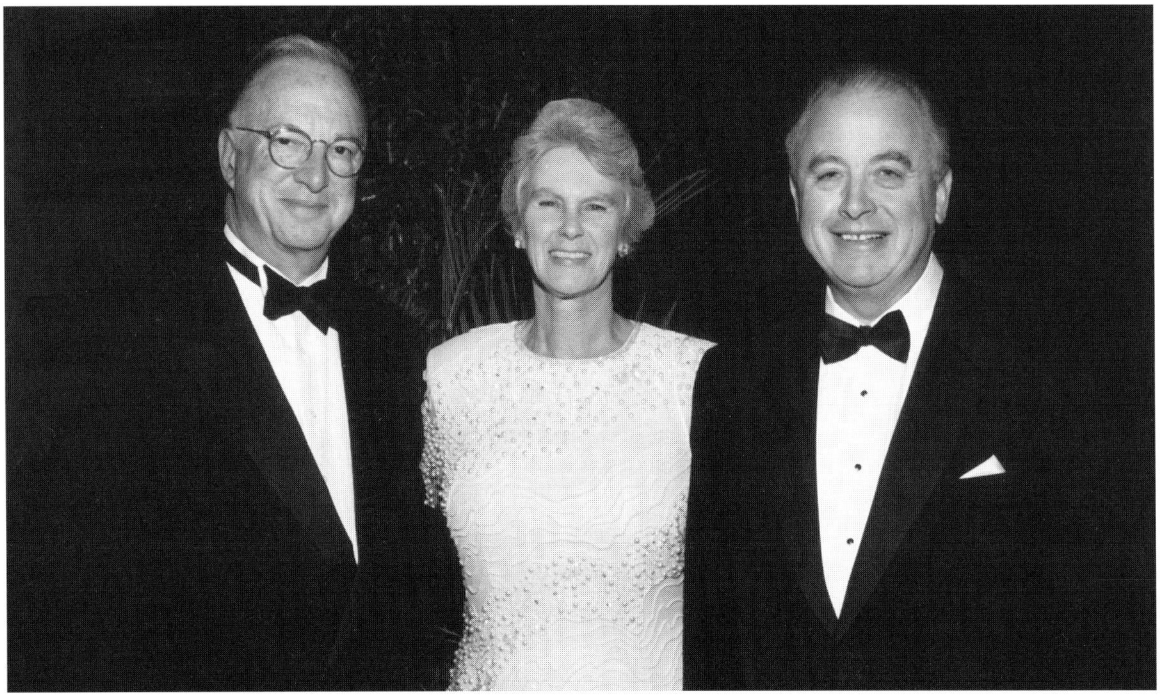

FIGURE 24-17
Dr. William Tasman is with Mr. and Mrs. Tim Sear. Mr. Sear is CEO of Alcon.

Chapter 25
Vision and Art

Our 1988 Annual Report featured art and vision, and the effect one has on the other. This was one of the most popular pieces Wills has published, and I am indebted to Lynn Gartland and her staff for helping me reproduce a portion of it here. In addition, I have included a short review of the Battle of Hastings by noted Chaucerian scholar Thomas J. Garbaty, Ph.D., explaining how the outcome may have been influenced by an eye injury, and how the English defeat led to dramatic changes in the English language.

Art is not a simple process of reproducing an image of the world exactly as it is. Art transforms things through the artist's unique perspective and understanding and shows others a new and different vision of the world.

An impairment is, by definition, a problem that reduces the range of one's abilities or perceptions. Often, however, impairments can be turned to one's advantage. They issue a challenge one must rise to meet. They teach new sympathy for the troubles of others. Or they may offer a special experience of life that, through its unaccustomed vantage point, reveals features ignored by everyone else. Nowhere are the consequences of this more noticeable than in art.

A surprising number of famous artists have had serious eye problems, among them Cézanne, Degas, Dürer, Lautrec, Michelangelo, Monet, Piero della Francesca, Renoir, Turner, and da Vinci. Mary Cassatt, Daumier, and Sir Joshua Reynolds went blind. Edvard Munch suffered a hemorrhage in the macular area of his retina that left a birdlike shape in his visual field, and he began to include this image in his pictures. Camille Pissarro had a chronic inflammation of the tear ducts that forced him to avoid painting outdoors or to paint landscapes viewed through a windowpane, limiting his subject matter.

Disease is certainly not essential or even conducive to art, yet it is a conspicuous part of life that can leave a distinctive stamp on one's view of the world. It can therefore have a visible effect on the process of artistic creation.

In the field of art, eyes have been an intriguing anatomic feature for artists throughout the centuries. Leonardo da Vinci's "Mona Lisa," the eyes in El Greco's paintings, as well as the eyes in paintings of artists such as Picasso and Van Gogh often set the tone of the painting. And then, too, we have the artist's preoccupation with blindness as exemplified by a late 15th century stained glass window in the Frauenkirche in Munich showing Christ healing the blind, and Rembrandt's famous painting dealing with the same subject. As mentioned earlier, the post impressionist Edvard Munch suffered from macular degeneration, the most common cause of visual loss after age 60. In a self portrait he clearly shows that area of visual loss which appears to be a thumb print at the bottom of the picture.

And certainly, some mention of our own Benjamin Franklin is warranted. Philadelphia's first citizen was a multi-talented individual who among other things popularized the bifocal, a device almost all of us need sooner or later. Indeed, Franklin was shown wearing bifocals in one of the portraits painted by Charles Willson Peale.

"If Degas had died at fifty," said Renoir, "he would have been remembered as an excellent painter, no more. It is after his fiftieth year that his work broadens out and that he really becomes

Degas." In the late 1880s and early 1890s, in fact, Edgar Degas (1834–1917) began to shift from detailed oil paintings to looser, brighter pastels, and, later, almost exclusively to sculpture. His works concentrated on fewer and smaller subjects, tended to be more schematic and less dimensional, and were often left incomplete. Many of these changes may have been accommodations to the fact that, by this time, Degas was totally blind in one eye and had lost central vision in the other.

The last part of Degas' life was "a perpetual and tormenting exercise in circumvention," wrote one of his students, since he could only see around the spot at which he was looking and never the spot itself. Ophthalmologists of that time were unable to diagnose his ailment. Possibly he suffered from macular degeneration, which results in loss of central vision, or a retinal detachment, though another possible diagnosis may be solar retinopathy brought on by staring at sunlight on water while painting.

"I have just had and still have a spot of weakness and trouble in my eyes," he wrote in 1871, at the time when his eye problems first began. "It caught me at Chateau by the edge of the water in full sunlight while I was doing a watercolor and it made me lose nearly three weeks, being unable to read or work or go out much, trembling all the time lest I should remain like that."

Cataracts

In 1912, Claude Monet (1840–1926) learned that he had cataracts in both eyes. They developed slowly over the following decade, and he was able to continue his work, though his paintings demonstrated a progressive loss of detail and perspective and a gradual shift in color choice (Figs. 25-1 and 25-2). With dark-colored, senile cataracts such as his there is a reduction in the ability to distinguish blues and greens. By the early 1920s, it is said that Monet could neither accurately distinguish many colors nor read the labels on his tubes of paint, and others had to assist him. In 1923, with only 20/200 vision, or legal blindness, in one eye and light perception in the other, Monet had cataract surgery.

The operation was successful, but Monet developed a common post-cataract complication in which the capsule, left behind after lens removal, becomes cloudy. A second operation, a capsulotomy, was necessary. Monet recovered most of his vision, though for a time he was plagued by distortion, probably due to postoperative astigmatism. For several months after surgery, Monet suffered from xanthopsia, a rare but temporary disorder that makes everything seem excessively yellow, orange, and red. When the condition subsided, everything appeared to be "disgustingly" blue when viewed with his operated eye. His works from these months were overwhelmingly blue, green, and purple. Finally, special yellow-tinted lenses were prescribed that restored essentially normal vision. Several times during this difficult period Monet went back and attempted to correct the aberrant hues in earlier paintings.

Myopia

Myopia is a visual condition in which the image is focused in front of the retina. Near objects can be seen clearly, but beyond arm's length the world is a blur. In severe cases, such a disorder can have significant effect on the sufferer's personality and interests. Children with uncorrected myopia grow up in a world that is limited by vision. Studies have shown they are often more interested in details, intricacies, and intellectual pursuits, and less interested in sports or other more outgoing activities that require a distant focus of attention.

Among myopic painters one tends to find a great attention to fine detail when portraying near objects, but a much broader artistic rendering of more distant scenes, emphasizing color and form over realistic detail. Cézanne and Degas, both of whom also had retinal problems, were myopic, as were Lautrec, Pissarro, Renoir, and Rodin. Lautrec wore corrective glasses, but Renoir did not: He claimed that they would alter his artwork.

A myopic ophthalmologist described his uncorrected impression of an orchestra viewed 70 feet from the stage, which reads like a description of an Impressionist painting: "The conductor holds the centre of interest, gyrating in strange contortions like some fearful wizard before a medley of misshapen geometric patterns in blacks, greys, whites and brown and gold; there are no details anywhere, merely blurred outlines of colour, form, light and movement."

Astigmatism

The elongated figures in paintings by Modigliani and El Greco have led many to suppose that they suffered from astigmatism, an eye disorder in which there may be a distortion of the visual field so that figures seem stretched or tilted in one direction. In both cases this suspicion appears not to be true, since figures are consistently distorted in all directions.

El Greco's possible astigmatism was debated for many decades. Some pointed out the intriguing fact that if El Greco's paintings are photographed through a corrective lens, they can be rendered more normally proportioned and lifelike, though admittedly with considerable loss of artistic effect. Refuting suggestions of astigmatism, most critics claim that El Greco's preliminary sketches were normal, and that stylistic distortions were introduced only in the final execution. Moreover, there are paintings by the workshop of El Greco, on which the master never worked himself, that show the same characteristic elongations.

The contemporary painter Francis Bacon, who has diagnosed horizontal astigmatism, once remarked that early in his career he painted without his corrective glasses, but that when he looked at his paintings later, with his glasses, the vertical strokes "seemed too coarse, and broken-up,

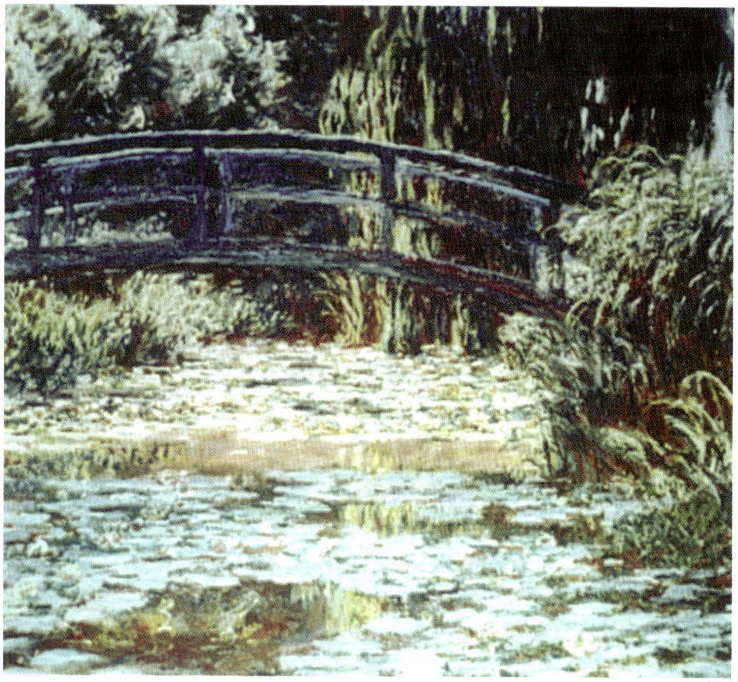

FIGURE 25-1
Claude Monet, Japanese footbridge at Giverny: 1899. (Courtesy of Philadelphia Museum of Art)

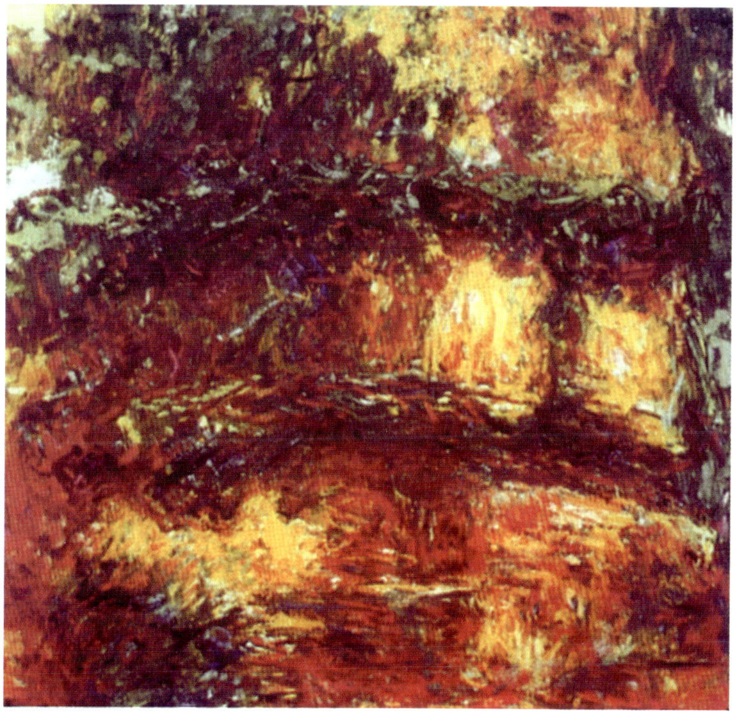

FIGURE 25-2
Claude Monet, Japanese footbridge at Giverny: c. 1918–26 after cataracts developed. (Courtesy of Philadelphia Museum of Art)

so that the images had lost their compactness." Another artist with a similar disorder always drew vertical lines at a slight slant, since otherwise they tended to shimmer and he could not judge the overall effect.

Form in Art

In July 1988, the Wills Eye Hospital lobby was transformed into an art gallery, with the "Form in Art" exhibit, which featured 31 colored sculptures created by visually impaired artists in a unique art study course sponsored by the Philadelphia Museum of Art.

Begun in 1972, at the Philadelphia Museum of Art the "Form in Art" program has touched the lives of hundreds of visually impaired men and women, from the ages of 20 to 98, providing opportunities for self-expression through art. The students work in a studio at the Art Museum, under the direction of independent artists who act as instructors.

Alice Lea Tasman, a former staff member of the Philadelphia Museum of Art who several years ago envisioned Wills Eye Hospital to be the perfect venue for the Form in Art exhibitions, along with the support of Robert Montgomery Scott, then President of the Museum, brought these works to our hospital lobby marking the first time the exhibit was ever shown outside of the Art Museum. At the 9th Annual Exhibition Mr. Scott commended the artists for their inspirational exhibit, adding that displaying it at Wills was a "natural union" of two great institutions with a common commitment to the visually impaired.

The exhibit has inspired others with visual impairments, since many people with vision problems pass through Wills to receive care. Now approaching its fifteenth year, "Form in Art" remains an inspiration to all.

The Battle of Hastings and How an Eye Injury Changed the Language

By Thomas Garbaty, Emeritus Professor of English, University of Michigan Ann Arbor, Michigan

During the occupation of Great Britain by the Romans, the Emperor Hadrian built a wall in the northern part of the country to contain the Picts. When the Roman Empire was declining in 500 A.D. the fifth Roman Legion left to go back home and there was no longer anyone to control the Picts. They breached Hadrian's wall and began to ravage the countryside. Some of the northern European Teutonic tribes such as the Saxons volunteered to come to England to help restore order and, indeed, they did. The language spoken at this time in England is known today as Old English. It is a difficult language for scholars to master, and, in the words of one critic, demands a certain amount of Prussian discipline for students to achieve a reading proficiency.

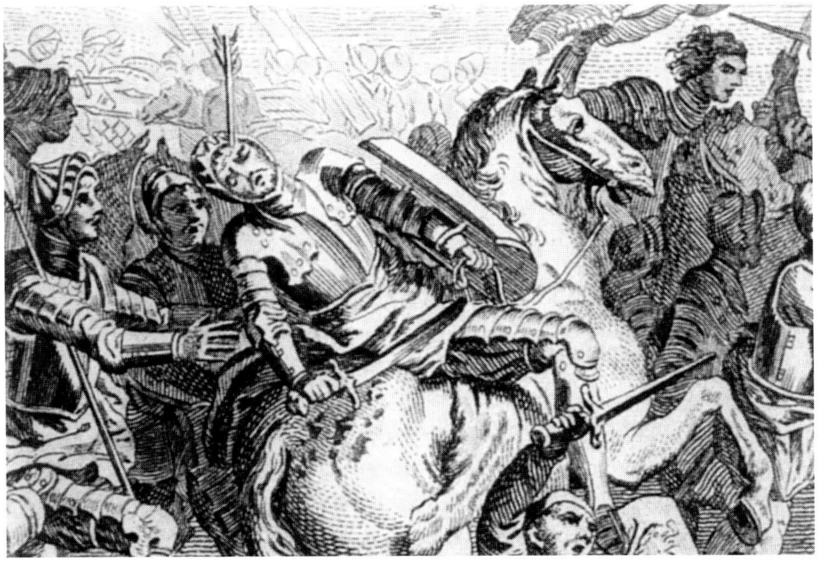

FIGURE 25-3
17th C. print depicting the death of King Harold at the Battle of Hastings.

A few centuries later during the reign of Edward the Confessor, there was no direct heir to the throne. Edward designated William of Normandy to succeed him, but at the same time also made overtures to Harold, one of his chief lieutenants, suggesting that he might be the next king. When Edward the Confessor subsequently died, Harold assumed the throne. This was not well received by William of Normandy and he thereupon proceeded to plan an invasion of England. This is depicted in the Bayeux tapestry where one can see troops gathered in ships on the Somme River. Actually, William's expedition turned out to be one of three successful cross Channel invasions, the other two being that of Julius Caesar and the Allied landing in Normandy in World War II.

Everyone knows that William landed in September, 1066. He was well-armed with cavalry and Norman knights who were professional soldiers. Harold had to rush back to engage William in the Battle of Hastings after repelling Viking incursions in the northern part of England. At that time it was customary for the English to pick up local militia so Harold's troops were not as well trained as the Normans. However, the English were at the top of the hill and were able to turn back several assaults by the Normans. They set up a shield wall but the Normans fired thousands of arrows over the wall, one of which pierced the eye of King Harold killing him instantly (Fig. 25-3). His brother had been killed previously so there was no remaining leadership.

William the Conqueror believed in the *ruse de guerre* and after Harold was killed, lured the leaderless English down the hill with a feigned retreat. They were then enveloped by the main body of William's army and were defeated. Had Harold lived, there is reason to believe that the English might have ultimately triumphed, since the numbers of men were relatively equal on both sides.

One third of the Saxon nobles sided with William from the beginning. The rest were slowly and efficiently eliminated by him. Since the Conqueror's army consisted largely of cadets (younger, landless sons whose inheritance in France went to their older brothers because of the Law of Primogeniture), William married the widows of the Saxon nobles to his Norman knights. The Saxon widows had to learn French or be rusticated from the court and the loyal Saxon nobles already knew French from the days of the Confessor. On the other hand, the common soldiers married into and were absorbed by the English lower classes (farmers, tradesmen, etc.) and the population pressure of language (not only by the farmer's daughter, but all her cousins and aunts) forced them to learn English. What developed were two languages spoken in England after the Conquest divided along socio/economic rather than national lines. In time the remaining ties to France were lost and the Norman nobility stayed in England not to return even to visit relatives. The many French "loan words" (as seen in the "table/field" splits: beef/cow, veal/cow, mutton/sheep, pork/swine; the table terms being Norman, the field terms English) which entered into the English language in the next 200 years show how the Norman nobility had to adapt to the population pressure of English. Old English with the addition of French evolved into Middle English (the language of Chaucer) and then Modern English.

References:

Baugh, Albert C., *A History of the English Language*, 2d ed. Appleton-Century-Crofts, Inc. 1957.

Garbaty, Thomas J., *Medieval English Literature*, 1984, reissued by Waveland Press, 1997.

Chapter 26

Women's Committee

Alice Lea Tasman

The Women's Committee for Wills Eye Hospital was formally organized in 1954. At this time, Mr. Ernest T. Trigg was President of the Wills Eye Committee of the Board of Directors of City Trusts. It was he who insisted that a Women's Committee was much needed and should be formed.

Three women were appointed to create this committee and each was asked to invite twenty friends to the Hospital for a luncheon. The original three were Mrs. Wilfred Fry (who later was a President), Miss Helen Kiley (who was in charge of public relations), and Miss Siegred Craig.

The original purpose of the Committee was to stimulate public interest in the Hospital which had been established in 1832 as a result of a bequest left in trust to the City of Philadelphia by James Wills, a grocer.

From the beginning the Women's Committee had the following categories of membership: Active, Associate, Honorary. The fundraising activities (which have been largely spent on hospital, medical, or surgical equipment and research) of the Women's Committee for the Wills Eye Hospital are and were as follows:

The **Wills Eye Ball** held each year in September or October is our major source of revenue. Our themes have been varied such as, "A Golden Opportunity" at the Hershey Philadelphia Hotel, "The Eyeland Ball" at the Four Seasons Hotel, "Hats Off to Philadelphia" at the Franklin Institute, "Gone With the Wind" at the Union League, "Roman Inspired" at the Hotel Atop The Bellevue, and "Wills Eye on Philadelphia" at the Philadelphia Museum of Art. These are just a few of the many wonderful Balls we have had.

Other major annual fundraising events have been the participation in the Annual **Philadelphia Charity Ball** in December. Our obligation is and was to provide advertising for their Ball program. The amount of advertising was based on the size of the organization and originally the business conditions of the community. All members of the Women's Committee were asked to attend each year. We, along with five or six other hospitals, are the beneficiaries of the proceeds from the Charity Ball.

Leap Into Spring Brunch was held every February and was a much anticipated event. Held at the Overbrook Country Club with a frog as our logo and with the cachet of Herb Clarke as Master of Ceremonies, wonderful prizes and dancing, it was always a great party. Later it was changed to a cocktail buffet due to the Committee's belief that to have another venue might spark the attendance. However, because of the time put in and proceeds realized, we decided to temporarily suspend this project.

Women's Committee Tea. Although not a fundraiser, the annual tea given by the Women's Committee for the doctors, residents, nurses and personnel has been a much anticipated event and is held every March or April.

Bite for Sight. In the past volunteers from the Wills family, the medical staff, Women's Committee and the Board of Directors of City Trusts helped recruit restaurants in Philadelphia and the entire Delaware Valley and asked them to contribute a percentage of their receipts obtained on a special day set aside for Bite for Sight Day in the Delaware Valley by the mayor. (This was usually in April.) We are proud to continue this tradition of our Bite for Sight campaign, and are indeed grateful to the many participating restaurants for helping Wills.

Form in Art held every July or August is now going on its 15th year. Wills Eye Hospital in conjunction with the Philadelphia Museum of Art hosts an annual display of blind artists' works in our Hospital's lobby. These works were created in a program at the Philadelphia Museum of Art and our Hospital is the only venue outside the museum where one can see and actually buy the original art works created by the visually impaired. This is a wonderful community outreach project and we host a cocktail buffet for the opening.

Our **Past Special Events** included the **Penn Valley Antique Show** held at the Philadelphia Marriott West. It benefited jointly the Wills Eye Hospital Women's Committee and the Penn Valley Women's Club. We had three categories for donations all of which received admission. It was a great show!

The **Emergency Aid Bazaar** was held each year a few weeks before Christmas. Women from our Wills Eye Women's Committee helped with the emergency aid workshop and created handmades to be sold at the Wills Eye booth at the Emergency Aid Bazaar. The venue was at a hotel and our booth was decorated and staffed by Wills Eye Committee members.

A **Bulb Sale** took place once a year, May through June. Orders were taken for superior quality Holland bulbs. These were delivered in the fall and made lovely gifts.

Our **Gift Shop**, which was expertly manned completely by volunteers of the Women's Committee and sold an array of gift items, used to have a cart which was taken to all patients in the Hospital when inpatients were the rule.

The creation of an **Ecumenical Meditation Room** was one of our most challenging and rewarding projects.

The Women's Committee has contributed over $2 million to Wills Eye Hospital. From the very beginning we have been a small energetic group of women dedicated to raising money as well as public awareness for Wills Eye Hospital, a facility which has no match in the world for its commitment and its execution of excellence in patient care, education and research.

Chapter 27

Looking Toward the 21st Century

Since the *History of Wills Eye Hospital* was last published in 2002 the revolution in health care delivery has continued at a rapid pace. Doctors are now forced to indirectly share financial responsibility in the care of patients and many decisions are made by non-physicians, most importantly the corporate executives in the various HMOs and insurance companies who often determine which doctor a patient must see.

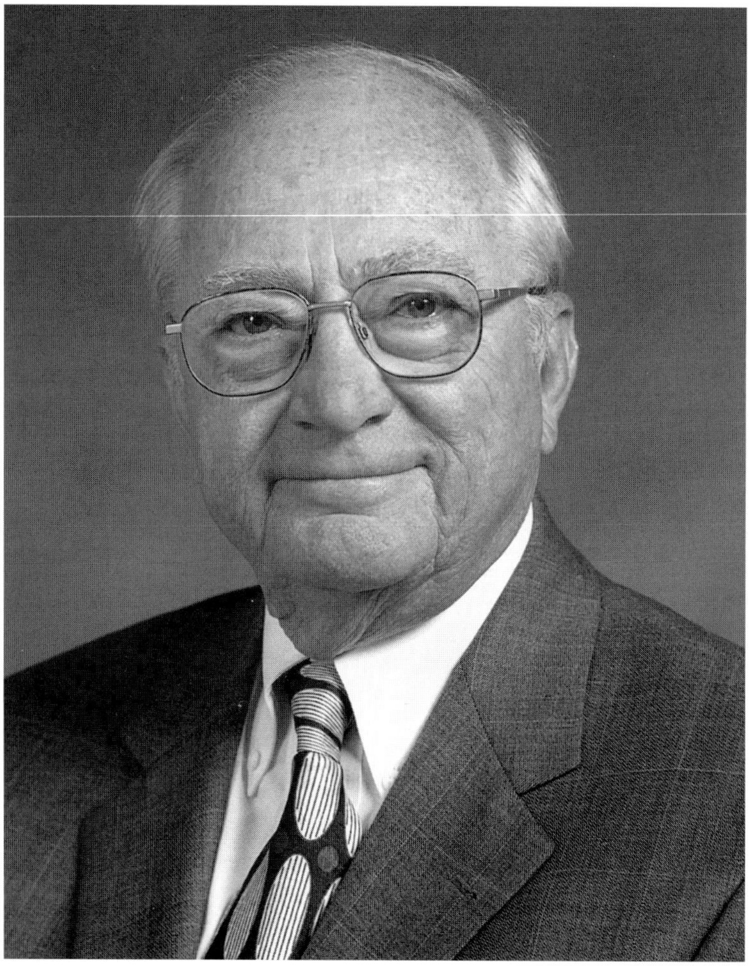

FIGURE 27-1
Edward Jaeger, M.D.

Ophthalmology has probably suffered as much if not more during this revolution than almost any other specialty. Whereas patients previously were hospitalized, since the early eighties ophthalmology has become an outpatient specialty.

Recognizing this, it became necessary to look at other revenue streams if Wills was to remain viable. In the recent past that depended in some part on keeping beds filled. Wills' solution was to diversify. Initially, this involved placing a Geropsychiatric Unit on the top floor of the hospital and then introducing neurosurgery. This transformed Wills, but through it all, Wills has maintained its preeminence in the delivery of eye care. It has continued to have one of the most outstanding staffs of any eye facility in the country if not the world, and the depth of talent on each service is a reason why Wills has remained on top.

Because of Wills' preeminence and its continued contributions to teaching, publications and presentations at meetings, I am confident about our future. In that vein let me say that there are several people who have contributed to Wills in different ways who are not chairmen of a subspecialty department and who have not been mentioned in the book. One of these is Dr. Edward Jaeger who has been a loyal supporter of Wills since he first went into practice. He and I edit *Duane's Clinical Ophthalmology* which was started by Dr. Jaeger and Dr. Duane. Clearly, however, without Dr. Jaeger the success of these volumes would not be what they are today. Dr. Jaeger has also been generous in his help with the outside medical student rotations as well as in our liaisons with Jefferson medical students.

In our new facility residents will be trained in a setting similar to the real world they will face when they leave Wills. As we now become more cost-competitive, Wills will continue to lead the way in how residents and fellows are trained.

Chapter 28

What's New Since Two Thousand Two

The major change over the last five years was the signing of an agreement in July 2006 between Wills Eye Hospital and Thomas Jefferson University Hospital that transferred ownership of the ophthalmology residency and inpatient programs from Wills Eye to Jefferson. Negotiations had been going on for close to two years, and it was nice to finally seem them come to fruition. The residency and fellowship programs will continue under the guidance of Wills Eye physicians. The Wills Eye Emergency Department will remain in the old Wills Eye building, now Jefferson Hospital for Neuroscience, for at least two more years. There are no plans beyond that time to move it elsewhere. It will remain open 24/7, 365 days a year.

As with most negotiated agreements, this one went down to the wire. There were numerous phone calls back and forth and emergency meetings, usually involving attorneys, before the deal was completed. It has now been nearly a year since the agreement was reached, and things seem to be proceeding nicely. Finally, with our inpatient programs under the aegis of Jefferson we have changed our name from Wills Eye Hospital to Wills Eye Institute.

Many of the other changes that have occurred at Wills Eye Hospital over the past five years have involved leadership. After serving as head of the Wills Glaucoma Service since 1968, Dr. George Spaeth stepped down as chairman in 2007. He will remain active in practice, both medically and surgically, so the term "retirement" is definitely to be avoided. A search committee identified Dr. L. Jay Katz, formerly a Co-Director of the Glaucoma Service, to succeed Dr. Spaeth.

Shortly after Dr. Spaeth's announcement, Dr. Joseph Flanagan stepped down as Chairman of Oculoplastics, a position that he held for 25 years. In May 2007, Dr. Robert Penne became Chairman of Oculoplastics. Dr. Flanagan will also remain active in practice.

In 2007 Dr. William Tasman plans to step down from his position as Ophthalmologist-in-Chief at Wills Eye and Professor and Chairman of the Department of Ophthalmology at Jefferson Medical College. In December 2004 he notified the Chairman of the Board of Directors of City Trusts and the Dean at Jefferson that they should look for a successor. A search committee was formed in October 2006 and is now working on a short list of candidates to be considered. Dr. Tasman will also continue in private practice.

Since 2002, when Wills Eye moved into its new facility, Dr. Gary Brown has become head of the Retina Service, succeeding former chairman, Dr. Bill Benson.

Dr. Peter Savino took over as Chairman of the Wills Eye Annual Conference in 2005, when Dr. Robert Penne's term expired. Dr. Penne had been the chairman from 2000 to 2005.

One of the most vital cogs in the Wills Eye machinery is the Director of Residency Education, a position held for years by Dr. Jack Jeffers, and then Dr. Marlon Maus, both of whom were superb. In 2002 Dr. Tara Uhler became Co-Residency

Director and in 2004 Director of the Residency Program. An ex-resident and glaucoma fellow, we are lucky indeed to have her. She is dedicated, extremely hard working, and beloved by both residents and staff.

In addition to these changes, a new named lectureship in honor of the late Dr. Paul Kenneth Nase has been added to the fall retina conference at Wills Eye. Ken was both a resident and a retina fellow at Wills Eye and was a well-respected vitreoretinal specialist in Reading, Pennsylvania. The lecture was endowed through the kindness of Ken's wife, Jane, who I am happy to say was present for the first Nase Lecture, given in October 2006 by Dr. Carmen Puliafito, Chairman of the Department of Ophthalmology at Bascom Palmer Eye Institute.

Dr. Richard Ellis has also endowed a lectureship, the first of which will be given in 2008.

The total number of residents has fluctuated over the last few years and is currently 24. This sometimes presents a challenge because of the Arizona surgical rotation and coverage at Cooper Hospital in Camden and Einstein in North Philadelphia. But the bottom line is that our residents continue to get the best clinical training available anywhere, and we continue to get the best clinical training available anywhere, and we continue to rank among the top three eye departments in the United States. The hundreds of applications that we receive each year are testimony to our outstanding teaching and quality of patient care. Complementing this achievement are the large number of applications we receive each year for our world-renowned fellowships in cornea, glaucoma, oncology, oculoplastics and retina.

Coincident with our academic mission Wills' presence throughout the Delware Valley has been enhanced by its evergrowing network of ambulatory surgical centers which now number nine.

Appendix A

The Board of Directors of City Trusts

President
John J. Egan, Jr.

Vice Presidents
M.W. Baehr, Sr.
Honorable Ronald R. Donatucci
Honorable Vincent J. Fumo

Directors
Ann G. Eisman
Louis J. Esposito
Michael P. Meehan, Esq.
Honorable Michael A. Nutter
Bernard W. Smalley, Esq.
Honorable Marian B. Tasco
Honorable Anna C. Verna*
Stephen R. Wojdak, Esq.

Ex Offico
Honorable John F. Street
Honorable Anna C. Verna

Marlene Brenner, *Secretary*

**City Council President Verna remains an active Board member.*
Because the City Council President is an Ex Officio member of the Board her name appears twice.

Appendix B
Medical Education

Ophthalmologist-In-Chief & Professor and
Chairman of Ophthalmology at Jefferson Medical College
William Tasman, M.D.
1985–2007

Executive Secretary to OIC
Diana Snyder

Director of Residency Program
Tara Uhler, M.D.

Coordinator for Residency Education
Margaret Harron

Coordinator for Resident Selection and
Administrative Assistant for Medical Education
Barbara Kephart

Director of Ophthalmic Pathology and
Continuing Medical Education (CME)
Ralph C. Eagle, Jr., M.D.

Executive Assistant CME
Lucia Manes

Director of Undergraduate Education
Edward A. Jaeger, M.D.

Course Coordinator and Administrative Assistant
Karen Carlucci

Audio Visual
Jack Scully
Roger Barone

Appendix C

Wills Eye Health System Officers

Chief Executive Officer
James J. Mulvihill

Managing Director, Wills Eye Health System
President, Wills Eye Surgical Network
Joseph P. Bilson

Chief Financial Officer (Jan. 2001 – July 2006)
Jeri Mogle
(Jeri transferred over to Girard Estate in July 2006; however, she still has an administrative role at Wills)

Director of Finance
Michael P. McKeever
(Michael started in Jan. 2005 – he took over most of Jeri Mogle's duties in July 2006)

Director of Human Resources and Compliance Officer
Cynthia Farano

Risk Manager / Administrative Assistant
Paula Marbach

Credentials
Toni Rachow

Appendix D

Administration and Board of Trustees of Thomas Jefferson University

President, Thomas Jefferson University
Robert L. Barchi, M.D., Ph.D.

Senior Vice President for Strategic Initiatives
Judith L. Bachman

Vice President and University Counsel
Cristina Cavalieri, B.S.N., Esq.

Dean, Jefferson College of Health Professions
James B. Erdmann, Ph.D.

Dean, Jefferson College of Graduate Studies
Vide President for International Affairs
James H. Keen, Ph.D.

Senior Vice President for Development
Davie R. Lepper

Vice President for Research
Steven E. McKenzie, M.D., Ph.D.

Chief Information Officer
Bruce Metz, Ph.D.

Dean, Jefferson Medical College
Senior Vice President for Academic Affairs
Thomas J. Nasca, M.D., M.A.C.P.

Director, Kimmel Cancer Center at Jefferson
Richard G. Pestell, M.D., Ph.D., F.R.A.C.P.

Vice President for Finance
Chief Financial Officer
Richard J. Schmid

Appendix E

Wills Attending Surgeons

1834-1852	Isaac Parrish, M.D.
1834-1864	Squier Littel, M.D.
1834-1854	Isaac Hays, M.D.
1834-1849	George Fox, M.D.
1849-1852	John Neill, M.D.
1852-1859	Edward Hartshorne, M.D.
1852-1857	Fitzwilliam Sargent, M.D.
1854-1861	Addinell Hewson, M.D.
1857-1864	William Hunt, M.D.
1859-1874	Thomas G. Morton, M.D.
1861-1901	George C. Harlan, M.D.
1863-1893	A. Douglas Hall, M.D.
1864-1869	D. Hayes Agnew, M.D.
1864-1872	Richard J. Levis, M.D.
1872-1895	H. Ernest Goodman, M.D.
1872-1873	Ezra Dyer, M.D.
1872-1897	Peter D. Keyser, M.D.
1872-1907	William W. McClure, M.D.
1872-1901	William F. Norris, M.D.
1872-1902	William Thompson, M.D.
1872-1890	George Strawbridge, M.D.
1877-1890	Henry S. Schell, M.D.
1890-1911	Charles A. Oliver, M.D.
1890-1916	Frank Fisher, M.D.
1890-1917	Samuel D. Risley, M.D.
1890-1898	Edward Jackson, M.D.
1893-1914	Conrad Berens, M.D.
1897-1900	John W. Croskey, M.D.
1898-1924	Peter N.K. Schwenk, M.D.
1901-1924	McCluney Radcliffe, M.D.
1901-1928	William Zentmayer, M.D.
1902-1916	S. Lewis Ziegler, M.D.
1902-1919	William C. Posey, M.D.
1907-1932	Paul J. Pontius, M.D.
1911-1919	William M. Sweet, M.D.
1916-1933	Burton Chance, M.D.
1917-1943	J. Milton Griscom, M.D.
1919-1949	Frank C. Parker, M.D.
1919-1924	Thomas B. Holloway, M.D.
1924-1938	B.F. Baer, Jr., M.D.
1924-1941	Thomas A. O'Brien, M.D.
1924-1939	Leighton F. Appleman, M.D.
1933-1937	Francis H. Adler, M.D.
1937-1952	Louis Lehrfeld, M.D.
1939-1957	Warren S. Reese, M.D.
1939-1961	Carroll R. Mullen, M.D.
1939-1966	James S. Shipman, M.D.
1939-1960	Edmund B. Spaeth, M.D.
1939-1953	William J. Harrison, M.D.
1939-1960	Isaac S. Tassman, M.D.
1943-1967	Wilfred E. Fry, M.D.
1949-1971	P. Robb McDonald, M.D.
1952-1964	Irving H. Leopold, M.D.
1953-1972	Patrick J. Kennedy, M.D.
1957-1958	Edward J. Donnelly, M.D.
1958-1981	Robert D. Mulberger, M.D.
1960-1968	William E. Krewson, M.D.
1960-1978	Joseph W. Hallett, M.D.
1966-1972	Harold D. Barnshaw, M.D.
1967-1973	Bernard C. Gettes, M.D.
1967-1976	Robison D. Harley, M.D.
1970-1981	Gerard M. Shannon, M.D.
1971-2002	William H. Annesley, Jr., M.D.
1972-1976	Albert F. Cleveland, M.D.
1972-1986	Oram R. Kline, M.D.
1973	Peter R. Laibson, M.D.
1973	George L. Spaeth, M.D.
1973-1981	Philip G. Spaeth, M.D.

1973	William Tasman, M.D.
1974	Lov K. Sarin, M.D.
1976-1980	Turgut N. Hamdi, M.D.
1976	Donelson R. Manley, M.D.
1978	Joseph H. Calhoun, M.D.
1979-1986	Malvin J. Dougherty, M.D.
1979-1981	Owen Belmont, M.D.
1979-1990	Richard A. Ellis, M.D.
1979	Vitaliano B. Bernardino, Jr., M.D.
1979-1981	Norman J. Schatz, M.D.
1979	Jerry A. Shields, M.D.
1981	Jay L. Federman, M.D.
1981	Joseph C. Flanagan, M.D.
1981	Edward A. Jaeger, M.D.
1981	William E. Benson, M.D.
1983-1988	Juan J. Arentsen, M.D.
1983-1987	E. Howard Bedrossian, M.D.
1983	Alfred C. Lucier, M.D.
1983-2000	Richard E. Goldberg, M.D.
1983	Peter J. Savino, M.D.
1983	Louis W. Schwartz, M.D.
1983-1989	Charles G. Steinmetz, III, M.D.
1984-2001	Raymond E. Adams, M.D.
1985-1995	Robert D. Reinecke, M.D.
1985-2000	Barry D. Galman, M.D.
1986	Ralph C. Eagle, Jr., M.D.
1987	John J. Siliquini, M.D.
1988	Richard P. Wilson, M.D.
1988	Robert C. Sergott, M.D.
1988	Winston M. Bryant, M.D.
1988	Stephen B. Lichtenstein, M.D.
1988-1999	Daniel M. Kane, M.D.
1989	Elisabeth J. Cohen, M.D.
1989	Leonard B. Nelson, M.D.
1990	Joseph I. Markoff, M.D.
1990-1999	James J. Augsburger, M.D.
1990	Gary C. Brown, M.D.
1992	Thomas M. Bosley, M.D.
1992	David J. Smith, M.D.
1993	Harold P. Koller, M.D.
1993	L. Jay Katz, M.D.
1994	Marlene R. Moster, M.D.
1994	David H. Fischer, M.D.
1995	Alan R. Forman, M.D.
1995	Michael L. Kay, M.D.
1997	Robert S. Bailey, Jr., M.D.
1997	Robert D. Behar, M.D.
1997	Mark H. Blecher, M.D.
1997	John B. Jeffers, M.D.
1997	Janine A. Matsko, M.D.
1997	S. Gregory Smith, M.D.
1998	Irving M. Raber, M.D.
1999-2002	David B. Soll, M.D.
1999	Michael A. Naidoff, M.D.
1999	Carol L. Shields, M.D.
2000	Sadeer B. Hannush, M.D.
2000	Sydney L. Tyson, M.D.
2001	Edward H. Bedrossian, Jr., M.D.
2001	Ignatius S. Hneleski, Jr., M.D.
2001	W. Reed Kindermann, M.D.
2001	Robert B. Penne, M.D.
2001	Christopher J. Rapuano, M.D.
2001	James F. Vander, M.D.
2002	Jonathan B. Belmont, M.D.
2002	J. Arch McNamara, M.D.
2004	Thaddeus S. Nowinski, M.D.
2004	Carl D. Regillo, M.D.
2005	Jurij R. Bilyk, M.D.
2006	Allen C. Ho, M.D.

Appendix F

Wills Eye Physicians and Their Faculty Rank at Jefferson

Alexander, Charles M.
Annesley, William H. – Professor
Armstrong, Thomas A.
Ayres, Brandon D. – Instructor
Bailey, Jr., Robert S. – Associate Professor
Bannett, Gregg A.
Beck, Sylvia R.
Bedrossian, Jr., E. Howard – Assistant Professor
Behar, Robert D. – Assistant Professor
Belmont, Jonathan B.
Benson, William E. – Professor
Bilyk, Jurji R. – Assistant Professor
Blecher, Mark H. – Clinical Assistant Professor
Bloom, Benjamin H. – Instructor
Brady, Luther W.
Brown, Gary C. – Professor
Brown, Leslie A.
Bryant, Winston M.
Calesnick, Jay L.
Calhoun, Joseph H. – Professor
Carrasco, Jacqueline R. – Assistant Professor
Carty, James B.
Caruso, Michael J.
Chaudhry, Iftikar M.
Christian, Colleen J. – Clinical Instructor
Chung, Christine A.
Clark, Francis J.
Coats, Thomas D.
Cohen, Elisabeth J. – Professor
Cohen, Marc S. – Assistant Professor
Cox, Mary Jude
Culp, Randall W.
Cutney, Carolyn A.
Davé, Nisha K.
DeFrancisco, David
DellaVecchia, Michael
Demirci, Hakan – Instructor
Dodds, H. Thomas
Dorfman, Alan M.
Dorfman, Neil H.
Dugan, John D.
Dunn, Eric S.
Eagle, Jr., Ralph C. – Professor
Effinger, Ellin B.
Ehrlich, Dion R. – Assistant Professor
Ellis, Steven P.
El-Mansoury, Jeylan A.
Federman, Jay L. – Professor
Fernandes, Eugene A.S.
Fineman, Mitchell – Assistant Professor
Fiol-Silva, Zoraida M.
Fischer, David H. – Associate Professor
Fisher, Joanna M.
Flanagan, Joseph C. – Professor
Forman, Alan R.
Forman, Jeffrey S.
Fung-Dante, Karen
Galiani, David L. – Clinical Instructor
Galib, Samuel H. – Assistant Professor
Garden, Marc D.
Garg, Sunir J. – Assistant Professor
Gault, Janice A. – Assistant Professor
Gerner, Edward W. – Associate Professor
Goel, Ravi D.
Goldman, Stephen M. – Clinical Assistant Professor
Goldstein, Scott M.
– Adjunct Clinical Assistant Professor

Grohsman, Jonathan
Grossman, Harry D.
Gunton, Kammi B. – Clinical Assistant Professor
Halevy, Jonathan D.
Hammersmith, Kristin M.
 – Clinical Assistant Professor
Hannush, Sadeer B. – Assistant Professor
Harris, Walter P. – Adjunct Instructor
Heist, Kenneth C.
Henderer, Jeffrey D. – Assistant Professor
Hirsch, Stuart E.
Hneleski, III, Ignatius S.
Hneleski, Jr., Ignatius S. – Assistant Professor
Ho, Allen C. – Professor
Jaeger, Edward A. – Professor
Jing, Jin
Kaiser, Richard S. – Assistant Professor
Katz, L. Jay – Professor
Kay, Michael L. – Assistant Professor
Kelly, Deborah J.
Kenney, Lawrence E.
Kimball, Ronald W. – Clinical Instructor
Kindermann, W. Reed
Kleiner, Robert C. – Clinical Associate Professor
Koller, Harold P. – Professor
Kresloff, Richard S.
Laibson, Peter R. – Professor
Lavrich, Judith B. – Clinical Instructor
Lee, Stephen Y. – Clinical Instructor
Lehman, Robert D.
Lehman, Sharon S.
Lennox-Thomas, Patricia
Lewis, James S.
Lichtenstein, Stephen B. – Assistant Professor
Lucier, Alfred C. – Clinical Associate Professor
Luminais, Steven K.
Luscavage, Lonnie
Maguire, Joseph I.
Manley, Donelson R.
Markoff, Joseph I. – Clinical Professor
Marr, Brian – Instructor
Martin, Melanie C.
Materin, Miguel
Matsko, Janine A.
McNamara, J. Arch – Assistant Professor
Miano, Michele A.
Miedziak, Anita I.
Mikaelian, Diran O.
Miller, Robert V. – Clinical Instructor
Milner, Ralph S.
Moster, Mark L.
Moster, Marlene R. – Clinical Professor
Murphey, Sheila A.
Myers, Jonathan S. – Assistant Professor
Nagle, Frank O.
Naidoff, Michael A. – Clinical Associate Professor
Naids, Richard E.
Nelson, Leonard B. – Associate Professor
Nowinski, Thaddeus S. – Associate Professor
O'Connor, Thomas J.
Ohnsman, Christina M.
Ortiz, Joseph M.
Pao, David S.C. – Clinical Instructor
Park, Carl H. – Assistant Professor
Penne, Robert B. – Assistant Professor
Pernelli, David R.
Pizzano, Joseph A.
Porter, Joel
Pro, Michael J. – Instructor
Pyfer, Mark F.
Raber, Irving M. – Assistant Professor
Racciato, Peter J.
Rapuano, Christopher J. – Professor
Regillo, Carl D. – Professor
Reilly, Theresa K. – Clinical Instructor
Reinecke, Robert D. – Professor
Repke, Carolyn S. – Clinical Instructor
Rizzo, John S.
Roat, Melvin I. – Clinical Associate Professor
Salvin, Jonathan H. – Clinical Instructor
Sammartino, John P.
Samuel, Michael A. – Instructor
Sando, Jr., Ralph S. – Instructor
Sando, Ralph S.
Sarin, Lov K. – Professor
Savino, Peter J. – Professor
Schmidt, Courtland M.
Schnall, Bruce M.
Schwartz, Geoffrey P.
Schwartz, Louis W. – Associate Professor
Sergott, Robert C. – Professor
Shields, Carol L. – Professor

Shields, Jerry A. – Professor
Siepser, Steven B. – Clinical Instructor
Siliquini, Jr., John J.
Sivalingam, Arunan – Associate Professor
Skovronsky, Mari
Slochower, Dennis
Smith, David J.
Smith, S. Gregory
Soll, Stephen M.
Spaeth, George L. – Professor
Spechler, Floyd F. – Clinical Instructor
Spina, Jr., Joseph – Clinical Assistant Professor
Stark, Bruce I. – Clinical Instructor
Stefanyszyn, Mary A. – Instructor
Stubbs, G. Winston
Sucheski, Brian M.
Sun, William Z. – Instructor
Swartz, Nancy G. – Instructor
Tabas, Janine G.
Tasman, William – Professor
Tassini, James C.
Tax, Richard L. – Instructor
Thomas, Tricia Lennox – Instructor
Tipperman, Richard
Tyson, Sydney L.
Uddoh, Cordelia N.
Uhler, Tara – Assistant Professor
Vander, James F. – Professor
Wasserman, Bruce N.
Weber, Amy E.
Webster, Guy F.
Weinstock, Floyd
Williams, Christopher A.
Wilson, Richard P.
Witherell, John C.
Wolf, Melvyn A.
Wong, Michael Y.
Yaros, Michael J.
Yasgur, Lee H.
Zeigen, Scott R.
Zolli, Christine L. – Clinical Instructor

Appendix G

Resident Surgeons

1839	John Neill
1841	Samuel L. Hollingsworth
1842	George N. Burwell
1843	William Spear
	John Curwin
1844	Robert O. Norris
1845	Robert Newton
1846	Daniel G. Heylman
1847	William R. Bancock
	Alfred M. Slocum
1848	I.A. Young
1849	Henry G. Graham
1850	Archibald J. Mcintyre
1851	James S. Green
1852	Theophilus Parvin
1853	Norval W. Littell
1854	John C. Homan
1855	John S. Kitchen
	William J. Davison
1856	Isaac N. Kerlin
	T. George Morton
1857	George C. Harlan
1858	Edward Livezey
1859	Charles C. Lee
1860	Charles E. Hackley
1861	William Savery
1862	Joseph G. Richardson
	Thomas Wister
1863	Charles T. Palmer
1865	Charles H. Thomas
1866	William W. McClure
1867	John C. Campbell
	Elliott Richardson
1868	Marshall Paul
	George Roberts
1869	J.C. Wilson
	Morris Longstreth
1870	William C. Cox
1871	N.G. Macomber
1872	E.Y. Burroughs
	H.D. Zendt
1873	J.A. Lippincott
1874	A. Stockhan
1875	Frank Fisher
1876	W.M. Mastyn
	G.W. Zeigler
1877	W.C. Henderson
1878	F.P. Perkins
1879	J.J. Owens
1880	J.H. Carrier
1881	B.L. Millikin
1882	George R. Rohrer
1883	Charles W. Kollock
1884	George T. Lewis
1885	Henry Sykes
1886	C.A. Woodnut
1887	S. Lewis Zeigler
1889	Joseph Ott
1890	M.W. Zimmerman
1891	Paul J. Pontius
1892	Edward C. Ellett
	Walter R. Parker
1893	Paul Guilford
	A.S. Wilson
1894	G.E. Curry
	Burton Chance
1895	D.E. Esterly
1896	James C. Bloomfield
	Edward R. Roderick
1897	Clinton J. Kistler
	Edmund D. Shortlidge

1898	Frank A. Ford
	Albert C. Snell
1899	Charles Lukens
	Walter B. Weidler
1900	Clarence Van Epps
	Frank C. Parker
1901	Harold G. Goldberg
1902	Homer J. Rhode
	Arthur J. Bedell
	W.L. Carrol
1903	John R. Taylor
	Robert I. Bullard
1904	James A. Kearney
	Owen M. Deems
1905	William G. Schlindwein
	J. Clyde Markel
1906	Samuel B. Hayes
	G.A. Briggs
1907	J. Milton Griscom
	Carl Boardman
1908	Charles W. Jennings
	Emory Hill
1909	Frank E. Detling
	Nelson S. Weinberger
1910	Thomas H. Cates
	John A. Kenney
1912	F.B. Moore
	C.M. Buckner
1913	Samuel Marshall
	H.C. Schmitz
1914	Paul H. Kleinhjans
	W.E. Carson
	J.W. Thompson
1915	Otis J. Simonds
	Harry V. Judge
1916	Frederick A. Schlanger
	Joseph V. Connole
1917	Warren S. Reese
	William F. Holzer
1918	R.S. Pendexter
	O.H. Yereman
1919	Ernest L. Posey
	Orla J. Parks
1920	Lee W. Hughes
	Joseph E. Beideman
1921	Cecil S. O'Brien
	Cecil P. Clark
1922	Charles A. Young
	Ivan J. Koenig
1923	Frank C. Smith
	Walter H. Fink
1924	Howard F. Hill
	Thurber LeWin
	John S. Plumer
	Hayward L. Blackmon
1925	George J. Dublin
1926	Wilfred T. Gratton
	Leo W. Funk
	James S. Shipman
	Wilfred E. Muldoon
1927	Maurice E. Marcove
	Walter C. Mott
	Lewis P. Glover
1928	William J. Burdashaw
	Pierre G. Jenkins
	James H. Delaney
1929	Noel T. Simmonds
	Thomas G. McLellan
	I. Jenkins Mikel
1930	John B. Moore
	William C. Ostrom
	Raymond N. Berk
	Stacy C. Howell
1931	Ethelburt B. Fairbanks
	James M. Baird
	William H.M. Thomson
	E. Leonard Goodman
1932	Walter L. Forster
	Benjamin Wolpaw
	Noel S. McBride
	Louis D. Gomon
	Carl D.F. Jensen
1933	E.R. Anderson
	James S. Jordan
	Ronald A.Cox
	Alvin W. Howland
	Robert F. Rohm
1934	John M. Wotring
	James E. Wilson
	James F. Finegan
	Samuel Philipps
1935	Roscoe J. Kennedy
	Robert S. Minton
	Henry K. Erwin
	William D. Angle
1936	L.M. Gurley

	P. Robb McDonald
	Van M. Ellis
	Irvin Levy
1937	James V.D. Quereau
	John S. Goldcamp
	Daniel B. Esterly
	Warren C. Phillips
1938	John L. Matthews
	Samuel Wenger
	Carl A. Hoefer
	James M. O'Brien
	Clyde H. Jacobs
1939	Carl F. Breisacher
	Kenneth L. Roper
	Walter J. Romejko
	E. Franklin Carol
1940	Arthur S. Clay
	Norbert W. Humpage
	Charles Ruggeri
	Ned Schwartz
	John W. Deichler
1941	Daniel F. Fisher
	Harold M. U'Ren
	Charles L. O'Neill
	Frank T. Cultrona
	Henry Abrams
1942	Theodore Long
	Harvey C. Ennis
	Irving L. Pavlo
	Samuel J. Altman
	Robert E. Shoemaker
	Garland M. Johnson
1943	Harry J. French
	James B. Vaughan
	Stanley W. Boland
	Ruth Leonard
1944	Juan A. Diaz
	Elbert C. Anderson
	Joseph F. Morrison
	Francis X. Budd
	Norbert F. Alberstadt
	Raphael Allan Fawcett
	Dorothy Campbell
1945	August J. Podboy
	Reuben G. Alexander
	Harvey D. Wright
	George E. Martz
	I. Harvey Plain
	Thomas C. Naugle
	Peter Sykowski
1946	W. Paxson Chalfant
	H. Gordon Anderson
	Marvin N. Lymberis
	Edwin R. Irgens
	Paul E. McFarland
	Albert F. Cleveland
	Levon K. Garron
	Frederick C. Kohlmeyer
	Octavius Capriotti
	Russell N. Brown
1947	Robert E. Duprey
	Emile M. Ravdin
	John L. Goff
	Robert A. Brown
	Ernest H. Heydt
	William L. Hoon
	Turgut Hamdi
	Joseph W. Taylor
1948	James H. Parker
	Isadore Eisenberg
	William E. Pickett
	James F. Ward
	George B. Hobach
	John P. Hobach
	Merrill H. Woolmington
	Edward C. Wolston
1949	Clemens Kirchgeorg
	Thomas G. Cogswell
	James E. Purnell
	Oram R. Klilne, Jr.
	Alan J. Rosenberg
	Arthur H. Keeney
	Albert E. Leggett
1950	Thomas G. Dickinson
	Paul Kahn
	Albert W. McDally
	Richard H. Seely
	Owen Belmont
	Edward J. Cannon
1951	Karl M. Aijian
	Charles G. Steinmetz, III
	William H. Annesley, Jr.
	Robert A. Anthony
	Cyril M. Luce
	William H. Kratka
	Florian R. Maylath

1952 Mila J. Ashodian
James F. O'Rourke
Emery E. Royce
1953 Thomas J. McKenna
William K. Wheatly
Robert E. Murto
Paul A. Gold
Philip G. Spaeth
John T. Gocke
Robert E. Lee Shumate
William M. McCarthy
1954 Irwin S. Terner
1955 *Change to 2 year residency with class starting July 1. This ended the 18 month residency with a new resident every 3 months.*
1956 Stanley A. Capper
Enrique Wudka
Khalida Naib
Arthur R. Labell
Gerard M. Shannon
1957 Emma C. Mueller
Arthur F. Calnan
Walter A. Fairfax
Howard K. Clough
Leonard Apt
Robert E. Maynard
Harry W. Camp
Francis J. Kanofsky
1958 Oswald C.C. De Melo
Reginald J. Raban
Edward C. Shrader
William L. Eubanks
Kenneth I. Michaile
Jerome Dersh
Robert C. Lee
Samuel W. Knisley
1959 *First class to have a Chief Resident(s)*
Milton Boniuk
E.R. Gonzalez Jiminez
Ralph S. Hamilton*
Myron A. Portenar
Arnold G. Kushner
Alex D. MacAskill
Joseph Amdur
1960 Arnold L. Rose
Romeo V. Fajardo
William Kamerling
Malvin J. Dougherty
Jerome A. Montana*
Lloyd W. Bailey
Charles D. Kelman
1961 John J. Martin
David M. Warner
Edwin U. Keates
Ernest H. Coleman
Clay W. Evatt
William Tasman*
Daniel I. Weiss
1962 Jonathan A. Holloway*
Edward G. Dailey
Robert H. Fessler
Louis X. Viggiano
Arthur M. Spiegleman
Gerald J. Chessen
Philip L. Levy
1963 George L. Spaeth*
Donald J. Praeger
Horry Heriot Kerrison
Basil Manley
W. Richard Green
Ronald B. Vittone
Robert E. King
Change over to 3 year residency.
1964 Raymond E. Adams*
I. Allen Chirls
Thomas L. Gorman
Ralph N. Goulston
Sanford D. Hecht
Peter R. Laibson
Stanley L. Spielman
1965 Stanley W. Boland
Line Chevrette
John J. Coyle
William F. Grant
Philip C. Hughes*
Philip M. Levy
Ronald L. Spielman
1966 Robert W. Connor
Richard E. Goldberg

Donelson R. Manley*
Morton W. Richman
Norman J. Fisher
John W. Tomlinson
Cyril J. Walsh
1967 Michael D. Cefaratti
William J. Kustrup
Joseph C. Flanagan
David Meyer
Barbara Mitchell
P. Kenneth Nase
Hunter R. Stokes*
1968 H. Thomas Dodds
Bert R. Estlow
Barry D. Galman
Kurt A. Gitter
Richard D. Hyman*
Kenneth R. Jaegers
David J. Singer
M. Madison Slusher
1969 Joseph H. Calhoun
James E. Copeland
Burton M. Cunin
Ben P. Houser*
Donald P. Lewin
Alfred C. Lucier
Cyrus L. Mineo
Donald F. Perkins
1970 William R. Griffith*
Pierre Guibor
William K. Harris
Martin B. Kaplan
Michael D. McManus
Joel Porter
Jerry A. Shields
Robert H. White
E. Randolph Wilkerson
Samuel Miller Winn
1971 William Alton Bohart
Brenton C. Burgoyne†
Henderson J. Cleaves
John B. Jeffers
Neil M. Krosney
David H. Miller
Robert V. Miller
Larry M. Piebenga
Robert E. Searle
Robert L. Shindler
Richard W. Sonntag*
Bruce C. Taylor
John H. Weaver
James E. Wilson
1972 Robert L. Alan
Samuel S. Amoni
Ann E. Barker
William Alden Blank
Theodore Buckner
J. Sidney Cotner
Thomas F. Drake
Eyck W. Fintelmann
Patrick D. Moore
William N. Offutt, IV
Hyman William Ross
Vincent A. Sanderson
Jonathan D. Trobe*
Ira Gary Weiner
1973 Bruce R. Berg
Stephen G. Cook
Joseph J. DeVenuto
Ido Egerer
Neil H. Joseph
Stephen M. Moehlman
John F. Moretti
Moira B. Murphy
Louis W. Schwartz
J.H. Stokes
John R. Trittschuh
George O. Waring, III
Edward J. Zobian*
1974 G.R. Barvinchak
James B. Carty*
Richard A. Getnick
R. H. Goodwin
William J. Jordan
Charles E. Letocha
John N. Negrey
Robert H. Nicholson
Harold I.R. Sawelson
Edward Mark Sorr
William V. Tillery
1975 Joshua N. Babad
Bernhard Heersink

**Chief Resident or Co-Chief Resident*

James E. Heeter
Douglas A. MacLeod
David B. Mallory
Bernard E. Patty
John D. Polansky
John J. Purcell*
Michael L. Steiner
Sanford Ullman
1976 Andrew Davidson
Daniel M. Kane
Philip H. McKinley*
Jerry W. Maida
James L. Mims
Paul R. Mitchell
D. Parker Stokes
Richard L. Tax
Stephen W. Wong
1977 Robert S. Baxter
Craig H. Douglas*
Jorge A. Godinez
Marnix E. Heersink
Alan E. Irwin
Joseph B. Michelson
Ronald R. Reed
Paul Remer
Ralph S. Sando
David J. Smith
James C. Tassini
1978 Thomas O. Burkholder
Edward C. Clark
Steven N. Cohen
Cono M. Grasso
Stephen B. Lichtenstein*
Joseph I. Markoff
Peter J. Racciato
Leon L. Remis
Richard S. Rowley
Robert F. Stephens
Richard P. Wilson
1979 Dennis J. Arinella
Susan C. Benes
Gary C. Brown*
Elisabeth J. Cohen
David S. Hyman
W. Reed Kindermann
Thomas L. Manzo
Richard P. Marcello
Joseph F. Morrison
David J. Randell
Robert C. Sergott
1980 Alexander A. Aimette
F. Jane Barton
Jonathan B. Belmont
Geoffrey Broocker
Stephen M. Felton
Robert Folberg
Andrew J. Levin
Richard K. Parrish, II*
Paul M. Pender
Mark C. Ruchman
Joseph J. Scuderi
Gerald J. Jacobs†
1981 Dominick A. Benedetto
Charles J. Castoro*
William J. Degenhardt
George E. Fava
Gregory G. Gensheimer
William G. Martin
Elizabeth A. Miller
John S. Rizzo
Michael S. Zamore
1982 Robert D. Behar*
James B. Dickson
Zoraida Fiol-Silva
W. David Kiser
Don G. Koepsell
Edward F. McCarthy, Jr.
Kenneth P. Moffat
Andrew J. Philips
Bruce I. Stark
Mary A. Stefanyszyn
Douglas J. Symes
Martin B. Wax
Michael Y. Wong
1983 Andrew W. Eller
Alan R. Erickson
Paul C. Ezell
Mark S. Keisler
Patrick T. Lally
Bruce C. Larson*
O. Duane Ragland
Michael X. Repka

**Chief Resident or Co-Chief Resident*
†Deceased during training

	Elizabeth A. Rocco*
	Kevin L. Sullivan
	Floyd Weinstock
	Norman F. Woodlief
1984	Robert S. Bailey*
	Roxana F. Barad
	Gary H. Cassel
	Neil G. Dreizen
	Marc D. Garden
	Debra A. Hamby
	Tyrie L. Hiller
	Robert D. Lehman, Jr.
	James G. Nachbar
	Thaddeus S. Nowinski
	Cynthia J. Parlato
	Jerome A. Peters
	John R. Stechschulte*
1985	Jeffrey F. Brown
	Michael A. Gruber*
	Linda Hsueh
	James F. Kapustiak
	Robert J. Mandel*
	Michael E. Margulis
	Judith E. Melick
	Richard S. Ross
	Alan G. Salz
	Mark A. Staffaroni
	Gregory C. Tesluk
	Catherine C. Ulasewicz
	Richard H. Wong
1986	Kent W. Baumann
	Sylvia R. Beck
	Jeffrey L. Bezier
	Mark H. Blecher*
	Joanna M. Drela-Fischer
	Richard L. Jahnle*
	Joseph H. Krug, Jr.
	Benita P. Kurtzman
	John J. Martin, Jr.
	David J. Seidman
	Saul Ullman
1987	Sandor M. Cohen*
	Matthew I. Ehrlich
	Mary M. Gilbert
	Alana L. Grajewski
	Paul W. Hiss
	Jonathan C. Javitt
	Judy T. Lin*
	Joseph I. Maguire
1988	Ryan F. Boland
	Thomas E. Clinch
	Marc S. Cohen*
	Cathy A. Colt
	Jay S. Duker*
	Stephanie A. Jones
	Gilbert H. Kliman
	Kent G. Leavitt
	Anne V. Parker
	Robert E. Penne
	Steven R. Schwartz
	Michael R. Seybold
	Robb R. Shrader
1989	Steven E. Brady
	Karen L. Fung
	Stephen E. Higgins
	Joseph J. Kesselring
	Alex V. Levin
	Marlon Maus
	Samuel R. Pesin
	Harvey J. Reiser
	Reginald J. Sanders*
	Courtland M. Schmidt, Jr.
	Arunan Sivalingam*
	Tamara Vrabec
	Mark R. Wieland
1990	Melissa M. Brown
	Catharine J. Crockett
	Bret L. Fisher
	Patrick M. Flaharty
	Mark A. Friedberg
	James T. Handa*
	Victor A. Holmes
	Bruce J. Keyser
	Ronald L. McKey
	Christopher J. Rapuano
	Paul A. Raskauskas
	Eric P. Suan*
1991	Robert L. Bergren
	Jurij R. Bilyk*
	Leslie A. Brown
	Ann M. Chien
	Carrie B. Davis

**Chief Resident or Co-Chief Resident*
†Deceased during training

Andrew J. Michael
Hunter R. Stokes, Jr.
Richard Tipperman*
Sydney Tyson
Barbara D. Wolock
Tien P. Wong
1992 Mary Louise Z. Collins
Allen Ho*
Mary Ellen P. Knapp
Isaac A. Lose
David A. Mittleman
Marjorie A. Murphy
William B. Phillips
Carl D. Regillo*
R. David Reynolds
Mark A. Verra
Christopher A. Williams
1993 Mark C. Austin
Jerry R. Blair
Benjamin Chang*
R. Douglas Cullom
C. Byron Faulkner*
Thomas I. Margolis
Wynne A. Morely
Florentino E. Palmon
Mark R. Stokes
Janine G. Tabas
John R. Trible
1994 John D. Dugan
Forrest J. Ellis
Mary Elizabeth Gallivan
J. William Harbour
Paul M. Herring*
Carol J. Hoffman
Mark L. Mayo*
Michele A. Miano
Timothy J. O'Brien
Asit S. Pruthi
Scott H. Smith
1995 Neal H. Atebara
Thomas S. Boland
David G. Buerger*
Christine A. Chung
Janice A. Gault
Steven J. Gedde*
Angela G. Houser
Kenneth C.M. Lee
Terrence D. McCanna
Carolyn S. Repke
Gregory L. Vaughn
1996 Warren J. Chang
Phillip H. Choo
Thomas D. Coats
Elizabeth A. Farr*
David S. Friedman
Faramarz Hidaji
Ignatius S. Hneleski, III
Jonathan S. Myers*
Scott J. Paulman
Emil I. Shieh
Ming X. Wang
1997 Ahmad A. Amir*
Michael J. Banach
Daniel E. Buerger
Eric S. Dunn
Geoffrey T. Emerick
Mitchell S. Fineman
Kenneth R. Jaegers, Jr.*
Anita I. Miedziak
Julian D. Perry
Matthew R. Runde
Steven B. Thom
1998 Steve Cohen
Suzanne K. Freitag
Christopher J. Kelly*
Mark R. Miller
Ketan H. Patel*
Niraj P. Patel
John J. Siliquini, Jr.
Prashanth Vallabhanath
John C. Witherell
Joseph M. Zobian
1999 Kammi K. Bisla
Christine W. Chung
Brian P. Connolly
Vincent A. Deramo
Ralph E. Oursler, III
Mark F. Pyfer
Douglas J. Rhee*
Jay Charles Rudd
Brian Sucheski*

**Chief Resident or Co-Chief Resident*

2000	Anthony J. Aldave
	Christopher D. Brown
	Tehmina Haque
	Mark J. Iacobucci
	Junhee Lee
	Shahzad I. Mian*
	Franco M. Recchia*
	Amy E. Weber
2001	Carlo R. Bernardino*
	Mary Jude Cox*
	Richard S. Davidson*
	Rod Foroozan
	Richard U. Kim
	Anna Park
	Raminder K. Saluja
	Tara A. Uhler
2002	Anya Bitterman
	Brandon G. Busbee*
	Garvin H. Davis
	Marc F. Jones
	James M. Klancnik, Jr.
	Brett Rosenblatt*
	Geoffrey P. Schwartz
	Mari Skovronsky
2003	Jacqueline R. Carrasco*
	Robert K. Chiang
	Carolyn A. Cutney
	Henry C. Lee
	Tricia L. Lennox
	Mimi Liu
	Heather A. Maust*
	Parveen K. Nagra*
	Christine E. Speer
2004	Brian D. Dudenhoefer
	John A. Epstein
	Stephen S. Hwang
	Kunal D. Kanitkar
	Derek Y. Kunimoto*
	Mary S. Makar
	Michael A. Negrey
	Karen S. Nipper
	Mark A. Rezac
	Robert P. Sambursky*
	Daniel E. Shapiro*
2005	Seema Aggarwal
	Brian C. Bigler
	Vatinee Bunya*
	Sandra Y. Cho
	Colleen P. Halfpenny*
	ThucAnh T. Ho
	Anson T. Miedel*
	Vasudha A. Panday
	Nicholas A. Pefkaros
	Derrick W. Shindler
2006	Shaleen L. Belani*
	Kevin B. Cranmer
	Bhairavi V. Kharod
	Andrew Lam*
	Joselito Navaleza
	Sagun J. Pendse*
	Richard Scartozzi
	Bradley T. Smith
	Vikas Tewari
2007	Shawn Chhabra
	Chrishondra Curry McCoy
	David Fintak
	Nicole R. Fram*
	Omesh P. Gupta*
	Dara Khalatbari
	Matthew R. Kirk*
	Katherine A. Lane
	Maria C. McNeill
2008	Justis P. Ehlers*
	Gregory L. Fenton
	Michael A. Malstrom
	Susan M. Gordon
	Eliza N. Hoskins*
	Chirag P. Shah*
	Heather N. Shelsta
	Allison P. Young*
2009	Paul S. Baker
	John M. Cropsey
	Emily A. DeCarlo
	Michael S. Ehrlich
	Robert E. Fintelmann
	Jesse B. McKey
	Avni H. Patel
	Garth J. Willis

**Chief Resident or Co-Chief Resident*

2010	Katherine E. Gres
	Suzanne Jadico
	Jennifer H. Kim
	Caesar Luo
	Melissa Neuwelt
	Linda Ohsie
	Julie Rosenthal
	Rachel K. Sobel
2011	Behin Barahimi
	Christopher M. Fecarotta
	Adam T. Gerstenblith
	Sebastian B. Heersink
	Anne M. Nguyen
	Michael P. Rabinowitz
	Gary Shienbaum
	Eileen Wang

Chief Residents for 2009 – 2010
have not yet been selected.

Appendix H

Postgraduate Fellows

Cornea Fellows

1963	Tadeu Cvintal, M.D.
1967	Guilherme Ortolan, Jr., M.D.
1968	Shashi Dhiri, M.D.
1969	Jose T. Oconer, M.D.
	Emanuel Tanne, M.D.
	Jack Wolper, M.D.
1970	Wendell E. Willis, M.D.
	H. Thomas Dodds, M.D.
1971	Pratima Tolat, M.D.
1972	Larry Piebenga, M.D.
1974	Jay Krachmer, M.D.
	George Waring, M.D.
	Neil H. Joseph, M.D.
1975	Jack Kabak, M.D.
	Juan Arentsen, M.D.
1976	George W. Stubbs, M.D.
	Aisha Simjee, M.D.
1977	Richard Eiferman, M.D.
	Walter Mazzanti, M.D.
1978	Michael Ference, III, M.D.
	James Allen, M.D.
	Rollande Michaud, M.D.†
1979	Irving M. Raber, M.D.
	Barton Halpern, M.D.
1980	Humberto Belloso, M.D.
	Marc Michelson, M.D.
1981	Peter Berkowitz, M.D.
	Robert Cykiert, M.D.
	William Yeakley, M.D.
1982	Todd Fladden, M.D.
	Lewis Groden, M.D.
	Carolyn Sakauye, M.D.
1983	Charles Adams, M.D.
	Paul Galentine, M.D.
	Carlos Traverso, M.D.
1984	Harry Buchanan, M.D.
	Stephanie Croll, M.D.
	Patricia Laughrea, M.D.
	Yaacov Rozenman, M.D.
1985	Gail Genvert, M.D.
	Cynthia Parlato, M.D.
	Eric Donnenfeld, M.D.
	Jed Rabinovitch, M.D.
1986	Carol S. Clemons, M.D.
	Steve Poleski, M.D.
	Thom Thomassen, M.D.
1987	Mark Speaker, M.D.
	Roy Rubinfeld, M.D.
	Raymond M. Stein, M.D.
	Miguel Lugo, M.D.
1988	Casmir Napora, M.D.
	Wilson Ko, M.D.
	Frank Bowden, M.D.
	Roger Luskind, M.D.
1989	Stephanie J. Marioneaux, M.D.
	Anne V. Parker, M.D.
	Holly Kent, M.D.
	Kent J. Leavitt, M.D.
1990	Adam Altman, M.D.
	Steven Brady, M.D.
	Gregory Doren, M.D.
	Cenina Gonzalez, M.D.
1991	Catherine Crockett, M.D.
	Marta Lopatynsky, M.D.

†*Deceased*

Scott Strelow, M.D.
Helia Angotti, M.D., PhD.
Annamaria Martini, M.D.
1992 Ann C. Guidera, M.D.
Rajesh Rajpal, M.D
Laurence Sperber, M.D.
Israel Kremer, M.D.
1993 Lin Chou, M.D.
Christopher Blanton, M.D.
Jonathan Silbiger, M.D.
Harminder S. Dua, M.D.
1994 M. Reza Dana, M.D.
Matthew B. Goren, M.D.
Vera O. Kowal, M.D.
Jose Alvaro P. Gomes, M.D.
Yoonwon Myong, M.D.
1995 Oscar Pineros, M.D.
Stephen Y. T. Lee, M.D.
Carol J. Hoffman, M.D.
Marc A. Honig, M.D.
Regis de Figueiredo, M.D.
Andrea Gomes, M.D.
1996 Piet van Rensburg, M.D.
Stephanie B. Levey, M.D.
Jodi Ian Luchs, M.D.
David Varssano, M.D.
Jorge Luis Dias, M.D.
Noemi Lois Puente, M.D.
1997 Christian Santa Cruz, M.D.
Monica Cunha-Monteiro, M.D.
Jatupol Kositsawat, M.D.
Terry Kim, M.D.
Richard C. Rodman, M.D.
Rene Dinh, M.D.
Germano A.R. Ferreiro, M.D.
1998 Jo-Ann Haney-Tilton, M.D.
Matthew R. Jones, M.D.
Tina C. Lucas Glass, M.D.
Anita I. Miedziak, M.D.
Fabiana Paula Tambasco, M.D.
Jy-Been Liang, M.D.
1999 Harvey U. Fracht, M.D.
Sanjeev Grewal, M.D.
Sudha Sudesh, M.D.
Manapon Lekskul, M.D.
Luis G. Paparo, M.D.
Marco A. G. Tanure, M.D.
Thidanan Rattanatam, M.D.
Ricardo Sampaio, M.D.
2000 Christine W. Chung, M.D.
Evan Lee Held, M.D.
Wee Jin Heng, M.D.
Paulo T.S. Alvim, M.D.
Rose Mary Santim, M.D.
2001 William A. Sray, M.D.
Beth A. Handwerger, M.D.
Srilata S. Naidu, M.D.
M.S. Sridhar, M.D.
Cemille Banu Cosar, M.D.
Ming-Cheng Tai, M.D.
2002 Jonathan S. Weyne, M.D.
Anna J. Park, M.D.
Elizabeth M. Hofmeister, M.D.
Alexandre S. Marcon, M.D.
Maria A. Carrasco, M.D.
Jen-Chieh Lin, M.D.
Gulderen Aktan, M.D.
2003 Uchoandro B.C. Uchoa, M.D.
Renata A. de Rezende, M.D.
Kristin Hammersmith Matelis, M.D.
Andrew J. Epstein, M.D.
Dany Najjar, M.D.
Jeane Haidee G. Mah-Sadorra, M.D.
2004 Stephanie Anne Baxter
Leslie Emmet-Buck
Parveen Nagra
2005 Federico Badala, M.D.
Vatinee Y. Bunya, M.D.
Steven [Buck] J. Rogers, M.D.
2006 Faris R. Ghosheh, M.D.
Brett A. Levinson, M.D.
Christine G. Saad, M.D.
2007 Hall Fenn Chew, M.D.
Elad Feldman, M.D.
Dean Yon Mah, M.D.

Neuro-Ophthalmology Fellows

1977	Tulay Kansu, M.D.
	Robert Osher, M.D.
1978	Walter Cobbs, M.D.
	Jan Hilliker, M.D.
1980	Susan Benes, M.D.
1981	Edwin R. Swann, M.D.
1982	Roy W. Beck, M.D.
	Craig H. Smith, M.D.
1983	Thomas M. Bosley, M.D.
	John Guy, M.D.
1984	Robert C. Harbour, M.D.
	Mark L. Moster, M.D.
1985	Saunders L. Hupp, M.D.
	Sarkis M. Nazarian, M.D.
1986	David A. Cohen, M.D.
1987	Mitchell D. Drucker, M.D.
	Luis Becerra-Cabal, M.D.
	Aziz S. Abdul-Rahim, M.D.
	Susan Ksiazek, M.D.
	Motohiro Kiyosawa, M.D.
	Dermot Roden, M.D.
1988	Marc Cohen, M.D.
	Robert Granadier, M.D.
	Robert Penne, M.D.
1989	Hitoski Okabe, M.D.
	Harry Stumm, M.D.
	Patrick Kilhenny, M.D.
	Marlon Maus, M.D.
1990	Patrick Flaharty, M.D.
	William Cantore, M.D.
	Sunita Yedavally, M.D.
	Charles Cantor, M.D.
1991	Stephen Best, M.D.
	Matthew Kay, M.D.
1992	Nancy G. Schwartz, M.D.
	Mary Ellen Cullom, M.D.
	Neil Aburn, M.D.
1993	Edsel Ing, M.D.
	Amy Jeffrey, M.D.
	David Weinberg, M.D.
1994	Louis Blumenfeld, M.D.
1995	Barry Schanzer, M.D.
1997	Vipul Lakhani, M.D.
1998	David B. Auerbach, D.O.
1999	Helen V. Danesh-Meyer, FRACO
	Kenneth C. Kubis, M.D.
2001	Ivan Castillo, M.D.
2002	Lawrence M. Buono, M.D.
	Rod Foroozan, M.D.??
2003	Michaela Mathews, M.D.
2004	Pragati Shukla, M.D.
	Raed Behbehani, M.D.
2006	Molly Gilbert, M.D.

Retina Fellows

1962 L.K. Sarin, M.D.
1964 Vicente T. de la Paz, Jr., M.D.
Herman J. Hunter, Jr., M.D.
1965 Sheldon P. Braverman, M.D.
Stephen S. Elgin, M.D.
A. Raymond Pilkerton, Jr., M.D.
1966 Hugh L. Morris, M.D.
1967 Guilherme Ortolan, Jr., M.D.
Albert W. Zimmerman, Jr., M.D.
1968 William S. Gilbert, M.D.
David Meyer, M.D.
Paul K. Nase, M.D.
Myron Yanoff, M.D.
1969 Richard E. Goldberg, M.D.
Joseph C. Patti, M.D.
1970 Donald P. LeWin, M.D.
Alfred C. Lucier, M.D.
Peter V. Palena, M.D.
1971 Stanley Carson, M.D.
Jay L. Federman, M.D.
Donald E. Roy, M.D.
1972 Kenneth R. Jaegers, M.D.
Antonio Ramos-Umpierre, M.D.
Jerry A. Shields, M.D.
Bruce C. Taylor, M.D.
1973 Ira B. Fuller, III, M.D.
Hyman William Ross, M.D.
Reid F. Schindler, M.D.
Alvin Weiner, M.D.
1974 Joseph J. DeVenuto, Jr., M.D.
David S.C. Pao, M.D.
Joseph J. Timmes, M.D.
John R. Trittschuh, M.D.
1975 Robert L. Lewandowski, M.D.
Carol G. Reinert, M.D.
Edward M. Sorr, M.D.
Richard L. Winslow, M.D.
1976 Edward A. Deglin, M.D.
Brian C. Leonard, M.D.
Larry E. Magargal, M.D.
Harold Weiss, M.D.
1977 David S. Boyer, M.D.
Christopher L.B. Canny, M.D.
Stephen W. Wong, M.D.
1978 Jorge A. Godinez, M.D.
Leonard Joffe, M.D.
Richard C. Lanning, M.D.
Joseph B. Michelson, M.D.
Thomas R. Pheasant, M.D.
1979 Larry A. Donoso, M.D.
Garry D. Grant, M.D.
George E. Miller, M.D.
S. Richard Ombres, Jr., M.D.
Raymond E. Townsend, M.D.
1980 James J. Augsburger, M.D.
Robert F. Stephens, M.D.
Santiago Perez, M.D.
1981 Gary C. Brown, M.D.
David H. Fischer, M.D.
Jeffrey L. Shakin, M.D.
1982 John R. Gonder, M.D.
Miriam E. Ridley, M.D.
George E. Sanborn, M.D.
1983 Alan F. Cruess, M.D.
William L. Decker, M.D.
Wayne M. Grabowski, M.D.
1984 Fox M. Boswell, M.D.
Andrew P. Schachat, M.D.
Harshad G. Shah, M.D.
1985 William A. Britton, Jr., M.D.
Ernest G. Guillet, M.D.
J. Arch McNamara, M.D.
Stephen T. Petty, M.D.
1986 James P. Bolling, M.D.
Steven R. Leff, M.D.
John T. Minturn, M.D.
Michael P. Varenhorst, M.D.
1987 Mark E. DeSantis, M.D.
Michael A. Gruber, M.D.†
Hermann D. Schubert, M.D.
John C. Welch, M.D.
1988 Rajiv Anand, M.D.
H. Logan Brooks, Jr., M.D.
Mark T. Chiu, M.D.
Robert P. Schroeder, M.D.
1989 Craig M. Greven, M.D.

†*Deceased*

	Joseph I. Maguire, M.D.
	Raul J. Moreno, M.D.
	Eric P. Shakin, M.D.
1990	Jay S. Duker, M.D.
	Jarl C. Nielsen, M.D.
	David M. Pon, M.D.
	James F. Vander, M.D.
1991	Emad B. Abboud, M.D.
	Neil D. Brourman, M.D.
	Rickey D. Medlock, M.D.
	Arunan Sivalingam, M.D.
1992	Bruce J. Keyser, M.D.
	Tamara R. Vrabec, M.D.
	R. Trent Wallace, M.D.
1993	Robert L. Bergren, M.D.
	Gordon A. Byrnes, M.D.
	Tien P. Wong, M.D.
1994	Thaddeus J. Krolicki, M.D.
	William B. Phillips, M.D.
	Carl D. Regillo, M.D.
1995	Prema Abraham, M.D.
	Michael J. Borne, M.D.
	Dan P. Montzka, M.D.
1996	Philip G. Hykin, M.D.
	John O. Mason, III, M.D.
	Vernon K.W. Wong, M.D.
1997	Jeffrey P. Blice, M.D.
	Justin L. Gottlieb, M.D.
1998	Caroline R. Baumal, M.D.
	Scott J. Paulman, M.D.
	Sanjay Sharma, M.D.
1999	Mitchell S. Fineman, M.D.
	Gaurav Shah, M.D.
2000	Jennie Sung, M.D.
	Kenneth Jaegers, Jr., M.D.
	James H. Whelan, M.D.
2001	Brian P. Connolly, M.D.
	Frank J. McCabe, M.D.
2002	Luigi Borrillo, M.D.
	Magdalena F. Schuler, M.D.
2003	Kent A. Blade, M.D.
	Mark L. Nelson, M.D.
	Matthew T. Tennant, M.D.
2004	Gary Lane
	Sunir Garb
2005	Nick Anderson, M.D.
	Eric Weichel, M.D.
	Mimi Liu, M.D.
2006	Derek Kunimoto, M.D.
	Bernard Hurley, M.D.
2007	Jason Hsu, M.D.
	Eric Chen, M.D.
	Amitabh Bharadwaj, M.D.
2008	Andrew Lam, M.D.
	Marc Spirn, M.D.
2009	Anita Prasad, M.D.
	David Rhee, M.D.
	Omesh Gupta, M.D.

Clinical Glaucoma Fellows

1973	Munawar Ahmad, M.D.
1974	Richard Daniel, M.D.
1975	Antonio Montalbo, M.D.
	Nibondh Vacharat, M.D.
1976	Roger Hitchings, M.D.
1977	Kinnari Bakshi, M.D.
	Carlos de Figueredo, M.D.
	Julius Satish, M.D.
1978	Nirmal Kanal, M.D.
	Ralph Sando, M.D.
1979	Richard Wilson, M.D.
	Suzanne Li, M.D.
	Tharmalingam Sivendran, M.D.
1980	William Whelan, M.D.
	Lawrence Hurvitz, M.D.
1981	Edna Z. Mahmood, M.D.
	Isam Zakhour, M.D.
1982	Kevin C. Greenidge, M.D.
	Carlo Traverso, M.D.
1983	Ronald L. Fellman, M.D.
	Zoraida M. Fiol-Silva, M.D.
	James A. McAllister, M.D.
	Richard J. Starita, M.D.
1984	Joseph Caprioli, M.D.
	Marlene R. Moster, M.D.
	John D. Walker, M.D.
1985	Louis B. Cantor, M.D.
	Neil T. Choplin, M.D.
	Leslie J. Katz, M.D.
1986	Dan A. Nichols, M.D.
	Mark B. Sherwood, M.D.
	Steven T. Simmons, M.D.
	Ronald L. Gross, M.D.
1987	Janet Betchkal, M.D.
	E. Randy Craven, M.D.
	Shari Roth, M.D.
	Detlev Spiegel, M.D.
1988	James Brandt, M.D.
	Lawrence Jindra, M.D.
	Robb Shrader, M.D.
1989	Fred Orlando, M.D.
	Michael Stiles, M.D.
	Courtland M. Schmidt, Jr., M.D.
1990	Stephen J. Best, M.D.
	Y. Grace Oh, M.D.
	Tom Samuelson, M.D.
1991	Silvia Orengo-Nania, M.D.
	J. Brent Bond, M.D.
	Andrew J. Michael, M.D.
1992	Fritz Paul, M.D.
	Annette Terebuh, M.D.
	Martha Leen, M.D.
1993	David Boes, M.D.
	Brian Caputo, M.D.
	Stephen Wahl, M.D.
1994	Mark Lesk, M.D.
	Scott Stoller, M.D.
	Patrick Tiedeken, M.D.
1995	Denise Dudley, M.D.
	Anup Khatana, M.D.
	Ines Lanzl, M.D.
1996	Ioannis Aslanides, M.D.
	Augusto Azuara, M.D.
	Sai Gandham, M.D.
1997	Augusto Azuara-Blanco, M.D.
	Ioannis Aslanides, M.D.
	Tarek Eid, M.D.
	Ines Lanzl, M.D.
	Lavkumar Panchal, M.D.
	Kirti Singh, M.D.
1998	Nathan Congdon, M.D.
	Renato deCarvalho Costa, M.D.
	Anastasios P. Costarides, M.D.
	David D. Kim, M.D.
	Hany S. Habib Rizk, M.D.
1999	Graciela Blanco, M.D.
	Marcia Gomes, M.D.
	Jeffrey Henderer, M.D.
	Erkan Mutlukan, M.D.
	Karl J. Siebert, M.D.

2000	Helen Danesh-Meyer, M.D.
	Marcia Lucy Marques Pereira, M.D.
	Madhure Tamhankar, M.D.
	Richard D. Ten Hulzen, M.D.
	Chryssa Terzidou, M.D.
	Asher Weiner, M.D.
2001	Undraa Altangerel, M.D.
	Atilla Bayer, M.D.
	Paul Harasymowycz, M.D.
	Leslie S. Jones, M.D.
	Lorenzo J. Pecora, M.D.
2002	Undraa Antangerel, M.D.
	Mary Jude Cox, M.D.
	Andrea C. Goldberg, M.D.
	Muge R. Kesen, M.D.
	Rajesh Shetty, M.D.
	Tara A. Uhler, M.D.
2003-2004	Heather A. Maust
	Christina I. Tam
	Sophia Wamsley
2004-2005	Marc B. Mydlarski
	Chandrasekharan Krishnan
	Grace Lee
2005-2006	Kalpana Jatla
	Anna Junk
	Jerome Ramos-Esteban
2006-2007	Corey Batiste
	Albert Lin
	Sheila Bazzaz

Oculoplastic Fellows

1969	Emanuel Tanne, M.D.
1970	John G. Yassin, M.D.
1971	Robert H. White, Jr., M.D.
	Ignatius S. Hneleski, Jr., M.D.
1973	Herbert S. Greenwald, Jr., M.D.
1974	Jean-Claude Pilet, M.D.
	Jose Carlos Zenha, M.D.
	German S. Mendez, M.D.
1975	Christine Zolli, M.D.
	John N. Negrey, Jr., M.D.
1976	Gerald C.R. Cullen, M.D.
	Rutheva Dizon, M.D.
1977	David H. Saunders, M.D.
1978	Ernest Nicolitz, M.D.
1979	Daniel L. McLachlan, M.D.
1980	Gary L. Aguilar, M.D.
1981	Charles B. Campbell, III, M.D.
1982	Mark C. Ruchman, M.D.
1983	Joseph A. Mauriello, Jr., M.D.
1984	Mary A. Stefanyszyn, M.D.
1985	David C. Larned, M.D.
1986	Daniel P. Schaefer, M.D.
1987	James B. Dickson, M.D.
1988	George Alter, M.D.
1989	Robert H. Kennedy, M.D.
1990	Robert B. Penne, M.D.
1991	William J. Bigham, M.D.
1991-1992	Robert A. Mazzoli, M.D.
1993	Andrea Nowotny Hass, M.D.
1994	Peter J. Sneed, M.D.
1995	Ameet Goyal, M.D.
1996	David G. Buerger, M.D.
1997	Ignatius S. Hneleski, III, M.D.
1998	Andrew Eiseman, M.D.
	Michael A. Johnson, M.D.
2000	Daniel Elizondo, M.D.
2001	Byron A. Long, M.D.
2003	John J. Lee, M.D.
2005	Jacqueline R. Carrasco, M.D.
2007	Omaya H. Youssef, M.D.

Pediatric Ophthalmology Fellows

1969	Joseph H. Calhoun, M.D.
	Everett A. Moody, M.D.
1970	Ronald M. Hughes, M.D.
	Robert H. White, M.D.
1971	Robert A. Sargent, M.D.
	James E. Wilson, Jr., M.D.
1972	Sidney Cotner, III, M.D.
	Ira G. Weiner, M.D.
	Maynard B. Wheeler, M.D.
1973	Stephen B. Levine, M.D.
	Luis J. Oms, M.D.
	Zane F. Pollard, M.D.
1974	Anthony R. Caputo, M.D.
	James B. Carty, Jr., M.D.
	I. Matthew Rabinowicz, M.D.
1975	Paramjit S. Fagoora, M.D.
	Joao R. Franco, M.D.
1976	William E. Hutton, M.D.
	John M. Koors, M.D.
	James L. Mims, III, M.D.
	Brian D. Altman, M.D.
1977	Craig H. Douglas, M.D.
	J. Bruce Hess, M.D.
	Ralph S. Milner, M.D.
1978	Miles J. Burke, M.D.
	Pamela V. Ombres, M.D.
	Robert L. Schwartz, M.D.
	Epaminondas Branco-Neto, M.D.
1979	W. Reed Kindermann, M.D.
	Joseph J. Kubacki, M.D.
	Alan Richards, M.D.
	Renee Vasquez, M.D.
1980	Rebecca J. Adams, M.D.
	John W. Simon, M.D.
1981	Douglas A. Freeley, M.D.
	Lauri D. Ervin Mulvey, M.D.
1982	Steven E. Rubin, M.D.
	Rudolph S. Wagner, M.D.
1983	Susan M. Szmyd, M.D.
	Robert N. Troia, M.D.
1984	Jeylan El-Mansoury, M.D.
	Herbert D. Goldman, M.D.
1985	Trudi R. Grin, M.D.
	Robert A. King, M.D.
1986	Robert Catalano, M.D.
	David J. Seidman, M.D.
1987	Anne Clark, M.D.
1988	James A. Deutsch, M.D.
	Mary A. O'Hara, M.D.
1989	Colleen J. Christian, M.D.
	William Potter, M.D.
1990	Judith B. Lavrich, M.D.
	Mark A. Steele, M.D.
1991	Michael J. Bartiss, M.D.
	Daniel T. Weaver, M.D.
1992	Lucy L. Chen, M.D.
	Scott E. Olitsky, M.D.
1993	Donna B. Ornitz, M.D.
	William O. Young, M.D.
1994	Ann V. Arthur, M.D.
	Linda K. Nakanishi, M.D.
1995	Robin L. Grendahl, M.D.
	Bradley A. Schwartz, M.D.
1996	Louis E. Furlan, M.D.
	Hulya Nurgun Orer, M.D.
1997	Louis E. Furlan, M.D.
	Hulya Nurgun Orer, M.D.
1998	Ilene B. Pardon, M.D.
1999	John Forbes, M.D.
	Thomas Metz, M.D.
2000	Kammi B. Gunton, M.D.
	Gerasimos Livir-Rallatos, M.D.
2001	Maher Attia, M.D.
	Anita L.W. Breckenridge, M.D.
2002	Ekaterini C. Karatza, M.D.

Oncology Fellows

1985	William Mieler, M.D.
1987	Michael Giblin, M.D.
1988	Hugh Parsons, M.D.
1989	Wolfgang Lieb, M.D.
1990	Laurence Roseier Diallo, M.D.
	Zhongyao Wu, M.D.
1992	Sung Bok Cha, M.D.
	Tai Won Lee, M.D.
	Arun Singh, M.D.
1993	Hayyam Kiralti, M.D.
1995	Ahmed Abdalla, M.D.
	Fernando Arevalo, M.D.
	Andre Hamada, M.D.
	Sundeep Kheterpal, M.D.
	Alegria Totah, M.D.
1996	Chaim Edelstein, M.D.
	Noemi Lois, M.D.
	Aichun Zhou, M.D.
	Dayou Zhao, M.D.
1997	Ahmet Kaan Gunduz, M.D.
	Noemi Lois, M.D.
	Zelia Melling, M.D.
	Gary J.V. Mercado, M.D.
1998	Fabio B. Nogueira, M.D.
	Jose S. Pulido, M.D.
	Young Doo Yoon, M.D.
	Dayou Zhao, M.D.
1999	Cynthia de Allmeida Carvalho, M.D.
	Waltenio V. Diniz Filho, M.D.
	Ihab S.M. Othmane, M.D.
	Paul A. Rundle, M.D.
	Maria C.M. Santos, M.D.
	Susan Schnieder, M.D.
2000	An-Ning Chao, M.D.
	Santosh G. Honavar, M.D.
	Muhammed H. Krema, M.D.
	Miguel A. Materin, M.D.
	Masood Naseripour, M.D.
2001	Hakan Demirei, M.D.
	Arman Mashayekhi, M.D.
	Noel Perez, M.D.
2002	Michele R. Piccone, M.D.
	Abd Allah El-Hussainy Shelil, M.D.

Foerderer Eye Movement Center for Children Fellows

1986	Suqin Guo, M.D.
1987	Yong Han Jin, M.D.
1988	Alina Zubcov, M.D.
	Irene Gottlob, M.D.
1989	Jong Bok Lee, M.D.
1990	Louis Blumenfeld, M.D.
1991	Genjiro Ohmi, M.D.
	Takao Hayashi, M.D.
1992	Hyosook Ahn, M.D.
1993	Sang Chul Park, M.D.
1994	Joa Jing Fu, M.D.
1995	Libe Gradstein, M.D.
1996	Basil A. Pakeman, M.D.
1997	Basil A. Pakeman, M.D.
1998	Libe Gradstein, M.D.

Academic Positions Held by Former Residents & Fellows

James Augsburger, M.D.
Chairman, Ophthalmology
University of Cincinnati
Cincinnati, OH

Alan Cruess, M.D.
Chairman, Department of Ophthalmology
Dalhousie University
Halifax, Nova Scotia
Canada

Richard Davidson, M.D.
Plastics, Ophthalmology Department
University of Colorado
Denver, Colorado

Craig Greven, M.D.
Chairman, Department of Ophthalmology
Bowman School of Medicine
Wake Forest University
Winston-Salem, NC

Shahzad Mian, M.D.
Ophthalmology Residency Director
University of Michigan
Ann Arbor, MI

Franco Recchia, M.D.
Retina Ophthalmology Department
Vanderbilt University
Nashville, TN

Douglas Rhee, M.D.
Glaucoma Research
Massachusetts Eye and Ear Infirmary
Boston, MA

Andrew Schachat, M.D.
Vice Chair for Clinical Affairs
Cole Eye Institute
The Cleveland Clinic
Cleveland, OH

Christine Speer, M.D.
Ophthalmology Department
Duke University
Durham, NC

Jennifer Sung, M.D.
Retina Service
Wilmer Eye Institute
Baltimore, MD

Myron Yanoff, M.D.
Chairman of Ophthalmology
Hahnemann University Hospital
Philadelphia, PA

Appendix I

Bedell Memorial Lecturers, Wills Eye Annual Conference

May 6, 1949	Arthur J. Bedell, M.D. (Albany, NY) "The Destruction of the Macula, Commonly Called Coloboma"
1950	Francis Heed Adler, M.D. (Philadelphia, PA) "Factors Determining the Choice of Operative Procedures in Squint"
March 7, 1951	Conrad Berens, M.D. (New York) "Some Preferred Techniques in Ophthalmic Surgery"
March 22, 1952	Derrick T. Vail, Jr., M.D. (Chicago, IL) "Zonule Membrane and Cataract Extractions"
March 21, 1953	John H. Dunnington, M.D. (New York, NY) "Sutures in Cataract Surgery"
1954	Daniel B. Kirby, M.D. (New York, NY) "Various Means of Direct Separation of the Zonule in Extracapsular Cataract Surgery" (Dr. Kirby died prior to the Conference; his paper was read by a member of the medical staff.)
Feb. 19, 1955	Algernon B. Reese, M.D. (New York, NY) "Diagnosis and Treatment of Orbital Tumors and Simulating Lesions"
Feb. 18, 1956	Albert D. Ruedemann, M.D. (Cleveland, OH) "Progressive Bilateral Exophthalmos Differential Diagnosis and Treatment"
Feb. 9, 1957	John McLean, M.D (New York, NY) "Management of the Primary Glaucomas"
Feb. 22, 1958	Paul Chandler, M.D. (Boston, MA) "Problems in the Diagnosis and Management of Lens Reaction"
Feb. 21, 1959	Brittain F. Payne, M.D. (New York, NY) "Complications Following Cataract Surgery"
Feb. 20, 1960	Peter C. Kronfeld, M.D. (Chicago, IL) "The Glaucomas Secondary to Cataract Operations"
Feb. 11, 1961	Michael J. Hogan, M.D. (San Francisco, CA) "Cyclitis"
Feb. 17, 1962	Frank Walsh, M.D. (Baltimore, MD) "Some Considerations Regarding Occlusive Vascular Disorders"

Feb. 23, 1963	Professor Hans Goldmann (Bern, Switzerland) "Senile Changes of Lens and Vitreous"
Feb. 15, 1964	Edmund B. Spaeth, M.D. (Philadelphia, PA) "Surgical Pathology of the Lids and the Orbit in Children"
Feb. 20, 1965	Donald J. Lyle, M.D. (Cincinnati, OH) "Observations of Degeneration and Regeneration of Sensory and Motor Nerves Serving the Eye in Animal Experimentation and Clinical Observation"
Feb. 5, 1966	A.E. Maumenee, M.D. (Baltimore, MD) "Lesions Produced by Alterations in the Vitreous"
Feb. 11, 1967	Joaquin Barraquer, M.D. (Barcelona, Spain) "Microsurgery, Keratoplastics, and Keratoprostheses"
Feb. 10, 1968	Professor Gerd R.E. Meyer-Schwickerath (Essen, West Germany) "Ophthalmology and Photography"
Feb. 8, 1969	Harvey E. Thorpe, M.D. (Pittsburgh, PA) "Management of Penetrating Wounds and Retained Ocular Foreign Bodies"
Feb. 7, 1970	David G. Cogan, M.D. (Boston, MA) "Internuclear Ophthalmoplegia: Typical and Atypical"
Feb. 13, 1971	P. Robb McDonald, M.D. (Philadelphia, PA) "Retinal Detachment—Then and Now"
Feb. 5, 1972	Lorenz E. Zimmerman, M.D. (Washington, DC) "Problems in the Diagnosis of Malignant Melanoma of the Choroid"
Feb. 3, 1973	Harold G. Scheie, M.D. (Philadelphia, PA) "Proliferative Angle Closure and Secondary Glaucoma"
Feb. 16, 1974	John C. Mustarde, F.R.C.S., D.O.M. (Glasgow, Scotland) "Widening Horizons in Ophthalmic Plastic Surgery"
Feb. 1, 1975	Irving H. Leopold, M.D. (Irvine, CA) "Clinical Immunology for the Ophthalmologist"
Jan. 31, 1976	David Shoch, M.D. (Chicago, IL) "Thyroid Ophthalmology"
Feb. 5, 1977	Charles E. Iliff, M.D. (Baltimore, MD) "The Surgical Management of the Retractors of the Upper and Lower Lids"
March 3, 1978	Frederick C. Blodi, M.D. (Iowa City, IA) "Squamous Cell Carcinoma of the Conjunctiva"
March 2, 1979	Norman S. Jaffe, M.D. (Miami, FL) "The Changing Scene of Intraocular Implant Lens Surgery"
April 25, 1980	Cornelius D. Binkhorst, M.D. (The Netherlands) "Lens Implantation in the Mutilated Anterior Segment"
April 24, 1981	Stephen M. Drance, M.D. (Vancouver, BC) "The Early Psychovisual Disturbance in Open-Angle Glaucoma"
April 16, 1982	J. Lawton Smith, M.D. (Miami, FL) "Neuro-Ophthalmology, 1982"

Feb. 18, 1983	G. Richard O'Connor, M.D. (San Francisco, CA) "Therapeutic and Experimental Aspects of Ocular Toxoplasmosis"
March 30, 1984	Claes H. Dohlman, M.D. (Boston, MA) "The Skin and the Eye—An Important Correlation"
March 22, 1985	Edward W.D. Norton, M.D. (Miami, FL) "The Evolution of Vitreous Surgery"
March 14, 1986	John E. Wright, M.D., F.R.C.S. (London, England) "Diagnostic and Therapeutic Dilemmas in Orbital Disease"
April 3, 1987	H. Dunbar Hoskins, M.D. (San Francisco, CA) "Glaucoma: Problems and Pleasures"
March 18, 1988	Professor Franz Fankhauser (Bern, Switzerland) "Ophthalmic Laser Surgery—Past, Present and Future"
March 9, 1989	W. Richard Green, M.D. (Baltimore, MD) "Cytopathologic Evaluation of Ocular Fluid Specimens"
March 29, 1990	Simmons Lessell, M.D. (Boston, MA) "Traumatic Optic Neuropathies"
April 11, 1991	Charles D. Kelman, M.D. (New York, NY) "Ophthalmic Innovations: Seeds and Deeds"
April 2, 1992	Carl Kupfer, M.D. (Bethesda, MD) "Ophthalmology in the Year 2000"
April 1, 1993	George W. Weinstein, M.D. (Morgantown, WV) "The Future of Ophthalmology"
April 21, 1994	B. Thomas Hutchinson, M.D. (Boston, MA) "Perspectives on Changing Ophthalmic Practice"
March 16, 1995	Robert Ritch, M.D. (New York, NY) "Rethinking Glaucoma: A New Beginning"
March 14, 1996	Alfred Sommer, M.D., M.H.S. (Baltimore, MD) "Outcomes Research and Its Impact on Clinical Management"
March 20, 1997	Stanley Chang, M.D. (New York, NY) "Perflucarbon Liquids—Present and Future"
March 12, 1998	J. Donald M. Gass, M.D. (Nashville, TN) "The Fleck Retinal Syndrome"
Feb. 18, 1999	Daniel M. Albert, M.D. (Madison, WI) "The Retinoblastoma Story Revised and Revisited"
March 9, 2000	Richard P. Mills, M.D., M.P.H. (Lexington, KY) "Glaucoma Imaging—Same Song, New Verse"
March 29, 2001	Neil R. Miller, M.D. (Baltimore, MD) "New Concepts in the Diagnosis and Management of Leber's Hereditary Optic Neuropathy"
March 21, 2002	Carmen A. Puliafito, M.D., M.B.A. (Miami, FL) "Imaging in the 21st Century"

2003	W. Bruce Jackson, M.D. "How Has Excimer Laser Surgery Changed Ophthalmology?"
2004	Lawrence A. Yannuzzi, M.D. "Retinal Imaging: Today and Beyond"
2005	Robert N. Weinreb, M.D. "Reflections From the Optic Nerve: Past and Future"
2006	Harry W. Flynn, Jr., M.D. "Complications of Cataract Extraction: Pearls for Successful Management"
2007	Kenneth Rosenthal, M.D. "Combining Refractive Surgery with Cataract Surgery"

Appendix J

Silver Tray Recipients

1962	James S. Shipman, M.D.
1963	James H. Delaney, M.D.
1964	Edmund B. Spaeth, M.D.
1965	Isaac Tassman, M.D.
1966	Wilfred E. Fry, M.D.
1967	Warren S. Reese, M.D.
1968	Patrick J. Kennedy, M.D.
1969	P. Robb McDonald, M.D.
1970	Kelbin A. Kasper, M.D. (ENT)
1971	Harold D. Barnshaw, M.D.
1972	Albert F. Cleveland, M.D.
1973	James S. Jordan, M.D.
1974	G. Curtis Pritchard (Administrator)
1975	Robert D. Mulberger, M.D.
1976	Robert E. Shoemaker, M.D.
1977	Arthur H. Keeney, M.D.
1978	Joseph W. Hallett, M.D.
1979	Nathan S. Schlezinger, M.D. (Neurologist)
1980	Robison D. Harley, M.D.
1981	Thomas D. Duane, M.D.
1982	Oram R. Kline, Jr., M.D.
1983	Owen Belmont, M.D.
1984	Philip B. Spaeth, M.D.
1985	William H. Annesley, Jr., M.D.
1986	Samuel Blank, M.D. (Anesthesiologist)
1987	Malvin J. Dougherty, M.D.
1988	Joseph C. Flanagan, M.D.
1989	William Tasman, M.D.
1990	George L. Spaeth, M.D.
1991	Hunter R. Stokes, M.D.
1992	John J. Siliquini, M.D.
1993	William N. Offutt, IV, M.D.
1994	Raymond E. Adams. M.D.
1995	John B. Jeffers, M.D.
1996	Peter R. Laibson, M.D.
1997	James J. Augsburger, M.D.
1998	Edward A. Jaeger, M.D.
1999	William E. Benson, M.D.
2000	Joseph H. Calhoun, M.D.
2001	Robert C. Sergott, M.D.
2002	Elisabeth J. Cohen, M.D.
2003	Ralph C. Eagle, Jr., M.D.
2004	Gary C. Brown, M.D.
2005	Peter J. Savino, M.D.
2006	Jerry A. Shields, M.D.
2007	Cono Grasso, M.D.

**Served as Chairman of the Annual Conference*

Appendix K

Annual Irving H. Leopold Lecture

A new lectureship honoring Dr. Irving H. Leopold, the first Ophthalmologist-in-Chief at Wills, was inaugurated in April 1987 during the Annual Wills Eye Conference. Endowed by the Allergan Division of SmithKline Beckman and the late Mrs. Leopold, it focuses on ocular pharmacology and therapeutics. Most appropriately, the first lecture was presented by Dr. Leopold.

April 2, 1987	Irving H. Leopold, M.D.* "Ocular Therapeutics Through the Retro-Spectroscope"
March 19, 1988	George O. Waring, III, M.D. "Refractive Corneal Surgery—Promises and Pitfalls"
March 10, 1989	Richard L. Lindstrom, M.D. "Current Concepts in Posterior Chamber Lens Implantation"
March 30, 1990	Manus C. Kraff, M.D. "Complications and Problem-Solving in Cataract and Intraocular Lens Surgery"
April 12, 1991	Paul R. Lichter, M.D. "Interpretation of the Medical Literature: What's There and What's Not"
April 3, 1992	Brian C. Leonard, M.D. "Alternative Reimbursement Plans: The Canadian Experience"
April 2, 1993	Richard K. Parrish, II, M.D. "The Evolution of Glaucoma Filtering Surgery"
April 22, 1994	Jay H. Krachmer, M.D. "How to Decide Whether or Not to Do Refractive Surgery"
March 17, 1995	Kenneth L. Abrams, D.V.M. "When Your Patients Have Four Legs: An Overview of Veterinary Ophthalmology"
March 15, 1996	R. Doyle Stulting, M.D., Ph.D. "The Science and Sociology of Refractive Surgery"
March 21, 1997	Norman Medow, M.D. "Great Moments in Ophthalmic History"
March 13, 1998	Richard J. Mackool, M.D. "Megatrends in Microsurgery: Managed Care and the Big Bang Theory"
Feb. 19, 1999	Marguerite M. McDonald, M.D. "Excimer Laser Surgery: A Decade of Progress"
March 10, 2000	Robert H. Osher, M.D. "Challenging Cases in Cataract Surgery"

**Dr. Leopold is the only one to have also delivered the Bedell Lecture.*

March 30, 2001	Gilbert H. Kliman, M.D., M.B.A. "The New Economy of Ophthalmology"
March 22, 2002	Douglas D. Koch, M.D. "Update in Wavelength-Guided Ablation"
2004	Paul P. Lee, M.D., J.D. "Do We Practice What We Know? Clinical Trials and Community Care"
2005	Henry Jampel, M.D. "Medical Management of Glaucoma: Integrating Perspectives from Patients, Physicians, and Trials"
2006	Donald D'Amico, M.D. "Neovascular AMD — The Current Treatment Landscape"
2007	Ike Ahmed, M.D. "Cataract Surgery from the Glaucoma Specialist's Viewpoint"

Appendix L

Ophthalmologists-in-Chief

1960-1964	Irving H. Leopold, M.D.
1964-1973	Arthur H. Keeney, M.D.
1973-1981	Thomas D. Duane, M.D.
1981-1985	Robert D. Reinecke, M.D.
1985-2007	William Tasman, M.D.

Appendix M

Wills Eye Annual Conference Chairpersons

1949	Carroll R. Mullen	(1 Year)
1950-1960	Isaac S. Tassman, M.D.	(11 Years)
1961	Carroll R. Mullen	(1 Year)
1962-1963	Patrick J. Kennedy, M.D.	(2 Years)
1964-1966	Harold D. Barnshaw, M.D.	(3 Years)
1967-1969	Albert F. Cleveland, M.D.	(3 Years)
1970-1973	Robert D. Mulberger, M.D.	(4 Years)
1974-1976	Gerard M. Shannon, M.D.	(3 Years)
1977	Malvin J. Dougherty, M.D.	(1 Year)
1978-1980	Oram R. Kline, Jr., M.D.	(3 Years)
1981-1983	John J. Siliquini, M.D.	(3 Years)
1984-1986	Raymond E. Adams, M.D.	(3 Years)
1987-1989	Owen Belmont, M.D.	(3 Years)
1990-1994	James J. Augsburger, M.D.	(5 Years)
1995-1999	Christopher J. Rapuano, M.D.	(5 Years)
2000-2005	Robert B. Penne, M.D.	(5 Years)
2005-	Peter J. Savino	

Appendix N

Wills Eye Society Presidents

1927-1929	J. Milton Griscom, M.D.
1929-1931	Edward Jackson, M.D.
1931-1933	Paul J. Pontius, M.D.
1933-1935	Walter R. Parker, M.D.
1935-1936	Paul J. Pontius, M.D.
1936-1938	Arthur J. Bedell, M.D.
1938-1940	Edward C. Ellett, M.D.
1940-1942	Albert C. Snell, M.D.
1942-1946	Frank C. Parker, M.D.
1946-1948	Burton Chance, M.D.
1948-1950	James S. Shipman, M.D.
1950-1952	James S. Jordan, M.D.
1952-1954	Charles A. Young, M.D.
1954-1955	Thurber LeWin, M.D.
1955-1956	James H. Delaney, M.D.
1956-1957	Warren S. Reese, M.D.
1957-1958	Lee W. Hughes, M.D.
1958-1959	Noel S. McBride, M.D.
1959-1960	Roscoe J. Kennedy, M.D.
1960-1961	Joseph E. Beideman, M.D.
1961-1962	Kenneth L. Roper, M.D.
1962-1963	Lycurgus M. Gurley, Jr., M.D.
1963-1964	P. Robb McDonald, M.D.
1964-1965	Alvin W. Howland, M.D.
1965-1966	Levon K. Garron, M.D.
1966-1967	Pierre G. Jenkins, M.D.
1967-1968	James V.D. Quereau, M.D.
1968-1969	Robert F. Rohm, M.D.
1969-1970	R. Alan Fawcett, M.D.
1970-1971	James H. Parker, M.D.
1971-1972	Joseph Morrison, M.D.
1972-1973	Clyde H. Jacobs, M.D.
1973-1974	Hunter R. Stokes, M.D.
1974	Albert F. Cleveland, M.D.
1975	Philip C. Hughes, M.D.
1976	Robert E. Shoemaker, M.D.
1977	William R. Green, M.D.
1978	William H. Annesley, Jr., M.D.
1979	Clay W. Evatt, Jr., M.D.
1980	William Tasman, M.D.
1981	Kenneth R. Jaegers, M.D.
1982	Owen Belmont, M.D.
1983	John D. Polansky, M.D.
1984	Malvin J. Dougherty, M.D.
1985	William Offutt, IV, M.D.
1986	Oram R. Kline, Jr., M.D.
1987	Raymond E. Adams, M.D.
1988	Joseph C. Flanagan, M.D.
1989	Stephen B. Lichtenstein, M.D.
1990-1992	Joseph I. Markoff, M.D.
1992-1993	Jonathan B. Belmont, M.D.
1994-1995	Richard P. Wilson, M.D.
1996-1998	Gary Brown, M.D.
1999-2002	Robert Bailey, M.D.
2003-2004	Robert C. Sergott, M.D.
2005-2006	Elisabeth J. Cohen, M.D.
2007-	Cono M. Grasso, M.D.

Appendix O

James S. Shipman Award

1967 Kurt A. Gitter, M.D.
1968 Ben P. Houser, Jr., M.D.
1969 Donald P. Lewin, M.D.
1970 Jerry A. Shields, M.D.
1971 Jonathan D. Trobe, M.D.
1972 George O. Waring, III, M.D.
1973 Ido Egerer, M.D.
1974 John J. Purcell, Jr., M.D.
1975 John J. Purcell, Jr., M.D.
1976 Joseph B. Michelson, M.D.
1977 Ronald R. Reed, M.D.
1978 Robert C. Sergott, M.D.
1979 William G. Martin, M.D.
1980 Stephen M. Felton, M.D.
1981 Norman F. Woodlief, M.D.
1982 Andrew W. Eller, M.D.
1983 Thaddeus S. Nowinski, M.D.
1984 Robert D. Lehman, Jr., M.D.
1985 Gregory C. Tesluk, M.D.
1986 Carol L. Shields, M.D.
1987 Eric P. Shakin, M.D.
1988 Marc S. Cohen, M.D.
1989 Tamara R. Vrabec, M.D.
1990 Christopher J. Rapuano, M.D.
1991 Richard Tipperman, M.D.
1992 Carl D. Regillo, M.D.
1993 John R. Trible, M.D.
1994 Ming X. Wang, M.D.
1995 David G. Buerger, M.D.
1996 Jonathan S. Meyers, M.D.
1997 Julian D. Perry, M.D.
1998 Brian P. Connolly, M.D.
1999 Vincent A. Deramo, M.D.
2000 Anthony J. Aldave, M.D.
2001 Rod Foroozan, M.D.
2002 Brandon G. Busbee, M.D.
2003 Heather Maust, M.D.
2004 Robert P. Sambursky, M.D.
2005 Bradley T. Smith, M.D.
2006 Kate A. Lane, M.D.
2007 Nicole R. Fram, M.D.

Appendix P

P. Robb McDonald Award

1992	Andrew Michael, M.D. (Glaucoma)
1993	Mary Ellen Cullom, M.D. (Neuro-Ophthalmology)
1994	Jose A.P. Gomes, M.D. (Cornea)
1995	Silvana V. Araugo, M.D. (Glaucoma)
1996	Tarek Eid, M.D. (Glaucoma)
1997	Richard Rodman, M.D. (Cornea)
1998	Nathan Congdon, M.D. (Glaucoma)
1999	Kenneth Kubis, M.D. (Neuro-Ophthalmology)
2000	Helen Danesh-Meyer, M.D. (Cornea)
2001	Beth Handwerger, M.D. (Cornea)
2002	Mary Jude Cox, M.D. (Glaucoma)
2003	Dany M. Najjar, M.D. (Cornea)
2004	Parveen Nagra, M.D. (Cornea)
2005	Eric Weichel, M.D. (Retina)
2006	Noel Hoirgan, M.D. (Oncology)
2007	Pedro F. Salazar, M.D. (Oncology)

Appendix Q

The Convocation

The Opening

of

the new Wills Eye Hospital

Friday, November first

Two thousand and two

at two-thirty o'clock

Wills Eye Hospital Auditorium

840 Walnut Street

Philadelphia, Pennsylvania

The Wills Eye Hospital Opening Ceremony
November 1, 2002

PROCESSIONAL
Vivaldi: Concerto in C for
Two Trumpets and Strings

THE NATIONAL ANTHEM
Stephen S. Hwang, M.D.

INVOCATION
The Reverend Edward C. Bradley, S.J., M.D.
Clinical Associate Professor of Medicine
Jefferson Medical College

CONVOCATION
Paul C. Brucker, M.D., *President*
Thomas Jefferson University

CONFERRING OF HONORARY DEGREES

President Brucker

Andrew Wyeth, *Doctor of the Fine Arts*
Presented by: William Tasman, M.D.
Professor and Chairman
Department of Ophthalmology
Jefferson Medical College

Alan C. Bird, M.D., FRCS, FRCOpth., *Doctor of Science*
Presented by: William E. Benson, M.D.
Professor of Ophthalmology
Jefferson Medical College

ADDRESS
Doctor Tasman
"Vision and Art"

BENEDICTION
Reverend Bradley

RECESSIONAL
Purcell: Voluntary in C for
Two Trumpets and Strings

ACKNOWLEDGEMENTS

Marshal
Allen C. Ho, M.D.
Associate Professor of Ophthalmology
Jefferson Medical College

Program Coordinators
William Tasman, M.D.
Lynn Sobolewski

Musicians
Joseph I. Markoff, M.D., Ph.D., trumpet
Clinical Associate Professor of Ophthalmology
Jefferson Medical College

Jason DePue, violin
Zachary DePue, violin
Priscilla Lee, violincello
Daniel E. Shapiro, M.D., trumpet
Richard Tang, viola

Andrew Noel Wyeth

Doctor of the Fine Arts

Born July 12, 1917 in the home of his parents in Chadds Ford, Pennsylvania, Andrew Wyeth was educated at home by tutors from 6 years of age until he was 9 years old. By 1932, his father, N.C. Wyeth, a distinguished illustrator, took 15-year-old Andrew into his studio as an apprentice. Soon thereafter, Andrew had his first one-man exhibition at the McBeth Gallery in New York.

His future wife, Betsy James, who in turn introduced him to model Christina Olsen, became Mrs. Wyeth in 1940. They had two sons, Nicholas and Jamie.

Mr. Wyeth became the youngest member of the American Water Color Society when he was elected at the age of 23. As his career progressed he participated in a major group of exhibitions at the Museum of Modern Art in New York, which were entitled "American Realist and Major Magic Realists."

In 1948, Mr. Wyeth painted "Christina's World" using Christina Olsen as his model, a painting that was later acquired by the Museum of Modern Art in New York City.

Mr. Wyeth's first honorary degree was from Colby College in Waterville, Maine. His curriculum vitae lists 24 honorary degrees in recognition of his major contributions to the art world. Thus, the Jefferson-Wills honorary degree would make his 25th. Among others, awards have been given by Harvard, Princeton and Dartmouth. In the Delaware Valley area, Penn, Temple, Delaware, Swarthmore College, Dickinson, Franklin and Marshall, LaSalle, Lincoln, and Ursinus have also honored Mr. Wyeth.

In 1955, Mr. Wyeth was made a member of the American Academy of Arts and Letters and the National Institute of Arts and Letters in New York. The American Academy is composed of only 50 individuals who elect their own members and Mr. Wyeth was the youngest ever elected. He is also the youngest member-elect to the American Academy of Arts and Sciences in Cambridge, Massachusetts.

At President John F. Kennedy's suggestion Mr. Wyeth received the Presidential Medal of Freedom. Because of President Kennedy's tragic assassination, the Medal was presented by President Lyndon B. Johnson in December 1963, just one month following the death of President Kennedy.

In 1970, Mr. Wyeth had the distinction of having the first major solo exhibition of art ever held in the White House. From 1971–1985 he painted the major body of his work, which later became known as the "Helga Collection." Then in 1977, Mr. Wyeth was elected as an associate member of the Estatute de France Academy des Beaux Arts, Paris, France. He was elected to membership in the Soviet Academy of the Arts in Leningrad, USSR in 1978, and in 1989 he received the award for distinguished achievement from the Philadelphia Art Alliance along with his son, Jamie Wyeth. Another tribute to Mr. Wyeth was the awarding of the Congressional Gold Medal by President George Herbert Walker Bush at a White House ceremony in October 1990. He was the first artist to be so honored.

No stranger to Philadelphia, Mr. Wyeth received the Founder's Day medal at the Pennsylvania Academy of Fine Arts as part of its 193rd anniversary celebration in 1998. More recently on June 8, 2001, the John Singer Sargent medal was awarded to Andrew and Jamie Wyeth in New York City at the Metropolitan Museum of Art by the American Society of Portrait Artists Foundation. Interestingly, John Singer Sargent's father, Fitzwilliam Sargent, had been a surgeon at the Wills Eye, which strengthens the bond between art and the Will's Eye Hospital and lends additional appropriateness to honoring Mr. Wyeth today.

Alan Charles Bird

Doctor of Science

Professor Alan Charles Bird was born in Bromley, Kent on July 4, 1938. He was graduated from Bromley Grammar School in 1956 and from Guy's Hospital Medical School in London in 1961. He completed his residency at Moorfields Eye Hospital in London in 1967. Initially most interested in Neuro-ophthalmology, he came to the United States in 1968 for a fellowship at the Bascom Palmer Eye Institute in Miami, Florida, under Dr. J. Lawton Smith. During his year there, he became interested in the then-new technique of fluorescein angiography which Drs. J. Donald M. Gass and E.W.D. Norton were using to greatly further our understanding of macular diseases. Returning to London, he joined the staffs of the Institute of Ophthalmology and the Moorfields Eye Hospital. Gradually, his main interests shifted to retinal diseases. In recognition of his outstanding academic and teaching achievements, he rose to become Professor of Clinical Ophthalmology at the Institute of Ophthalmology and Consultant at the Moorfields Eye Hospital.

Professor Bird is one of the world's experts on age-related macular degeneration, having written important papers on its pathophysiology, prognosis, and treatment. He has helped to elucidate the role of Bruch's membrane in retinal pigment epithelial dysfunction. He was the first to recognize tears of the retinal pigment epithelium. For many years he has traveled to the Caribbean to study sickle cell retinopathy. He has also written many valuable papers on retinitis pigmentosa and other tapetoretinal diseases, macular dystrophies, retinal vascular disease, and numerous other inherited diseases.

What has made Professor Bird great is that he is a perpetual student, always asking about the "why of things." Not satisfied with simply describing a condition, he seeks its histopathologic, genetic and molecular basis. His 39 research grants reflect this interest in both clinical and basic science research. Professor Bird enjoys sharing his knowledge with others. He has given 37 named lectures around the world, including the Duke Elder Lecture, the Doyne Lecture, the Proctor Lecture, the Paul Henkind Lecture, the Jackson Lecture, the Ernst Custodis Lecture, and the Bowman Lecture. He has written 64 chapters and has 340 papers in peer-reviewed journals. His curiosity shows no signs of abating: he currently has 13 papers submitted for publication.

For his many achievements, Professor Bird is widely recognized as being one of the world's leading ophthalmologists. He is or has served on the editorial board of the *British Journal of Ophthalmology, Graefe's Archive for Clinical and Experimental Ophthalmology,* the *Japanese Journal of Ophthalmology* and *Investigative Ophthalmology and Vision Science*. He has received many of our profession's prestigious honors and awards including the Hermann Wacker Prize from the Club Jules Gonin, the Gass Medal of the Macula Society, the William Mackenzie Medal of Glasgow University, and the Jules François Medal of International Council of Ophthalmology.

Professor Bird is married to Sarah. They have two children.

The University Mace

The Thomas Jefferson University mace, carried for the first time in the 1986 commencement ceremonies by Grand Marshal Robert Mandle, Ph.D., was designed and cast by Howard Serlick, member of the Guild of Mastercraftsmen, Winterthur Scholar, and Chief Conservator (Gilding) of the Historical Society of Pennsylvania. It was crafted by silversmith Eugene Zweigle and woodturner Michael Copeland.

The four-foot-long, fourteen-pound mace is made of ebony highlighted with lapis lazuli to reflect Jefferson's colors (black and blue). It features a miniature of Henry Mitchell's sculpture, The Winged Ox, symbol of St. Luke the Physician, the original of which stands beside the Scott Building on Walnut Street. The miniature was cast in silver by Mister Zweigle, who also fabricated the University seal, the profile of Thomas Jefferson, mounted at the base of the staff. The J.E. Caldwell Company coordinated the project.

Mister Mitchell's original statue of The Winged Ox, adopted by the University in 1976 as its symbol of clinical excellence, is mounted on a column containing the names of fifty medical scientists who have most advanced the art of healing. It also reflects the historical evolution of Thomas Jefferson University from its beginnings as Jefferson Medical College in 1824 to its current status as an academic health center comprising the Medical College, the College of Health Professions, the College of Graduate Studies, and the Thomas Jefferson University Hospital, a part of the Jefferson Health System.

The mace, a grand emblem of the University's heritage, is carried at the head of all formal academic processions.

History of Wills Eye

Index

Page numbers followed by *f* indicate figures.

D

E

F

G

P

Q

R

S

X

Y

Z